Glimpses from History

Respiratory Medicine in India

From Antiquity to Future

Glimpses from History
Respiratory Medicine in India
From Antiquity to Future

Surinder K Jindal
MD FAMS FNCCP FICS FCCP
Emeritus Professor and Former Head
Department of Pulmonary Medicine
Postgraduate Institute of Medical Education and Research
Chandigarh, India

Medical Director
Jindal Clinics
Chandigarh, India

Foreword

PS Shankar

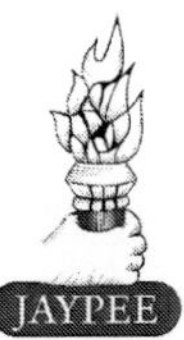

JAYPEE BROTHERS MEDICAL PUBLISHERS
The Health Sciences Publisher
New Delhi | London

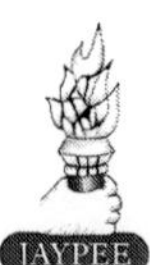

Jaypee Brothers Medical Publishers (P) Ltd

Headquarters
EMCA House, 23/23-B
Ansari Road, Daryaganj
New Delhi 110 002, India
Landline: +91-11-23272143, +91-11-23272703
+91-11-23282021, +91-11-23245672
e-mail: jaypee@jaypeebrothers.com

Corporate Office
4838/24, Ansari Road, Daryaganj
New Delhi 110 002, India
Phone: +91-11-43574357
Fax: +91-11-43574314
e-mail: jaypee@jaypeebrothers.com

Overseas Office
JP Medical Ltd.
83, Victoria Street, London
SW1H 0HW (UK)
Phone: +44-20 3170 8910
e-mail: info@jpmedpub.com

EU GPSR Authorised Representative
Logos Europe, 9 rue Nicolas Poussin
17000, La Rochelle, France
Phone: +33 (0) 6 67 93 73 78
e-mail: contact@logoseurope.eu

Website: www.jaypeebrothers.com
Website: www.jaypeedigital.com

Inquiries for bulk sales may be solicited at: jaypee@jaypeebrothers.com

Glimpses from History: Respiratory Medicine in India—From Antiquity to Future / Surinder K Jindal

First Edition: **2026**

ISBN: 978-93-7202-535-4

Printed at: Samrat Offset Pvt. Ltd.

FOREWORD

Respiration forms the essence of life. The first breath taken by a new born a few seconds after birth marks the beginning of a process that will continue until death. Professor Surinder K Jindal, a distinguished professor of pulmonary medicine, renowned researcher and investigator of large multicentric studies, outstanding educator, noted author/editor, and recipient of national and international awards, has written this treatise on historical developments in India on this vital function of all living beings.

It is a great pleasure to write foreword to this book "*Glimpses from History: Respiratory Medicine in India—From Antiquity to Future*" in which Professor Jindal has provided a glimpse of the Indian history through 23 chapters. The initial 4 chapters deal with the historical anecdotes from the past. He has specifically elaborated Breathing as a sacred function. All faiths, religions, and civilizations have recognized it as the sign or essence of life. Since ancient times, breathing has been recognized as beginning of life and its cessation end of life. In ancient times, people knew various breathing techniques. *Sushruta Samhita* and *Charaka Samhita* had recognized the importance of breathing in maintenance of good health. Western and Eastern civilizations, faiths, and religions had considered breathing as an important event essential to life and well-being.

In subsequent chapters, the story of respiration enters the Renaissance period. It deals with different conditions affecting the respiratory system and their diagnosis with the use of physical signs such as inspection, palpation, percussion, and auscultation with a stethoscope. Introduction of X-ray and other imaging techniques made a revolution in the study of respiratory diseases. He has discussed in detail how Allopathic Medicine, Ayurveda, Homoeopathy, Unani, and Siddha system of medicine has formulated the methods to assess various respiratory diseases. He has discussed the development of medical education during the British (including Portuguese and French) rule of the country. India has witnessed significant advances during the post-Independence period in health care, education, and national programs to control and eliminate diseases, particularly tuberculosis, growth of pharmacologic industries, and development of postgraduate study of respiratory diseases including tuberculosis as a specialty.

The author has discussed in detail about tuberculosis, asthma, and allergy; tobacco smoking and respiratory diseases such as COPD and cancer; occupational lung diseases; and respiratory sleep disorders. He has been highly lucent to give historical perspectives of these disorders. The recent developments such as interventional pulmonary procedures, thoracic surgery, and lung transplantation have been also discussed. Oxygen is the essence of life. The author has given Indian perspectives on oxygen therapy, changing environment, and climate conditions. Heat waves, cold exposure, biomass fuels, depleting ozone shield, exposure to UV radiation, burning of fossil fuels, deforestation, and chlorofluorocarbon propellants affect the airways and alveoli. The author has discussed the developments in the background of Indian scenario.

In the recent years, ethics and end-of-life care in respiratory medicine have gained importance. The author has analyzed the complex moral and philosophical issues, and end-of-life care requiring critical decisions. He has analyzed life-sustaining treatment, organ transplantation, role of mechanical ventilation, and noninvasive ventilation. There is a separate chapter on developments in the Armed Force

Medical Services and high-altitude respiratory conditions affecting the level of oxygen in the body.

The author has not forgotten developments in the country in respiratory research, guidelines, and consensus statement on respiratory disorders. He has discussed research done on juxtacapillary (J) receptors, domiciliary antituberculosis chemotherapy, multidrug-resistant tuberculosis, BCG vaccine, asthma, COPD, interstitial lung diseases (ILD), and lung cancer. ILD, once considered rare in India, is frequently recognized due to an increased awareness and availability of different diagnostic procedures.

The author has devoted a chapter on the stalwarts who have worked in the field of respiratory medicine in the recent past in the country. The last chapter 23 deals with the future of respiratory medicine in India rising burden of respiratory diseases such as asthma, COPD, and cancer, air pollution, drug-resistant tuberculosis, respiratory critical care, and role of artificial intelligence.

Professor Jindal has crystallized in this book the historical development of respiratory medicine in India and abroad from pre-historic time till recent years. He has discussed succinctly various respiratory disorders encountered in the country and newer methods of diagnosis and treatment. He has used simple language which is understood by every reader. The sources of information listed at the end of each chapter have added value to the book.

The book is a welcome addition, which is interesting to read for all pulmonologists, physicians, postgraduate students, and practitioners. I congratulate Professor Jindal for producing such a handy book of great utility. It is a valuable addition to the respiratory medicine literature.

PS Shankar
Emeritus Professor, Rajiv Gandhi University of Health Sciences
Distinguished Professor, KBN University
Diamond Jubilee Professor, MR Medical College
Karnataka, India

PREFACE

The development of respiratory medicine to a form with which we are currently familiar since antiquity has been fitful, with several tumultuous stages interspersed with periods of stability. The history of medicine, including that of the respiratory system, has been extensively searched and much is now known of various developments in the Western World. Some of the older descriptions of Greek and Egyptian civilizations provide fairly significant information on how medicine was practiced in older times. Many researchers of modern medicine have eluded in their works as to how the practices of medicine have evolved in different fields.

There is general lack of a concise source of information on historical developments in the Indian continent. OP Jaggi's multiple volumes on "History of Science and Technology in India" provide valuable inputs about folk medicine, ayurveda, western medicine, and others. A recent history book, "The Golden Road: How Ancient India Transformed the World?", by William Dalrymple inspired me to look into the Indian developments and contributions in medicine specifically in the field of my own specialty, respiratory medicine. Both the pulmonologists and the medical historians often trace this history to a period when the physicians and philosophers started recognizing various medical and surgical disorders affecting the human body. It would, however, seem that the history of normal and abnormal breathing is even more ancient. Breathing was recognized by ancient man as a sign of life, its absence as the sign of death, and problems with breathing as a sign of an illness. There is enough evidence to support that the concepts about the importance of breathing were known in the ancient civilizations which existed several millennia earlier.

Breathing and breathing disorders have been repeatedly mentioned in the medical texts of the early periods. While *Tamka Swasa* (asthma), *Yakshma* (Tuberculosis), "*kasa*" (bronchitis), *yoga, pranayama*, and the core concept of *Tridosha* are commonly known since the early Vedic civilization, it is not often recognized that there were several other conditions which were known and/or came to be described in one or the other context or in one or the other form in later Indian texts. For example, a technique called "*mukha-mārga*,"—blowing air into the mouth of a person who has stopped breathing—was known as the earliest form of resuscitation. *Sushruta Samhita* also mentioned a similar technique called "*prāṇa-pratīkṣepa*" (restoring life force).

Numerous indirect references may be found in historical texts or travelogues of foreign travelers like the Chinese Faxian and Xuanzang of the ancient periods. During the post-Mauryan period, the Moroccan traveler Ibn Battuta wrote about witnessing Indian villagers using mouth-to-mouth resuscitation to revive people who had stopped breathing. There is a fair description of physical disability of workers engaged in building of stone monuments in the hymns and poetry related to the Pallava Dynasty of 7th century CE. Similarly, the Mughal era manuscripts such as "*Insha-i-Mahru*" mention about the challenging working conditions of workers involved in masoning and laboring activities in the building of the Taj Mahal, while the sufferings of textile workers of the 16th century are found in *Ain-i-Akbari*, 1590 CE.

I find it both interesting and educational to look for incidental examples related to respiratory medicine in India. One notices that the level of knowledge in the ancient past was generally similar in the Indian and the European continents. For example, the humoral theory was independently hypothesized in disease causation in both the continents. But the progress in India became rather stagnant in the later periods. It is only in the very recent times that we have again started regaining our position.

I have tried to collate the anecdotal information from secondary sources in a manner which is better understood by students of medicine and those interested in the Indian developments. One cannot deny the different interpretations by different readers and scholars. I shall feel highly satisfied if it stimulates at least a few to look into greater depth and clarity.

Surinder K Jindal

ACKNOWLEDGMENTS

I acknowledge the help and valuable additions made by several of my friends and colleagues who have provided inputs to different chapters. Reminiscences, personal notes, and photographs by colleagues such as SK Chhabra, Basil Varkey, Ashok Shah, Aloke Ghoshal, SK Sharma, Rajendra Prashad, V Thanasekaraan, C Ravindran, Uma Mohan Krishnaswamy, Nikhil Sarangdhar, and Abha Mahashur have greatly helped to recollect the contributions of some of the pulmonary stalwarts of the recent times. I also greatly appreciate the addition of a separate chapter "Saga of Developments in the Armed Forces" by Lt Gen (Retd) Dr BNBM Prasad. Some of the photographs were provided by Drs Vikram Jaggi, Srinivas Rajagopala, Apar Jindal, Col Vikas Marwah, Meenu Singh, and DJ Christopher for which I am very thankful. The great help in suggesting, editing, and painlessly correcting the manuscript was rendered by my son Aditya, himself a respiratory physician who possesses keen interest in and knowledge of history. He has also provided some of the photographs used in this book.

Finally, I am especially thankful to my publisher, M/S Jaypee Brothers Medical Publishers (P) Ltd, and the Development Editor Ankit Singh who have made it possible for this work to get into your hands.

Surinder K Jindal

CONTENTS

CHAPTER

1

Breathing: A Sacred Function

Roots in Theology and Religion

Respiration—Essence of Life

Respiration in lay terminology is synonymous with "breathing"—the essence of life. Breathing defines the onset of life and its cessation the end. The term "respiration" is derived from the root Latin word *"spir"* which means to breathe. In scientific nomenclature, breathing is defined as the physical process of inhalation of air (essentially, oxygen) in the lungs while respiration is a broader chemical process of transfer of oxygen from environment to the lungs and thereafter to the body cells for their normal function as well as the elimination of carbon dioxide, *"the waste product"* produced as a result of cellular metabolism. Respiration therefore includes two major processes: Inspiration, i.e., inhalation of air (primarily oxygen) in the lungs and; expiration, i.e., exhalation of carbon dioxide. Respiration at the level of lungs is sometimes referred to as "external" respiration which is visible while respiration at the level of the cells is "internal" respiration which is more a metabolic function and not externally visible.

"Breathing" essentially implies "external respiration"—the most important function identified in all ancient civilizations as the earliest recognized sign of life. In several ways, it is a sacred function for humans. It occupies the most prime position for survival of a living being. Breath and breathing, considered as fundamental to life were expressed in various forms in different religious texts and traditions. In a majority of world civilizations, the longevity of life is measured by the number of breaths which are predetermined in fate. Without doubt, breathing remains the most critical and manifested evidence of survival.

First Breaths

Life begins when the organism starts breathing. The first breaths of a newborn are crucial for transitioning from fetal to neonatal life. As the lungs expand and oxygen levels rise, the baby's body starts to adapt to the new oxygen-rich environment. The first breath has both spiritual and medical significance for survival. It symbolizes the beginning of a new life. In some cultures, the first breath is believed to be a moment when the soul enters the body, connecting the child to a higher power or divine force. It can be seen as a transition from a spiritual realm to the physical world, marking the child's entry into the world of humans. Many cultures perform rituals or ceremonies to welcome the newborn, often involving prayers, blessings, or sacred rituals.

According to modern history of anthropological development, the breathing apparatus in animals and humans appeared long before the noticeable act of breathing. While aquatic animals developed gills for simple gas exchange over a billion years earlier, the evolution of lungs, branching airways and functioning air sacs was much later in birds and mammals, yet a few hundred million years before the birth of modern man of the *Homo sapiens* species. In the more recent history, an image suggesting the structure of respiratory tract with a windpipe and a pair of lungs could be seen in an Egyptian hieroglyph of the 30th century BC.

Theological Concepts of First Breaths

Despite some differences, many ancient cultures shared common themes, such as the significance of the first breath as a moment of transition and transformation. The ancient Greeks believed that the first breath marked the beginning of life and the entry of the soul (psyche) into the body. In Hindu culture, the first breath was often associated with the *Jeevakarma or Jatakarma* ceremony to welcome the newborn and seek blessings for their well-being and prosperity. Rituals and prayers were (and are) often performed to purify and protect the newborn from negative influences. *Garuda Purana* discusses the soul's journey and its entry into the body, highlighting the significance of the first breath. In Ayurveda, *prana vayu* refers to the life force or vital energy that enters the body with the first breath while *Jiva pravesha* concept refers to the entry of the soul *(jiva)* into the body. The Ayurvedic text *Charaka Samhita,* described the importance of the first breath in initiating life and vitality.

In some Christian traditions, baptism is performed soon after birth, symbolizing the child's entry into the Christian faith and cleansing from original sin. It places significant spiritual importance on the first breath, highlighting the sacredness and significance of new life. In Islam, the *Azaan* (call to prayer) is recited in the newborn's ear, followed by the *Iqamah,* to introduce the child to the faith and invoke blessings. Some Muslims perform the *Tahnik* ritual, where a small amount of dates or honey is placed in the newborn's mouth, symbolizing sweetness and blessings. Sikhs recite *Gurbani* (Sikh scriptures) in the newborn's presence, seeking blessings and protection.

Theological and Spiritual Significance

Beyond its physical necessity to live, breathing holds profound religious and spiritual significance. It weaves the human experience with threads of spirituality, religion, and the scriptures. Breathing is also practiced as a fundamental spiritual ritual to cultivate life energy, balance, and harmony. For modern medical practitioners, it is somewhat difficult to define the spiritual and metaphysical goals and to appreciate the significance of breathing to achieve them. Nonetheless, different types of breathing significantly affect the psychological and physical states of mind. Clinical psychologists and psychiatrists commonly recommend different breathing techniques for some of the mental disturbances. It is also perhaps the only autonomous vital function of human body which can be partly controlled with voluntary efforts.

Sri Paramahansa Yogananda in his "Autobiography of a Yogi" wrote: "*The mystery of life and death, whose solution is the only purpose of man's sojourn on Earth, is intimately interwoven with breath. Breathlessness is deathlessness. Realizing this truth, the ancient rishis of India seized on the sole clue of the breath and developed a precise and rational science of breathlessness.*"

There are deep theological roots of breathing in different theological, historical, and philosophical contexts that shape our understanding of this vital function in the power of Creation of life and its sustaining presence. Theological understanding connects life to the divine. It is also integral to various practices such as the prayer, meditation, yoga, *pranayama,* and others in different religions and sects. It is a fundamental process to connect the human soul to the divine and achieve spiritual enlightenment.

Vedic or Hindu Foundations

There are different concepts about the origin of life in different religions. According to the Hindu scriptures, the *Puranas,* the universe was created by Lord *Brahma* and Goddess *Shatrupa* (or *Saraswati, Brahma's* consort) whose union gave birth to *Manu.* The human race originated from the union of *Manu* and his wife *Ananti. "Prana"* equated to "breath" mentioned multiple times in different contextual references in the ancient Hindu scriptures (such as the *Upanishads, Yajur-Veda, the Atharva-Veda, the Brahmanas,* and the *Sutras*), is considered as most essential of all the vital airs for survival.

The process of breathing is deeply rooted in theology and described in various forms in different scriptures. In Hinduism, the story of birth of *Lord Ganesha* characteristically impresses upon the importance of breathing "to be alive." *Mother Parwati,* the consort of *Lord Shiva* wanted to protect her privacy when the Lord was away. To keep a guard, she designed a model of clay and *blew breath into the nostrils* to give it life. When *Shiva* returned, He did not recognize the boy and killed him in a furious battle. *Parwati* was very angry and wanted him brought back to life. Shiva ordered his men to bring the head of any living being they met first. His men cut the head of an elephant which they first saw. The elephant's head was transplanted on to the corpse of the slain boy who was also blessed that He would be worshipped first in all future adorations. This is also often quoted as the first instance of "transplantation" in the medico-theological history.

There are several other stories about breath in Hindu mythology. Breath, considered as equivalent to air or wind (*Vayu*) is worshipped as a god in most religious functions and other ceremonies. Lord *Vishnu,* the God for protection of the universe among the Hindu trinity, who appears in different incarnations during crises, is said to remain suspended in the ocean. His

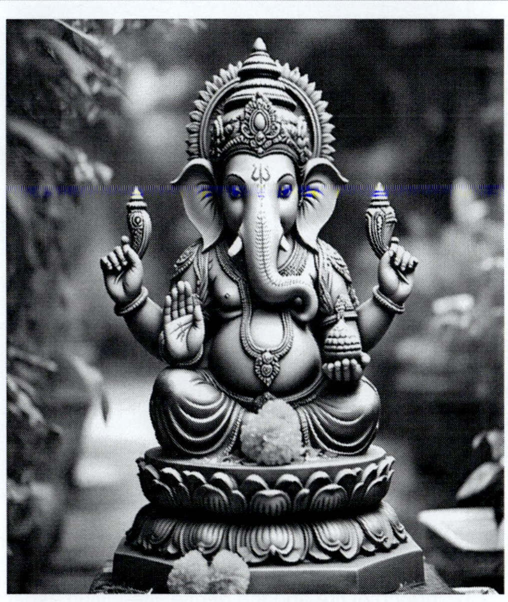

पर्वतीप्रियः शिवः प्राह तामिच्छन्तीं पुत्रम्
मृत्तिकापुत्रः स भविष्यति गणेशः
तेन प्राणाः प्रतिष्ठाप्या यथा जीवेति च
तद्वाक्ये पर्वती देवी प्राणाः प्रतिष्ठाप्य च

Shiva, dear to Parvati, told her:

- "This clay-son will be born.
  He will be Ganesha, born from clay."
- "Breathe life into him, so he may live."

As Shiva commanded,
Parvati breathed life into Ganesha

(Shiva Purana, Rudra Samhita,
Parvati Khandam, Ch 13).

Lord Ganesha came to being after mother goddess Parvati breathed life into a clay model created by Lord Shiva.

inhalation and exhalation destroy and create universes and other material elements. *Asvins Kumars* are twin deities considered as the divine healers of the gods. They are the sons of the sage *Kashyap* and his wife *Aditi*. They also represent the left and right nostrils.

There have been different theories in Hinduism on relation between *prāṇa* with the atmospheric air. In *Ṛigveda,* the atmospheric wind is identified with the breath of *Puruṣa,* the universal man. This is akin to the Egyptian god *Amun,* who is considered as identical to the wind, the source of life as breath in the living. *Prana* is the life-supporting nourishment for the mind and body. It is one of the most frequently mentioned entity in the Hindu philosophical text *Upanishads.* In *Upanishads, prana* is not just the air to breathe, but the energy which sustains the life until its death. *Prana* is equated to "self" and the main element of life and believed to survive as "last breath" until a future life.

Breathing protects the organs in the body, and also keeps them free from evil. A scholarly analysis of "The Hindu Conception of Functions of Breathing" by Arthur Ewing is available in an elegant treatise published in the beginning of the last century. The author identifies that *the Hindu concept of prana* had implied the dual breath processes of inhalation and exhalation as is now known. *Vedanta,* the ancient school of Hindu philosophy is based on three primary Hindu texts: the *Upanishads, the Brahma Sutras, and the Bhagavad Gita.* It includes several different terms which mean different types of breaths. Some of these terms which have been used include the *Prdna, Apana, Tyfna, Iddna, and Samdna.* They are all meant to serve different vital functions. The same have been also referred to as *prāna, udāna, samāna, apāna, and vyāna.*

Western Mythologies

Breathing was also given supreme importance in Roman, Greek, Egyptian, and other global mythologies. In Roman Mythology, breathing was associated with the creation of life and the universe. The myth of *Venus* describes how the goddess emerged from the sea, symbolizing the birth of life and the breath of creation. *Vitalis,* the Roman spirit of life was often depicted as a breath of air which represented the vital energy of living beings. *Flora, Anima, and Aquilus* were gods or goddesses who represented breath of life in one or the other form.

In Greek mythology, breathing was associated with the creation of life and the universe. For example, the myth of Prometheus describes how the titan stole fire from the gods and gave it to humans, symbolizing the spark of life and the breath of creativity. Breathing and the breath of life were associated with Zephyr, the Greek god of the west wind, often depicted as a gentle breeze. Zephyr represented the breath of life and the gentle, life-giving aspect of the wind. Pneuma, the Greek concept of breath or spirit was often associated with the soul or life force and was

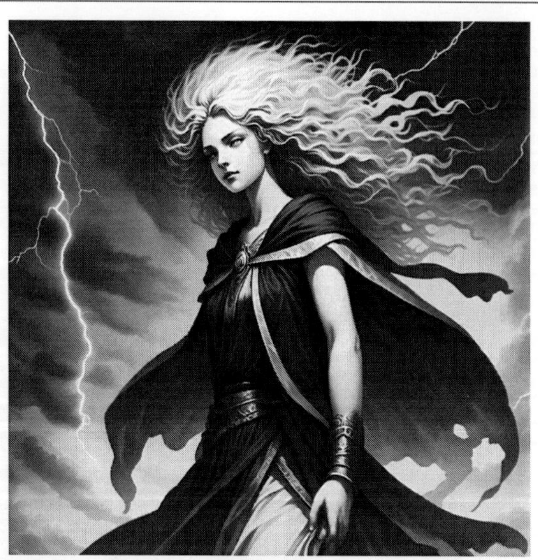

Zephyr, the Greek god of the west wind, often depicted as a gentle breeze represents the breath of life and the gentle, life-giving aspect of the wind.
Source: AI created photograph.

believed to be the vital energy that animated living beings. Psyche, the Greek goddess of the soul, often depicted as a butterfly or a winged goddess, was associated with the breath of life and the soul's connection to the divine.

The ancient Greeks laid great stress upon the importance of breath in understanding the human soul which was thought to combine different parts, with breath playing the most important role: The rational mind (*Nous*) connected to the divine through breath; the spirited aspect (*Thymos*) was energized by breath, and the desiring aspect (*Epithymetikon*) was influenced by breath. Breath was thought as a pathway to seek the union with the divine and achieve greater self-awareness and inner strength. Different breathing techniques (such as *Diaphonia, Prosoche, Askēsis*) had been variously practiced to achieve these objectives. Early Greek philosophers such as Plato and Aristotle also emphasized the divine importance of breathing for all spiritual and mental functions.

Ancient Egyptian mythology gave similar importance to breathing in maintaining life and vitality and connecting with the gods and the divine. The ancient Egyptians believed that breathing was a sacred act, and they developed various techniques, such as meditation and controlled breathing, to cultivate spiritual growth and connection with the divine. Breathing ensured the *pharaoh*'s immortality and preserved the balance and order of the universe (*ma'at). Shu, Ma'at, and Ankh,* the different Egyptian gods represented the life-giving power of air and the breath of life. They symbolized the breath of life and the gentle breeze, i.e., breathing. "*Ba*," the Egyptian concept of the soul, often depicted as a bird or a human-headed bird represented the life force and the breath of life.

Biblical Foundations

"Then the Lord God formed the man of dust from the ground and breathed into his nostrils the breath of life, and the man became a living creature."

(Genesis 2:7)

Breath has a great spiritual and existential meaning in Christianity. There are numerous references to breathing in Christian scriptures. It is a gift of God bestowed upon man to live. According to Judeo-Christian religious beliefs, God formed a man of dust and clay and breathed air into the nostrils and the man became a "living soul." "God breathes life into humanity, establishing a direct link between divine breath and human existence (Genesis 2:7). He was then placed in the Garden of Eden formed by the God. In some way, the story is similar to that of the birth of *Ganesha* in Hinduism.

Breathing has deep symbolism and is associated with the Holy Spirit, spiritual life, and prayer. The Spirit of God is described as the source of breath, highlighting the sacred nature of respiration (Job 33:4).

"Jesus breathes the Holy Spirit upon his disciples, signifying the transmission of divine life" (John 20:22).

"Every breath you take is a gift of life from the living God."

Ruach (the Hebrew word for the breath of God) gives life: *"And the breath of the Almighty gives me life."*

The practice of *insufflation* (i.e., the act of breathing upon a person) is identified with re-enacting the influence of the Holy Spirit. Insufflation rites in fact play a seminal role in Baptism in the Eastern Orthodox Church while these are *deployed for consecration by the Roman Catholics.* Jesus' breathing upon his disciples may represent "incarnation," the embodiment of divine life in Christian study of the Church and the origins of Christianity. Breathing also represents the community aspect of faith, connecting believers through shared spiritual practices. Similarly, Pneumatology (often associated with breath) in Christian theology refers to a discipline within that focuses on the study of the Holy Spirit exploring the divine presence within believers. The term "pneumatology" frequently used interchangeably with pulmonology, is derived from the Greek word Pneuma which designates "breath" or "spirit."

In later Christian beliefs, there are sporadic references to breath as emphasized in the "union of soul and body"—the soul is "born of the breath of God, immortal, corporeal, and representable" (Tertullian). "*Breath*" (pnoe) in the New Testament is mentioned as the vital principle, the Gift of God and "*Breathed*" is used as Lord's concrete symbolism of the giving of the Spirit.

Importance of Breathing in Jewish History

Judaism, which shares a common Abrahamic origin with Christianity, also considers breathing as a life-force. Breathing finds a significant mention in Jewish spirituality, philosophy, and daily life. While the ancient Jewish text *Torah* describes God breathing life into Adam as stated earlier, *Talmud* discusses breathing techniques for spiritual growth and *Kabbalah* emphasizes breath control for mystical experiences. The Jewish practices, *Shema, Amidah, and Kabbalistic Meditations* involve one or the other kind of breath control or a breathing exercise. Jewish Rabbi Abraham Isaac Kook wrote about role of breathings in spiritual growth and Rabbi Nachman of Breslov emphasized breathing in prayer. Rabbi Yehuda Halevi had linked breathing to divine inspiration. Breathing was also given great significance in Jewish Mysticism: *Merkabah Mysticism* advocated breath control for divine ascension while *Kabbalistic Meditation* taught breathing techniques for unity with God.

Breathing in Zoroastrianism

Zoroastrianism founded by the prophet *Zarathustra* in about 1500 BCE, attached great significance to breathing like most other religions. Ancient Zoroastrians (Persians commonly recognized as *Parsis* in India) emphasize the importance of breathing in spiritual and physical contexts. Breathing is seen as a divine gift which links humans to the creator, *Ahura Mazda*. While the sacred scripture, *Avesta* contains prayers, hymns, and philosophical discussions, *Vendidad* is a collection of laws and teachings, including those related to breathing and health. Breathing exercises and prayers help to purify the soul. Zoroastrian priests and practitioners used breathing exercises similar to *pranayama* by Hindu saints. Breathing also played a role in various Zoroastrian rituals. Zoroastrian breathing practices significantly influenced Islamic mysticism (*Sufism*).

Ancient Zoroastrian archeological artefacts found at *Persepolis* depict breathing-related rituals. The *Persepolis Fortification Tablets* also bear administrative texts which mention breathing exercises. The important Zoroastrian spiritual practices and rituals such as *Yasna, Vendidad,* and *Navjote* involve breathing exercises and prayers.

Chinese Theology

The ancient Chinese, like many other civilizations believed that there is a body and a spirit which are essential for existence on earth. Breath is intimately connected to the body's energy systems. *The "breath soul" (hun-ch'i)* returns to heavens at the time of death, while the *"body-soul" (hsing-p'o) turns to earth.* It is the breathing which stops when a person dies. While *Jing* is the essence, stored in the body and is nourished by breath, *Qi* is the life energy circulating through the body which is balanced by breath; the *Shen* is the spirit, which is connected to breath. In Taoism, breath is the source of life energy (Qi). Qi ("breath" or "dragon's breath") is the vital life force, like *prana* in Indian culture. It is an essential means to connect with the Tao. It is important for balancing and harmonizing the body's energy. Confucianism considered breath as essential to cultivate values and morality.

There are various spiritual practices based on breathing techniques: Zhuanqi (Rotating Qi, using breath to circulate energy); Tuna (Expelling and absorbing Qi, using breath to balance energy) and

Xiuzheng (cultivating correctness, using breath to align with the Tao). The embryonic breathing involves one inhalation (xī) and one exhalation (hū) to make one respiratory cycle. The practice involves breathing in through the nose, holding the breath for as long as possible, and then exhaling through the mouth. Tai *Chi* is the practice of deep breathing through the nose, using the full capacity of the lungs, and exhaling through the mouth. The movement of the diaphragm expands the lower abdomen during inhalation and contracts it during exhalation (abdominal breathing). The *"yin yang breathing"* is based on the Taoist (Daoist) concept of complementary energies of yin yang in which *Yin* is the inwards energy (equivalent of inspiration) and *Yang* is the energy being released which is equivalent to exhalation.

Religious Contexts

Breathing History in Buddhism

Gautam Buddha, also considered as the 9th incarnation of Lord Vishnu in Hinduism laid the foundation of Buddhism and greatly stressed upon the importance of breathing and meditation. According to the Buddhist teachings, respiration is essential for transformation of consciousness to closely link the mind with the body. Conscious control of breathing points to the realization of the conscious of—Self (atman). It is the fundamental practice for concentration, mindfulness, and wisdom.

Buddha taught the importance of breath in his teachings, *Anapanasati Sutta* and *Satipatthans Sutta.* Anapanasati *Sutta* describes the details of Buddha's breathing technique during meditation which is a crucial aspect of Buddhist meditaion. *Anapana,* the Pali word for breathing refers to inhalation and exhalation. *Anapanasati* is the basic meditation technique in Buddhism. It is described as "Experiencing the whole body, I shall breathe in and, experiencing the whole body, I shall breathe out." It is often practiced as deep abdominal inhalation and slow exhalation, often with counting. It constitutes one of the four foundations of mindfulness: Body, feelings, mind, and *Dhammas.* In multiple variations, the practice is also common to several other forms of Eastern Buddhism such as the Tibetan, Zen, Tiantai, and Theravada systems.

Jainism

Beyond theology, the process of breathing finds an equally important and upright position on moral, spiritual, and noble grounds in other important religions practiced in different parts of the world. In Jainism, breathing is critical for self-realization and liberation. Some of the most significant Jain texts which stress upon the significance of breathing are: *Tattvartha Sutra* (importance of breathing in spiritual growth); *Yogashastra* (on breathing techniques such as yoga and meditation) and *Dravyasamgraha* (on the role of breathing in achieving liberation).

There are three main types of breathing linked to the concept of *Prana,* the life force. These are: *Udana,* (the upward breath, associated with spiritual growth), *Prana* (the inward breath, linked to physical sustenance) and *Apana* (the downward breath, connected to elimination). Through different breathing techniques, the Jains tend to achieve their various interior and pure goals including *Ahimsa* (nonviolence); Self-control (for inner peace and balance); Meditation (*Dhyana,* to quieten the agitated mind and access higher states); Purification (to purify the body, mind, and spirit for spiritual growth), and Liberation, i.e., to achieve liberation (*Moksha,* freeing the soul from the cycle of rebirth).

Sikhism

Breathing is considered essential for spiritual growth and self-realization.

It facilitates meditation, mindfulness, self-control, and purification. The Holy *Guru Granth Sahib* includes several references to the importance of breath and breathing techniques:

"ਸੁਆਸ ਸੁਆਸ ਸਿਮਰਨਾ, ਪ੍ਰਭੁ ਨਾਮ ਜਪਨਾ" (*Su-aas su-aas simrana, Prabhu Naam japana*)
"With every breath, remember (the Lord), and chant the Name of the Lord."

(Guru Granth Sahib, Page 262)

"ਇਹੁ ਸੁਆਸ ਇਹੁ ਸੁਰਤਿ ਇਹ ਮੁਹਲਤ ਹੈ ਜੋਗੀ ਕੀ" (*Ihu su-aas ihu surti ih muhlat hai jogi ki*)
"This breath, this awareness, is the opportunity for the yogi (to unite with the Divine)."

(Guru Granth Sahib, Page 278)

"ਸੁਆਸ ਸੁਆਸ ਮੇਲੀਐ ਪ੍ਰਭੁ ਨਾਲਿ" (*Su-aas su-aas meleeai Prabhu naal*)
"Unite with the Lord with each breath."

(Guru Granth Sahib, Page 265)

Similarly, *Adi Granth* (an earlier version of the *Guru Granth Sahib*) also emphasizes the significance of breathing in spiritual growth. The *Sikh Rehat Maryada* (the Sikh code of conduct) also mentions the importance of breathing techniques in meditation and spiritual practice.

Breathing is a gift from God meant as a means to connect with the Divine, *Waheguru* (God). Conscious breathing helps to cultivate a sense of gratitude and devotion. It is also seen as a means to purify the body, mind, and spirit, preparing the individual for spiritual growth. Breathing techniques, such as focusing on the breath or using specific breathing patterns, are used in Sikh meditation (*Simran*) to quieten the mind and access the higher states of consciousness. Breathing is also believed to help control the mind and emotions and leading to inner peace and balance.

Importance of Breathing in Islam

Breathing in Islam is a sacred act which connects the man, the soul, and the spirit with Allah and the universe. Through breathing practices, Muslims deepen their connection to Allah and the universe, cultivate spiritual growth and self-awareness, and find inner peace and balance in daily life. Some of the practices in daily life which directly or indirectly employ breathing include: (1) *Salat* (conscious breathing during prayer to focus the mind and heart; (2) *Sawm* (fasting, which includes controlling breath to cultivate self-discipline), and (3) *Zakat* (charity, which includes sharing one's "breath" with others). Some of the important breathing techniques which are integral to Islamic spiritual practices include: (1) *Qalb* (focusing on the heart, using breath to cultivate love, and compassion); (2) *Nafas* (controlling breath to quieten the mind and; (3) *Sukoon* (finding satisfaction and inner peace through conscious breathing).

The Holy Quran emphasizes the importance of breath as a symbol of life and spiritual growth:

- *Surah Al-Hijr (*15:29): Allah breathes life into the clay, creating humanity.
- *Surah Al-Isra* (17:85): The Spirit of Allah is described as the breath of life.
- *Surah Al-Qiyamah* (75:38): The breath of life is a reminder of Allah's power and mercy.

Prophet Muhammad emphasized the significance of breathing in spiritual growth:

- *Hadith*: "Take slow, deep breaths, for it calms the heart and soul."
- *Hadith*: "The best of worship is to sit in solitude, breathing in the presence of Allah."

During 11th to 13th century, breathing became a fundamental aspect of Islamic spirituality in *Sufism*, a mystical form of Islam that emphasizes the spiritual search for God. Sufi saints emphasized the importance of breathing in spiritual growth and self-realization. In Sufism, breath is considered a manifestation of the divine life force (*Ruh*) and spiritual consciousness. Breathing techniques were believed to help purify the heart and soul. Sufi texts such as *The Mathnawi* by Rumi, and *Fusus al-Hikam* by Ibn Arabi explore breathing as a divine manifestation. The *Ihya Ulum al-Din* by Al-Ghazali covers breathing techniques for spiritual purification.

Of various *Sufi* breathing techniques, *Sufi Yoga* combines physical postures, breathing, and spiritual focus. The famous *Sufi* saint Hazarat Nizamuddin had adopted and advocated Yogic breathing exercises to keep the breathing in rhythm. Other *Sufi* practices include breath control, or *pas-e-anfas* to establish a deeper spiritual connection.

- *Dhikr*: The remembrance of Allah, often practiced through breath awareness and repetition of divine names.
- *Muraqabah*: Meditation, focusing on breath and heart, to cultivate love and devotion to Allah.
- *Tasbih*: The use of breath to recite praises and supplications to Allah.

Breathing occupies a special place not only because it is vital for life but also for its deep theological roots. It plays both the roles—the physical function to sustain life and a spiritual function to attain a higher state of mind and liberation. A variety of breathing techniques continue to be advocated and practiced in different religions and sects till date to live a healthier and peaceful life. Unlike the other essential and vital body functions (cardiovascular and neurological) which have autonomic regulation, breathing is one act which can be partly controlled on will and modified for shorter periods as a voluntary act.

Sources

1. Shiva Purana, Rudra Samhita, Parvati Khandam, Chapter 13. (Translation by J. L. Shastri, 1970). [Online] Available from https://hinduismdebunked.com/scripture/SivaPurana.pdf [Last accessed September, 2025].
2. Evangelical Review of Theology A Global Forum Volume 46, Number 1. Wipe & Stock Publishers, Eugene;2022. https://theology.worldea.org/wp-content
3. The concept of Breath of life in Christianity. https://www.wisdomlib.org/christianity/concept/breath-of-life
4. Dolansky, Shawna. Now You See It, Now You Don't: Biblical Perspectives on the Relationship Between Religion and Magic. Pryor Pettengill Press, Eisenbrauns; 2008.
5. Lisa E Dahill. Christian Worship and the Natural World. LIFE IN ALL ITS FULLNESS. Liturgy. 2016 31(4): 43–50.
6. Todd Weir. Breath of Life | John 20:19-23 | May 28, 2023. https://www.congochurchbbh.org
7. Easwaran E. The Upanishads. In: Easwaran E (Ed). US: Nilgiri Press; 2007.
8. Ravindra R. The Bhagavad Gita. In: Ravindra R (Ed). Mumbai: Jaico Publishing House; 2004.
9. Rambachan A. The Advaita Worldview - God, World, and Humanity. https://www.scribd.com/document
10. Burke AG. (Sami Nirmalanand Giri). The Breath of Life, The Practice of Breath Meditation according to the Hindu, Buddhist, Taoist, Jewish, and Christian Traditions, 2012.https://www.scribd.com/document/473801541
11. Thurman R. The Tibetan Book of the Dead. In: Thurman R (Ed). New York, U.S: Bantam Books Inc; 1994.
12. Halkias G. (2006). Breath awareness in world's religious traditions. [Online] Available from https://elinepa.org/breath-awareness-in-world-s-religious-traditions/ [Last accessed September, 2025].
13. Ahrens L. Importance of Breath. Reference:Yoga Teacher Training January 2011. [Online] Available from https://www.yogapoint.com/mainstory/TopstoryContents/importance_of_breath.html [Last accessed September, 2025].
14. Ewing AH. The Hindu Conception of the Functions of Breath. A Study in Early Hindu Psycho-Physics. J Am Oriental Society. 1901;22:249-308.
15. Singh DP. (2021). Air - A Classical Element of Life in Sikh Theology, Asia Samachar, Malaysia. [Online] Available from https://asiasamachar.com/2021/09/19/40575/ [Last accessed September, 2025].
16. Dundas P. The Jains, 2nd edition. London and New York: Routledge; 2002.
17. Dastagir G. "Nafs". Islam, Judaism, and Zoroastrianism. Encyclopedia of Indian Religions. Dordrecht: Springer Netherlands; 2018.
18. Cook D. "Mysticism in Sufi Islam". Oxford Research Encyclopedia of Religion. Oxford: Oxford University Press; 2015.
19. Ben-Sasson HH. A History of the Jewish People. In: Ben-Sasson HH (Ed). Cambridge, MA: Harvard University Press; 1976.
20. Goodman M. The Oxford Handbook of Jewish Studies. In: Goodman M (Ed). OUP Oxford: Oxford University Press; 2004.
21. Skjærvø PO. (2011). Zoroastrianism: An Introduction. [Online] Available from https://dokumen.pub/the-spirit-of-zoroastrian-ism-9780300181012.html [Last accessed September, 2025].

CHAPTER 2

Ancient India—Indus Valley Civilization, Birth of Ayurveda, and the Mauryan Era

Ancient Indian history can be dated back to 5–10 millennia from now although the periods are rather ill defined. The *Vedas*, the oldest Hindu scriptures, belong to antiquity. The Indus Valley civilization, sometimes referred to as the *Harappan* civilization of the Indian subcontinent, existed during the *Bronze age* from about 3300–1300 BCE for around two millennia. The Vedic period extended from the later part of the Indus Valley period to about 500 BCE covering the late Bronze Age and early Iron Age of the history of India. Mohenjo-Daro was a part of the Indus Valley Civilization which constituted an advanced urban civilization that flourished in North-western India, the modern-day Pakistan. Both the Indus Valley civilization and the Vedic Age generally belong to the prehistoric period.

Respirology during Indus Valley Civilization

Robert Arnott in his book, "Disease and Healing in the Indus Civilization" describes the knowledge of several diseases and medical practices of that period. There is good archaeological evidence in form of Terracotta Tablets with inscriptions of medical texts and prescriptions. Human skulls with holes suggestive of medical interventions such as trephination, i.e., skull-drilling, were found on excavation. Seals with medical symbols depicting diseases and treatments have been also found. But no specific information regarding respiratory or lung diseases can be derived from the available evidence.

Vedic Age

People of the Vedic period attached great significance to breathing in their daily rituals, prayers, music, dance, and athletics. There is an extensive use of breathing related terms such as "*prana*"(life force, breath), "*svara*" (breath, sound) and "*vayu*" (air or wind) in the available texts—*Rigveda* (c. 1500 BCE), *Yajurveda* (c. 1200 BCE), and *Atharvaveda* (c. 1000 BCE). *Agastya*, a Vedic sage of that period emphasized breath control while *Patanjali,* a yoga sage wrote *Yoga Sutras* about different breathing practices and *Pranayama* (breath control), *Yoga Nidra* (guided meditation), and *Bhastrika Pranayama* (bellows breath). From importance of the sacred act of breathing, the concepts had further moved on to its malfunctioning and recognition of disease. The Ayurvedic physician, *Charaka* who described different herbal drugs for different illnesses also belonged to that period.

Symptoms suggestive of pulmonary tuberculosis (*Rakta Pitta)*, an important lung disease (also known as *Phthisis* and *Consumption)* were described. References to tuberculosis were found in Rigveda (as *yaksma)* and Atharvaveda (as *balasa)*. Evidence of tuberculosis has been also found in skeletal remains of that period. Paleopathological examination of two individual skeletons from Harappa revealed findings which were highly suggestive of tuberculosis. Reference of "scrofula", i.e., tuberculous lymphadenopathy is found in *Atharvaveda*. Both *Yajurveda* and *Sushruta Samhita* recommended different forms of treatment for tuberculosis.

Classification of diseases having five types :

पञ्च गुल्मा इति वातपित्तकफसन्निपातशोणितजाः; पञ्च प्लीहदोषा इति गुल्मैर्व्याख्याताः, पञ्च कासा इति वातपित्तकफक्षतक्षयजाः, पञ्च श्वासा इति महोर्ध्वच्छिन्नतमकक्षुद्राः, पञ्च हिक्का इति महती गम्भीरा व्यपेता क्षुद्राऽन्नजा च, पञ्च तृष्णा इति वातपित्तामक्षयोपसर्गात्मिकाः, पञ्च छर्द्य इति द्विष्टार्थसंयोगजा वातपित्तकफसन्निपातोद्रेकोत्थाश्च, पञ्च भक्तस्यानशनस्थानानीति वातपित्तकफसन्निपातद्वेषाः, पञ्च शिरोरोगा इति पूर्वोद्देशमभिसमस्य वातपित्तकफसन्निपातक्रिमिजाः, पञ्च हृद्रोगा इति शिरोरोगैर्व्याख्याताः, पञ्च पाण्डुरोगा इति वातपित्तकफसन्निपातमृद्भक्षणजाः; पञ्चोन्मादा इति वातपित्तकफसन्निपातागन्तुनिमित्ताः (४);

10. Five *gulmas* (abdominal tumour) *Vātika, paittika, ślaiṣmika, sānnipātika* and *raktaja* (due to blood).

11. Five Splenic disorders (as above)

12. Five *Kāsas* (coughing), *Vātika, paittika, ślaiṣmika kṣataja* (due to ulceration) and *kṣayaja* (due to wasting).

13. Five *Śvāsas* (dyspnoea), *Mahāśvāsa, ūrdhvaśvāsa, chinnaśvāsa, tamaka śvāsa* and *kṣudra śvāsa.*

14. Five *Hikkās* (hiccup), *Mahāhikkā, gambhīrahikkā, vyapetā*

Classification of diseases having five types in *Charak Samhita* mentions five "*kasas*" and five "*swasa.*"
Source: From Agnivesa's "Carak Samhita" based on "Cakarapanidatta's Ayurveda Dipika" by Ram Karan Sharma and Vaidya Bhagwan Dash, Vol. I, Sutra Sthana, Chowkhamba Sanskrit Series Office, Varanasi.

Besides tuberculosis, other lung diseases which were commonly seen included asthma (described in Ayurvedic texts as *Tamaka Swasa*), bronchitis (described as *Kasa*) and pneumonia (*Shwasa Roga in* Ayurvedic texts). The Vedic-Age understanding of lung diseases and treatments demonstrates their advanced medical knowledge. Various lung diseases were attributed to environmental and lifestyle factors. Medical practitioners used different herbs and drugs to treat diseases. Medical practice of that period is the most likely source of ancient Indian medicine.

Birth of Ayurveda, Yoga, and Pranayama

It is difficult to date the exact period of the origin of *Ayurveda*. But for the stress on breathing to keep both physical and spiritual health, there are limited references made to the presence of diseases and their management both in the Western and the Eastern civilizations in the ancient period. In India, the birth of *Ayurveda* constituted an important part of the history of medicine. *Ayurveda,* now classified as an alternate system of medicine, continues to be widely practiced till date for the management of medical disorders including various respiratory illnesses. Some of the most common diseases and/or symptoms which attracted attention in the *Ayurvedic* system included the management of cough, fever, and tuberculosis.

The *Ayurvedic* system remains popular even now in various populations for different spectra of illnesses. It is believed to find its origin in *Atharvaveda* of Vedic medicine extending from 2nd millennium BCE to about 800 BCE. *Ayurveda* owes its birth to Dhanvantari, the Hindu physician of Gods who imparted the knowledge received from Lord *Brahma* to the Indian learned men. The story of Dhanvantari in Hindu medicine is as distinct as that of Asclepius—the Greek God of Medicine.

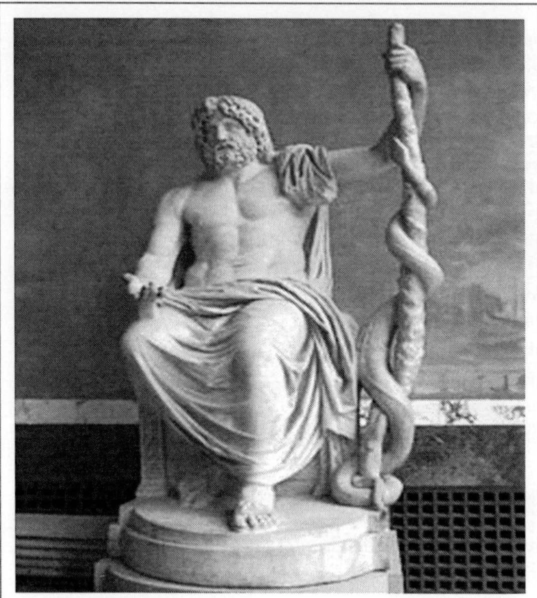

Asklepius—the Greek God of Medicine.

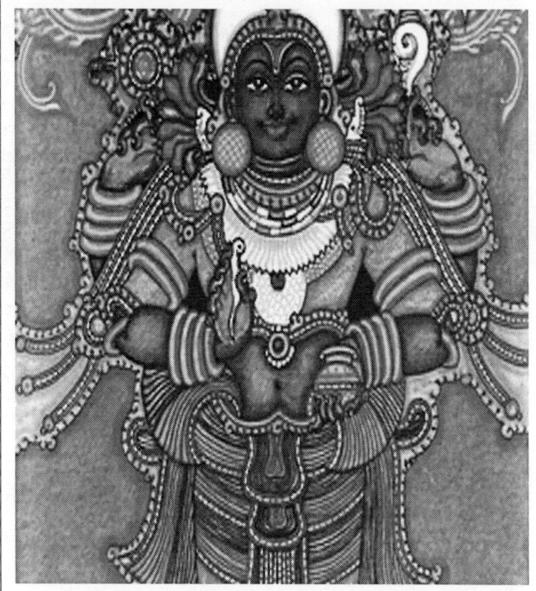

Dhanvantari—the ancient Vedic God of medicine to whom the Ayurveda owes its origin in Ancient India.

Dhanvantari

Dhanvantari's tale is entangled in layers of mystery of healing and treatment powers. There is mention of Dhanvantari in the *Vedas* as well as the *Puranas*, the Hindu religious texts. There are several different legends surrounding the birth and powers of Dhanvantari. There is a famous tale in "*Bhagavata Purana*" about the God of Medicine in Hinduism. On the advice of Lord Vishnu, both the gods (*devas*) and the demons (*asuras)* were looking for the nectar (*Amrita)* lying deep in the Ocean of Milk to gain immortality. They joined together to churn the sea with the help of a huge mountain (*Mandara*) as the axle and the serpent (*Vasuki*) used as the rope around the axle. A number of valuable items were churned out—a cow (*Kamdhenu*) which yielded enormous quantities of milk, the flying horse, the white elephant, moon, and nymphs. Finally emerged Dhanvantari, a handsome god with four hands, Clad in bright yellow silk, the god had a pitcher of nectar, a conch shell *(Sankha*), a wheel (*chakra*), and golden leech (*jalookaa*).

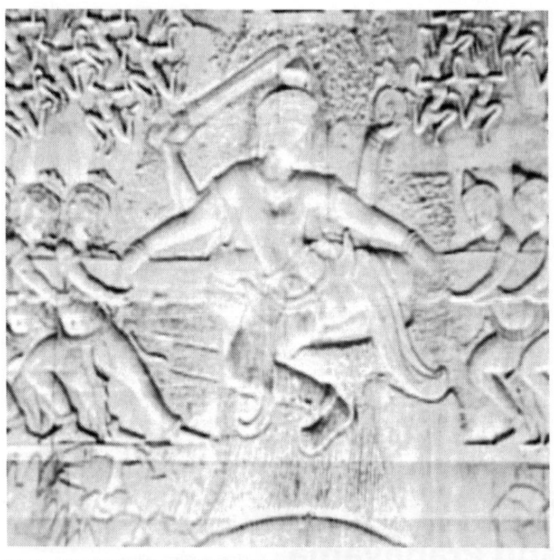

"*Samudramanthan*"—Carving on a wall in the ancient Angkor Wat temple in Cambodia, located in Siem, the ancient Khmer capital city of Angkor, originally constructed in 1150 CE as a Hindu temple dedicated to the God *Vishnu*.
Courtesy: Photo by Dr Aditya Jindal.

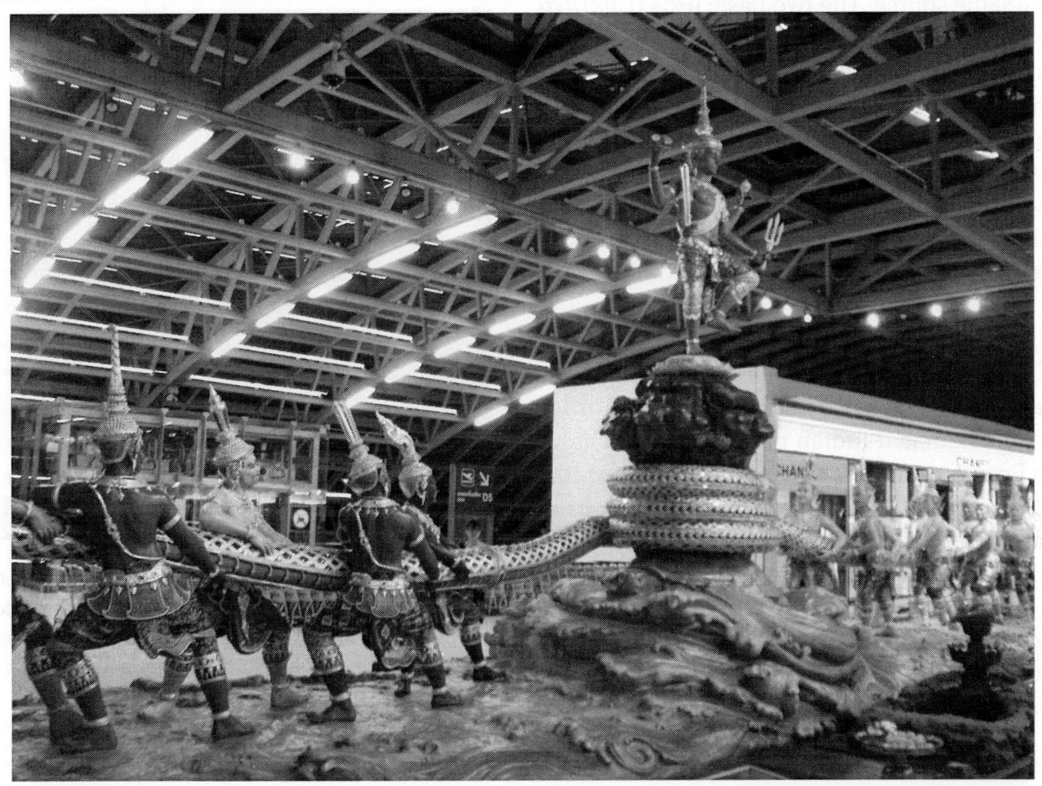

Samudralay—sculpture on Scene of the churning of the Milk Ocean *at* Svaranbhumi airport, Bangkok. *Courtesy*: Photo by Dr SK Jindal.

Dhanvantari carried a pitcher of nectar in his hand. The pot was snatched by the "*asuras*" potentially depriving the "devas" of immortality. Lord Vishnu therefore appeared after Dhanvantari in different incarnation of an enchanting damsel, Mohini, who tricked the *asuras* to distribute the nectar to the "*devas*" thus imparting them with immortality. Dhanvantari laid the foundation of Indian tradition of medicine—the *Ayurveda*.

He continues to be worshipped by a large number of Hindus on "*Dhanteras*"—2 days before the Hindu festival of Diwali. The day is considered as most auspicious for purchase of utensils or costly items of silver and gold to propagate prosperity. There are a number of Dhanvantari temples particularly in some of the states of Southern India. It is believed that Dhanvantari might represent a lineage of healers or a tradition of healing which passed on through generations since time immemorial. Dhanvantari is sometimes regarded as an *avatar* (incarnation) of *Lord Vishnu* who reigned as the King of Kashi during his incarnation on earth. He is also identified as the great-grandfather of *Divodasa*, the mythological King of Kashi (now Varanasi) in the *Vishnu Purana*.

Dhanvantari symbolizes the divine aspect of healing as well as *Ayurveda* and traditional Indian medicine. The term "*Ayurveda*" is derived from the Sanskrit words "*Ayur*" meaning "life" while *Vedas* are the ancient Indian scriptures, which contain references to medicinal plants, treatments, and health practices. The term *Vaid*, commonly used for an ayurvedic practitioner, also owes its origin to the same source. The two basic texts (*Charaka Samhita and Sushruta Samhita*) composed around 400 CE, laid foundations of *Ayurveda* with the core concept of *Tridosha* (three *doshas, Vata, Pitta, and Kapha*) which govern the human physiology and pathology. *Ayurveda* influenced by various cultures and traditions, has further evolved over centuries as a complementary system of medicine.

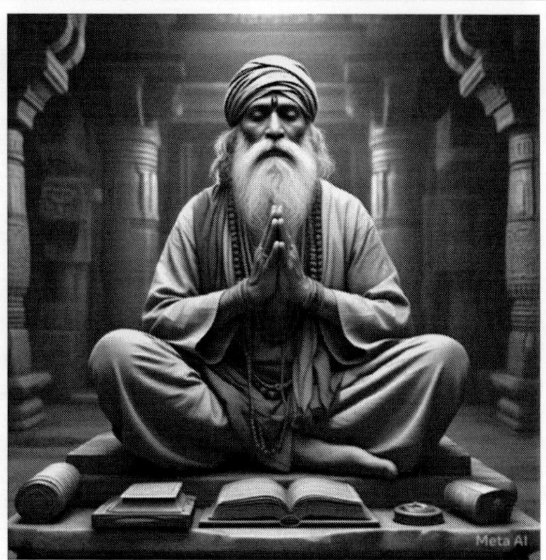

Sushruta – The ancient Indian physician and surgeon of the 6th century BCE, often referred to as "Father of Surgery". He made significant contributions to the field of various surgical fields, including thoracic surgery.
Source: AI created photograph.

Atreya Punarvasu

Atreya (or Atreyas) Punarvasu was another renowned ancient Indian physician and scholar who lived around 600 BCE. A descendant of *Atri* who is mentioned in the *Puranas* as one of the great Hindu sages, he is considered one of the earliest and most influential figures in *Ayurveda*. He was the personal physician of the king Nagnajita of Gandhara and taught Jivaka, the personal physician of Lord Buddha. He is also believed to be the author of the original contents of *Charaka Samhita*.

Sushruta Samhita

Sushruta, (6th century BCE) is considered as one of the earliest known surgeons in the world. His seminal work, the *Sushruta Samhita*, is a comprehensive medical text that covers various aspects of surgery, including those for lung diseases. *Sushruta Samhita*, composed in Sanskrit, is divided into six sections (*Sthanas*) and 186 chapters which cover various aspects of *Ayurveda*, including anatomy, physiology, pathology, diagnosis, treatment, and surgery. While the original text was likely written during the 6th–5th centuries BCE, several revisions and commentaries were added over the centuries. The major revisions were made by Nagarjuna (2nd century CE) and Dalhana (12th century CE). *Sushruta Samhita* has been translated into various languages and has influenced *Ayurvedic* and *Unani* medicine in India and elsewhere. The oldest surviving manuscript today dates back to the 10th century CE and is recognized by UNESCO as a "Memory of the World" document.

Charaka Samhita

The *Charaka Samhita* is another ancient *Ayurvedic* text that has a rich history spanning over 2000 years. The primary composition is attributed to Charaka, a renowned Ayurvedic physician during the Gupta Empire (320–550 CE). The *Samhita* is also composed in Sanskrit and includes eight sections (*Sthanas*) and 120 chapters which cover various aspects of *Ayurveda*. Commentaries were added to the primary text over the centuries and major revisions were made by *Chakrapani* (10th century CE) and *Vijayarakshita* (11th century CE). The oldest surviving manuscript dates back to the 10th century CE.

Both *Sushruta* and *Charaka Samhita* significantly contributed to respiratory medicine. They provide detailed descriptions of respiratory

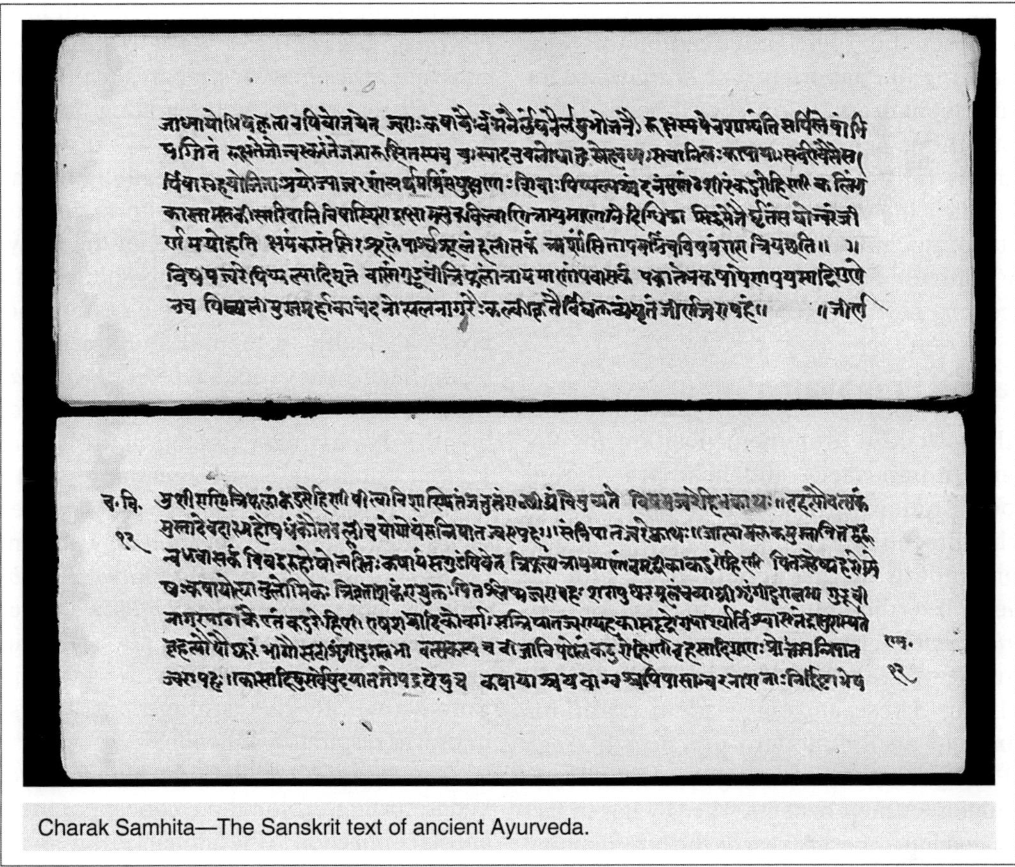

Charak Samhita—The Sanskrit text of ancient Ayurveda.

anatomy, including the lungs, trachea, and the bronchi as well as the examination techniques. *Sushruta Samhita* includes diseases such as *Dukhnak* with tuberculosis-like symptoms (characterized by cough, fever, weight loss, and weakness), *Kshayakshina,* i.e., pulmonary consumption (with symptoms such as cough, dyspnea, and chest pain), and *Swasakshaya*, respiratory disorders, including asthma and bronchitis. *Chakshushya* referred to eye and lung disease (conjunctivitis and pneumonia; may perhaps refer to vasculitis which we recognize now).

According to *both Samhitas,* it is the imbalance of the three *doshas or humors* (*Vata, Pitta, and Kapha*) which is responsible for these diseases. On the other hand, the exposure to cold, wind, and pollutants along with overexertion, stress, and poor sleep precipitate the problems or serve as risk factors. Various treatment modalities which were recommended included herbal remedies, dietary regimens, and regular exercises. Other interventions included *Panchakarma,* i.e., detoxification and rejuvenation therapies as well as surgical treatments such as the drainage of lung abscesses, tracheostomy, bronchotomy, and pneumonotomy. Charaka Samhita's descriptions of lung diseases subsequently shaped Ayurvedic pulmonology and greatly influenced the Ayurvedic respiratory practices.

Both *Charaka Samhita* and *Sushruta Samhita* *also* recognized the importance of breathing in maintaining physical and mental health and describe various breathing techniques. The *Charaka Samhita* emphasized the importance of nasal breathing, diaphragmatic breathing, and breath control for balancing *doshas* (energies).

The *Yoga Sutras* of *Patanjali*, although compiled later, reflect the Yogic practices of this era, emphasizing the importance of *Pranayama* for physical, mental, and spiritual well-being. Later, the breathing practices were further refined by various Tantric practices such as *Kundalini Yoga*, which incorporated complex rituals and meditation techniques during the early period of the Common Era (The *Hatha Yoga Pradipika*, 15th century CE).

Yoga and Pranayama

Breathing, held a prominent position for the ancient Indian sages and scholars of that period. Ancient India's developments in breathing techniques demonstrate a profound understanding of the human body and its connection to the universe. From the *Vedas* to *Tantric* practices, breathing played a vital role in spiritual growth, self-realization, and physical well-being. These ancient wisdom traditions continue to inspire modern practices of *Yoga and Pranayama*, which have gained worldwide recognition for their benefits. The UN has in fact designated June 21 every year as the International *Yoga Day* to signify the yoga's importance and capacity in enduring health, peace, harmony, and well-being. Recently in 2024, the UN General Assembly has also declared December 21 as the Meditation Day signifying the importance of combined mental and physical techniques, breathing exercises, quiet and calm breathing, and body awareness to promote relaxation and reduce stress.

Yoga places great emphasis on breathing, recognizing its profound physiological benefits and impact on physical, mental, and spiritual well-being. Besides several other benefits, *yoga* helps to regulate respiratory, mental, and nervous systems through enhanced emotional regulation. *Yoga* also increases lung capacity and improves sleep quality by reducing stress and anxiety through relaxation and calmness. Besides the physical and mental benefits, *yoga* is a method of achieving spiritual connection with life force (*Prana*), balancing energy (*Chakras*), and cultivate awareness. It prepares for meditation and self-realization by integrating body, mind, and spirit.

Pranayama is a set of breathing techniques in *Yoga* and Ayurveda that aim to control and regulate the life force (*Prana*) in the body. The practice of *Pranayama* is deeply connected to the art of breathing, and its benefits extend beyond physical health to mental and spiritual well-being. There are various types of *Pranayama*—*Ujjayi* (victorious breath), *Bhastrika* (bellows breath), *Kapalabhati* (breath of fire), *Anuloma Viloma* (alternate nostril breathing), and *Sitali* (cooling breath). In addition to the *yoga* methods mentioned earlier, *Pranayama* may also involve *Pranava (Om* chanting), *Bhaya Kumbhaka* (hold breath) and *Kevala Kumbhaka* (retention of breath). A large number of physical, spiritual, and psychosomatic benefits are derived from pranayama. It also strengthens lungs and improves respiratory function.

The *Upanishadic* Period which followed the Vedas, further explored the concept of breathing and its connection to the ultimate reality, *Brahman*. The *Chandogya Upanishad*, for instance, describes the five types of breath, emphasizing their role in achieving spiritual liberation. Yoga emerged further as a distinct philosophical school and marked a significant milestone in the breathing developments. Much later, *Patanjali's Yoga Sutras* (400 CE) systematically outlined various breathing techniques.

Mauryan Period

The historical Mauryan Era, from around 322–185 BCE, was founded by Chandragupta Maurya with the state capital at Pataliputra (now Patna). Mauryan Empire covered most of the Northern and North-Western India. Chandragupta was succeeded by his son Bindusara and then grandson, Ashoka. The Mauryan period was a well-developed era in the region in several fields including in medicine. The eminent history-author, William Dalrymple in his recent book, "*The Golden Road: How Ancient India transformed the World?*" vividly describes of the presence of an extensive economic development and contact for trade between Indian and the Western civilizations (via the sea routes). We can attribute some of the similarities about the concepts and treatments of diseases between the Indian, the Greco-Roman, Egyptian, and Arabic cultures on the basis of this exchange. Alexander's invasion of northern part of India via land-route in the 3rd century BCE during the Mauryan era had further augmented that contact.

This was also the time when Ayurvedic herbs, *yoga,* and *pranayama* firmly established their roots in medical practices. Both Buddhism and Jainism which originated in around 6th century BCE also laid great importance on breathing practices. Jivaka, who was Buddha's personal physician recommended that the Buddha screen people for diseases before ordaining (may be for fear of infectious disease such as tuberculosis).

Chanakya, (also known as Kautilya and Vishnugupta) the Prime Minister to the King Chandragupta, mentions a highly developed medical profession for both humans and livestock in his *Arthashashtra.* This is nicely deliberated upon by Patrick Olivelle in his recent article where he tells about the importance of Ayurveda in cleaning up the image of ancient Indian medical system against the charlatan practices. Emperor Ashoka (King Piyadasi) was a great patron of medical services and issued significant edicts.

"*.......everywhere the Beloved of Gods, King Piyadasi, has established two kinds of medical services: medical services for humans and medical services for domestic animals. Wherever medical herbs suitable for humans or animals are not available, I have had them imported and grown. Wherever medical roots or fruits are not available I have had them imported and grown. Along roads I have had wells dug and trees planted for the benefit of humans and animals. (Rock Edict II)*"

The Rock edict also suggests the existence of an international exchange particularly with Greece and other Mediterranean countries.

Siddha Medicine

Siddha medicine was another ancient traditional system of medicine which was commonly practiced in South India. It is believed to be founded by the legendary sage Agastya in 500 BCE who is popularly considered as the father of Siddha medicine. Almost a thousand years later, *Tirumantiram* wrote its foundational text; other works such as *Yogagnana, and Siddha Maruthuvam* were added. It continued to be popular during the medieval period but faced decline during the British Colonial Era. Tamil scholars and physicians have worked to revive *Siddha* medicine which remains in practice in Tamil Nadu

Siddha Medicine, like Ayurveda is based on the principles of three humors (*Vatham, Pittam, and Kapham*) and employs treatments with herbal and mineral-based medicine, *yoga*, meditation, *varma* therapy (acupuncture-like practice) and *Panchakarma* detoxification. In respiratory medicine, these treatments are frequently used for coughs, infections, tuberculosis, bronchitis, and asthma for their expectorant, antioxidant, and anti-inflammatory properties. *Yoga Nidra* (Guided meditation), *asanas,* and *pranayama* are often recommended for improvement of lung function and to reduce stress.

The medical practices during the Indus Valley civilization though primitive, were fairly well developed. Significant advancements took place in various fields, including in medicine, philosophy, and spirituality during the Mauryan era. This era also saw the rise of Buddhism and Jainism, which emphasized the importance of breath control and meditation. This was a transformative period for respiratory practices in ancient India with *Yoga, Pranayama,* and Ayurvedic herbs.

Sources

1. Arnott R. Disease and Healing in the Indus Civilisation. Middle Way Summertown Oxford: Archaeopress Publishing Ltd Summertown Pavilion; 2024. pp. 18-24.
2. Rao SR. Indus Valley Civilization. New Delhi: Archaeological Survey of India; 1962.
3. Griffith RTH. The Vedas. In: Griffith RTH (Ed); 1889.
4. Tracing the Timeless Journey of Yoga https://www.pib.gov.in/FeaturesDeatils.aspx?id=154674&NoteId=154674&ModuleId=2
5. Maina JN. The Evolution of Respiratory Systems. Cham, Switzerland: Springer International Publishing AG; 2018.
6. Kashinath Hadimur, RS Sarashetti. Physiological Aspects of Respiratory System in Ancient Indian Medicine (Ayurveda): A Review. Journal of Pharmaceutical and Scientific Innovation www.jpsionline.com (ISSN : 2277-4572).
7. Hudson DD. The Body of God: An Emperor's Palace for Krishna in Eighth-Century Kanchipuram. Oxford: Oxford University Press; 2008.
8. Gray LH. The Indian God Dhanvantari. J Am Oriental Society. 1922;42:323-37.
9. Olivelle P. (2024). Ancient Indian medical system had an image crisis. A new name fixed it. [Online] Available from https://theprint.in/opinion/theprint-purana/ancient-indian-medical-system-had-an-image-crisis-a-new-name-fixed-it/2247440/ [Last accessed September, 2025].
10. Mark JJ. Chanakya. [Online] Available from https://www.worldhistory.org/Kautilya [Last accessed September, 2025].
11. Madhavan C. Vishnu temples of South India, Volume two. Chitra Madhavan. 2008.
12. Meulenbeld GJ. History of Ayurveda by (1999-2002). [Online] Available from https://www.scribd.com/document/506176844/Meulenbeld-a-History-of-Indian-Medical-Literature-Vol-IA-1999 [Last accessed September, 2025].
13. PV Sharma. Susruta Samhita 1-3 Vols. 2013, https://www.amazon.in/dp/9381301255.
14. Sharma P. (1981). Charaka Samhita. [Online] Available from https://archive.org/details/Charaka Samhita Text With English Tanslation PV Sharma [Last accessed September, 2025].
15. Dalrymple W. The Golden Road: How Ancient India transformed the World? London: Bloomsbury Publishing plc; 2024.

CHAPTER 3

Contemporary Ancient History: Rest of the World

The ancient Indus Valley Civilization (3500–1500 BCE), the Vedic Period (1500–500 BCE) and the Mauryan Era (500–300 BCE) in India roughly corresponded to the Pre-Biblical and Biblical Periods in Western civilizations of Mesopotamia, Egypt, Greece, and Europe. The political, social, and cultural systems were well developed. Similar progress was found in the Eastern Chinese and Japanese civilizations. The developments in different parts of the world in different ancient civilizations were similar in several ways but could be largely considered as independent of each other. There was little known exchange of ideas because of the general lack of rapid means of communication during that period. The importance of breathing air as essential to life was well recognized in various theological texts, religious scriptures, and traditions. People of all these different civilizations considered respiration as a divine act or a "breath of life". But the functioning of the lungs, heart, or other organs was poorly understood.

Mesopotamia

Mesopotamian civilization, one of the oldest in the world, beginning around 3400 BCE existed in the area between the Euphrates and Tigris rivers to the north or northwest of Baghdad, in modern Iraq. While Sumeria spanned 5th–3rd millennia BCE in southern Mesopotamia, Assyria was another major ancient Mesopotamian civilization which existed from the 21st century BCE to the 14th century BCE. Mesopotamians believed that the gods breathed life into humans and linked breath to the soul and spiritual essence. Breath was seen as a life-giving force which also connected humans to the divine. Controlled breathing was considered essential for wisdom. Breathing rituals marked important life events (e.g., birth, death) while breath control was essential for musicians, dancers, and athletes. It was also given important medical and health significance, e.g., to help in diagnosis of illnesses as well as to treat with breathing exercises and inhalation therapies.

Breathing was believed to maintain balance in the body. The ancient Mesopotamian epic (1600 BCE), *Atra-hasis* (primarily derived from Akkadian clay tablets) and the epic of Gilgamesh (compiled by Sin-leqi-unninni around 1300–1000 BCE) describe some of the breathing related terms such as *"kalātu"* (*Akkadian*, Lung disease), *"napāhu"* (breath, wind), and *"šāpu"* (cough). Similarly, the Code of Hammurabi (1754 BCE), which features a code of law from ancient Babylon in Mesopotamia mentions breathing difficulties and lung diseases. The Assyrian Medical Texts (circa 700–600 BCE) also describe respiratory treatments. *Nergal* and *Gula*, the breathing-related gods were associated with respiratory diseases and invoked for respiratory health. The Sumerians also had breathing related gods such as *Enlil* (air god) and Enki (god of wisdom, associated with breath). The Sumerians practiced *Pranayama* such as breathing techniques and breath-control for meditation.

Egyptian Civilization: Ebers Papyrus

The most significant proof of the "presence" of the lungs is available from the Egyptian civilization of 3000 BCE. The Egyptians used to dissect the body after death and remove the organs (including the lungs), for embalming before mummification. Jakub Kwiecinski has described the respiratory tract from the Egyptian art of that period from a hieroglyph and depicted the presence of trachea, the cartilaginous rings, the two main bronchi, and the lung lobes. Ebers Papyrus, written in hieratic Egyptian is the best-known source of medical information of that period. In a recent article, the Papyrus also describes that there are four vessels to the lungs and to the spleen. Egyptians possibly possessed a sense of gross appearance of the lungs in normal as well as in various abnormal states such as abscesses, tumors, and trauma.

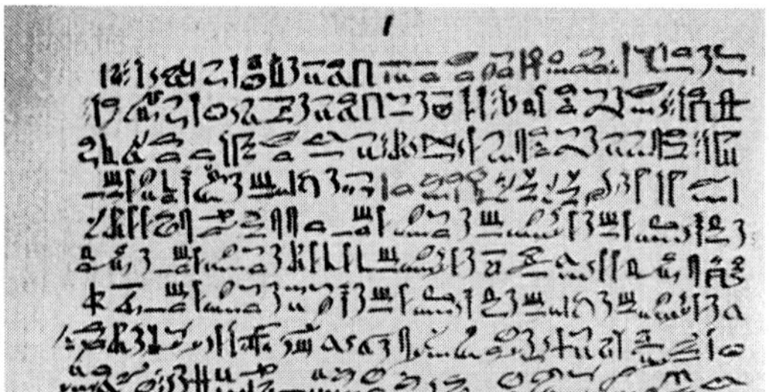

Ebers Papyrus—one of the earliest medical texts, written around 1500 BCE in Egypt. This was discovered by German Egyptologist and novelist Georg Moritz in 1873–1874.

The Ebers Papyrus also contains numerous magical formulas, folk remedies, and incantations meant to turn away disease-causing demons. For diagnoses, they employed observation of symptoms, examination of bodily fluids, and spiritual rituals. Treatments mostly consisted of herbal remedies, dietary regimens, prayers, and offerings to gods. Surgical procedure such as thoracentesis was also practised. Maintenance of a balance of *toxins, evil spirits, healthy diet*, regular exercise, and spiritual practices were advocated for disease prevention.

Ancient Egyptians acknowledged lung diseases as significant health issues and treated them with a focus on both spiritual and natural remedies. They believed in the *Wekhedu* (life force) concept and that imbalances led to various lung diseases, such as *Shw't* (pneumonia), *Hsb* (cough), *Sgr* (pleurisy), and *Mw't* (asthma). Evidence of skeletal deformities typical of tuberculosis, i.e., characteristic Pott's lesions have been found in the Egyptian mummies dating back to 2400 BC and similar deformities are clearly seen in early Egyptian art. But no such description or evidence of tuberculosis (TB) lesions is reported in Egyptian papyri.

Greek Civilization

Some major medical developments including those related to the respiratory system happened in Europe during the classical period. Many of these developments that happened in Greece were related to Hippocrates and his followers. Hippocrates was born in the Greek island of Kos around the year 460 BCE. His genealogy is often traced to his paternal heritage to Asklepius, the Greek god of medicine, and maternal ancestry to Heracles, (also known as Hercules in Roman mythology), the son of god Zeus and a mortal woman. Hippocrates coined the Hippocratic Oath which continues for its sanctity in today's medical practice. His major contribution, the Hippocratic Corpus, is a large collection of about 70 major works—textbooks, lectures, and essays on multiple medical subjects. The Corpus may perhaps also include contributions of different authors and philosophers of that time.

The Greek concept of causation of diseases at that time was attributed to the theory of humors, somewhat akin to the concepts of the Vedic and Mauryan periods in the Indian subcontinent. In *Ayurveda* too it was believed that disease is caused by an imbalance of three humors, or *doshas (defects)* known as *vata* (wind or air), *kapha* (water or phlegm), and *pitta* (fire and water or bile). The *kapha* in Ayurvedic and the phlegmatic (phlegm like) humor in Greek beliefs were related to the lungs while others owed their origin to the liver, gallbladder, and spleen or others.

The Greek humoral theory was first propagated by Hippocrates and subsequently by his followers, Plato and Aristotle (300 BCE). The concept continued to be believed for a prolonged period, further supported by Galen (2nd century CE) and later throughout the medieval and early renaissance periods in Europe. Galen in his treatise "On the Movements of the Heart and Lung", explained that the lung is a very soft and warm organ which is kept in constant motion. He also described about an interconnection between the heart and the lung and believed that the purpose of inspiration was to cool the heart while expiration was a means of ridding the body of heat.

Hippocrates is commonly referred to as "Father of Medicine" in view of his extensive contributions which laid the foundations of modern medicine. This had been especially so in the field of respiratory and lung diseases. He is credited with the recognition of the role of environment factors such as the climatic conditions, and of importance of physical examination for the diagnosis of diseases. There is good description of respiratory infections such as pneumonia, pleurisy, and thoracic empyema, as well as of other diseases like asthma and upper airway obstruction.

Hippocrates described pneumonia as a distinct clinical entity diagnosed by symptoms such as fever, cough, and difficulty breathing while pleurisy as an inflammation of the lining surrounding the lungs recognized in association with pneumonia from the characteristic symptoms of pleuritic chest pain and fever.

Asthma was mentioned as a disease characterized by wheezing, coughing, and shortness of breath due to an imbalance of bodily humors. Hippocrates employed physical examination including percussion and auscultation, to diagnose lung diseases. He had described the use of holistic treatments such as diet, exercise, and herbal remedies (as expectorants), for different pulmonary conditions such as asthma.

Hippocrates' contributions to the understanding of lung diseases are remarkable, considering the limited knowledge and technological advancements of his time. His work laid the foundation for future medical discoveries and remains an essential part of the history of pulmonary medicine. Humoral theory along with ancient ideas of Hippocrates, Galen, and others formed the basis of overall medical practice almost for the next millennium.

The period after the decline and fall of the Roman Empire in 5th century CE is often referred to as the Dark Ages. There was hardly any noticeable progress in philosophical, scientific, or medical ideas for almost a millennium. There were only occasional or sporadic discoveries, none of which can be categorized as significant in respiratory medicine.

Chinese Civilization

The Chinese civilization in antiquity was equally well developed in medical fields similar to the other contemporary civilizations. The classic medical writing, *Huangdi neijing* or the canon of internal medicine (*Yellow Emperor's Inner Classic*) is attributed to Huangdi (the Yellow Emperor)—one of the legendary founders of Chinese civilization. There are some other important Chinese compositions such as the medical writings of the Han dynasty (202 BCE–220 CE) and

Mojing (known as the "Pulse Classic") composed during the early period of the Common Era. The Chinese believed in the dualistic cosmic theory of *yin-yang*, the *yang* is the male principle, (active and light, represented by the heavens) and the *yin*, the female principle, (passive and dark, is represented by the earth). Health and several other issues are determined by the dominance of the *yin* or the *yang*. The ancient Chinese medicine aimed at the control their proportions in the body for a healthy life.

Ancient Chinese medical texts believed that *Qi* (life energy) and its balance were crucial for maintaining lung health while lung diseases were attributed to *Qi* imbalances. *Qi,* particularly in the teachings of Taoism and Confucianism, was seen as the fundamental energy believed to flow through the body, governing various physiological processes. *Qi* is constantly in motion, can transform into different forms, such as blood, body fluids, and energy. It is responsible for harmonious body functions for an optimal health. Several different types of *Qi* were described including the *Yuan Qi* (the innate energy present at birth), *Zhong Qi* (the energy governing digestion and respiration), *Zong Qi* (the energy inherited from ancestors) and *Wei Qi* (the energy protecting the body from external pathogens). When *Qi* is imbalanced or blocked, it can lead to various health issues, including fatigue, pain, digestive, and respiratory problems.

There is mention of several specific lung diseases known at that time: *Fei* (lung abscess), *Xuan yi* (pneumonia), *Chuan* (asthma), and *Ke-sou* (cough). For diagnosis, there was emphasis on pulse diagnosis, tongue analysis, and observation of symptoms to diagnose lung diseases. Traditional Chinese practitioners used different treatment modalities such as *acupuncture* (inserting thin needles into specific points on the body to stimulate the body's natural healing processes) and *moxibustion* (a traditional Chinese therapy with burning dried mugwort or moxa, a small, spongy herb, on particular points on the body). Other therapies included the herbal medicine (e.g., ginseng, licorice root), dietary therapy (e.g., avoiding cold foods), qigong, and breathing exercises.

The ancient Chinese concepts of lung health and disease continue to influence modern integrative respiratory care of traditional Chinese medicine. Besides herbal remedies, *acupuncture* remains one such common modality used in Chinese medical practice. *Acupuncture* is believed to restore balance and promote healing, relieve mental stress, and promote well-being. It is also believed to enhance immune function and body defenses as well as treat various lung diseases including asthma, chronic obstructive pulmonary disease (COPD), and lung cancer. There are specific *acupuncture* points (LU-7, LU-9, BL-13, and BL-23) which are targeted for lung diseases. *Acupuncture* is a valuable adjunct therapy for lung diseases, offering a safe and effective way to manage symptoms, improve lung function, and enhance overall well-being.

Japanese Civilization

The recognition and management of lung diseases in ancient Japanese civilization also demonstrate a unique blend of spiritual and natural approaches to respiratory health. Almost similar to the traditional Chinese and Korean medicine, the Japanese also believed in *Ki* (also spelled "Qi" or "Chi") which refers to the vital energy or life force that flows through the body. There are three different kinds of *Ki*—*Kokyu-ki* (breath energy), *Ketsu-ki* (blood energy), and *Shin-ki* (mind energy). Imbalances or blockages in *Ki* are responsible for different ailments including respiratory diseases while practices such as *Qigong, Taiji* (*Tai Chi*), and *Zen* meditation help to develop and balance Ki. Lung diseases were referred to in ancient Japanese civilization in the *Kojiki* (Record of Ancient Matters) and the *Man'yōshū* (Collection of Ten Thousand Leaves). Various respiratory problems which are mentioned include *Hai* (pneumonia), *Kaze* (cough), *Yuki* (pleurisy), and *Shō* (asthma). Management was focused on traditional herbal remedies *(Kanpō*), *acupuncture, moxibustion,* healthy diet, regular exercise, stress management, and spiritual practices (such as meditation and *Shinto* rituals).

Like the beliefs of many other traditional ancient civilizations, the Japanese concepts of lung health and disease continue to influence modern *Kampo* medicine and inspire research in integrative respiratory care.

Sources

1. Köcher F. Mesopotamian Medicine; 1963.
2. Heimerdinger JM. Breath and Soul in Mesopotamia; 2015.
3. Nunn JF. Ancient Egyptian Medicine. Norman: University of Oklahoma Press; 1996.
4. Kwiecinski J. First images of respiratory system in ancient Egypt: Trachea, bronchi and pulmonary lobes. Can Respir J. 2012;19(5):e33-5.
5. Ghalioungui P. The Ebers papyrus: A new English translation, commentaries and glossaries. Cairo: Academy of Scientific Research and Technology; 1987.
6. Hippocrates, (Stanford Encyclopedia of Philosophy): Overview of Hippocratic medicine.
7. Conarton RF (Ed). The Medical Legacy of Hippocrates; 2007.
8. Stefanakis G, Nyktari V, Papaioannou A, Askitopoulou H. Hippocratic concepts of acute and urgent respiratory diseases still relevant to contemporary medical thinking and practice: a scoping review. BMC Pulm Med. 2020;20(1):165.
9. Zhang Y, Lu P, Qin H, Zhang Y, Sun X, Song X, et al. Traditional Chinese medicine combined with pulmonary drug delivery system and idiopathic pulmonary fibrosis: Rationale and therapeutic potential. Biomed Pharmacother. 2021;133:111072.
10. Wang C, Xiao F, Qiao R, Shen YH. Respiratory medicine in China: progress, challenges, and opportunities. Chest. 2013;143(6):1766-73.
11. Danning Ma, Shanshan Wang, Yu Shi, Shenglou Ni, Minke Tang, Anlong Xu. The development of traditional Chinese medicine. Journal of Traditional Chinese Medical Sciences. 2021;8(Supplement 1): S1-S9.
12. Porter R (Ed). The Cambridge History of Medicine; 2006: Wellcome Institute for the History of Medicine, University College London, 2001. https://www.cambridge.org/in/universitypress/subjects/history/history-medicine/
13. Japanese Respiratory Society. The History of Pulmonology in Japan—A comprehensive overview of lung medicine in Japan; 2013.
14. Duglison R. Medical lexicon: a dictionary of medical science. Philadelphia: Blanchard and Lea; 1851. pp. 743-4.

CHAPTER 4

Medieval India

During the early part of the first millennium, there were significant developments in medicine in the Western world in Greece, Rome, and the rest of Europe. Several of these new findings were related to the understanding of respiratory medicine. These developments were largely built upon the foundational work of Hippocrates. Western physicians invested in research and development of a stepwise scientific approach. They followed a systematic approach of knowing the structure and function of body parts, abnormalities in the organ-function and possible causation and how to diagnose and manage the abnormality. It was not a systematically organized project. But a large number of independent or anecdotal discoveries did finally help to understand the difficult questions. More frequent and rapid communications helped in greater exchange and faster spread of ideas and inventions.

Early Post-Mauryan Period in India

Several important dynasties including the Sungas, Kanvas, Satavahanas, and Kushans ruled during the early post-Mauryan period between the fall of the Mauryas after the death of King Ashoka and the rise of the Guptas (2nd century BCE to 3rd century CE). There were significant developments in political, economic, and cultural fields. The art and architecture of that era were engraved in rock-cut caves, pillars, and *stupas*. Each dynasty introduced its own distinctive features reflecting the changing socio-political scenario. According to some of the Arabian and European travelers of around 600 CE, healthcare in general was well developed and hospitals had existed since the time of King Ashoka. These facilities were largely meant for the poor and the handicapped. Medical care generally included the treatment of common disorders such as tuberculosis, asthma, and injuries.

Medicine was taught alongside other subjects at some notable medical centers and universities (such as at the University of Nalanda) which emerged during this period. Nalanda University, located in present-day Bihar near the city of Rajagriha (now Rajgir) and established in the 5th century CE during the reign of Emperor Kumaragupta I of the Gupta Empire flourished for over 700 years. One of the oldest and greatest centers of learning in the ancient world, it attracted students and scholars from China, Korea, Tibet, Persia, and Central Asia. Even though healthcare was well provided for, little is known about the progress and developments in medical sciences, such as of any new research findings in fundamental physiology or pathology of diseases. India witnessed a significant progress in development of healthcare. But physicians in the Indian continent largely remained focused on treatments (with traditional herbal remedies, dietary regulation, yoga, and stress management). Unlike in the West, there was little progress in the basic understanding of organ structure and function in both normal and disease state.

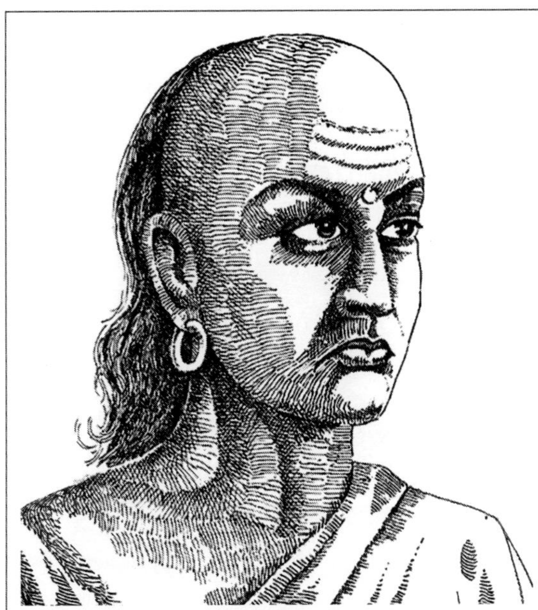

Chanakya, also known as Kautilya or Vishnugupta, and the author of *Arthashastra*, played a pivotal role in the establishment of the Mauryan Empire.

There were a few advancements in Ayurvedic lung medicine primarily through the contributions of earlier Ayurvedic texts. As discussed in the earlier chapter, *Charaka Samhita* had described respiratory diseases, including asthma, bronchitis, and pneumonia and *Sushruta Samhita* contained details of surgical procedures for lung conditions, such as empyema. There, however, were very few new additions to the disease understanding and treatment.

Medieval Period

India's medieval period (6th–18th century CE) saw some developments in lung medicine mostly restricted to herbal medicine and breathing techniques. Vagbhata's *Ashtanga Hridayam* was another addition which included classification of respiratory diseases and treatments. Madhava authored *Madhava Nidanam*, a text on disease diagnosis while Nagarjuna's *Yogaratnakara (1100 CE)* classified respiratory diseases and Ayurvedic treatments including for lung diseases. Sharangadhara made valuable additions and developed new treatments for lung conditions. The Ayurvedic pharmacopeia got expanded to include new herbal remedies for respiratory diseases. There was continued stress on *yoga, pranayama,* and respiratory health.

Breathing Concepts

The significant texts of this period included *Hatha Yoga Pradipika* (15th century CE) on yoga text emphasizing breathing techniques. That was a valuable addition to *Yoga Sutras* of Patanjali (4th century CE) on yoga philosophy of breath control. Some of the key concepts included *Prana* (life force), i.e., understanding of breath as vital energy; *Pranayama* (breath control techniques for regulating life force; *Nadi Shodhana* (nerve cleansing) breathing techniques for balancing energy; and *Kundalini* yoga, i.e., breathing and meditation for spiritual awakening.

There were some specific regional developments. For example, *Shaivism* and *Natha Sampradaya* emphasized breathing techniques in North India while *Siddha* tradition integrated yoga and breathing with Ayurveda in South India.

The *Vajrayana Buddhism* developed unique breathing and meditation practices.

Sharangdhara

Sharangadhara's Paddhati (13th century CE) was a significant addition to new herbal remedies for lung conditions. His comprehensive medical text, *Sarangdhara Samhita* consists of three different sections: *Sutra Sthana* dealing with general principles of medicine; *Nidana Sthana* on disease diagnosis and pathology, and *Chikitsa Sthana* which covers various aspects such as pharmacology, toxicology, and treatment of diseases. He also introduced innovative treatments, including the use of minerals and metals in medicine. Sarangdhara classified respiratory diseases into five categories—cough, asthma, bronchitis, pneumonia, and tuberculosis. Asthma was described as "*Svasa Roga*", characterized by difficulty breathing, wheezing, and coughing. He had also used inhalation therapy using herbal smoke for respiratory conditions.

Sarangadhara, explicitly described the physiological concept of respiration:

नाभिस्थ: प्राणपवन: स्पृष्ट्वा हृत्कभलान्तरम् ।।
कण्ठाद्बहिर्विनिर्याति पातुं विष्णुपदामृतम् ।
पीत्वा चाम्बरपीयूषं पुनरायाति वेगतः ।।
प्रीणयन्देहमखिलं जीवयश्चुठरानलम् ।

In summary, it translates that the "*vayu*" (air) located in the "*hrdaya*" (chest) goes out, and after drinking the "*Ambarapiyush*" (nectar), it goes back very quickly. It touches the interior of "*hrdaya*", promotes the "*Jatharanatha*" (life), and nourishes the entire body. Sarangadhara had described the sequences leading to the inhalation of ambrosia, the food of gods, or nectar-like substance vital to life, from the outside air, its circulation through the heart to the brain and all other parts.

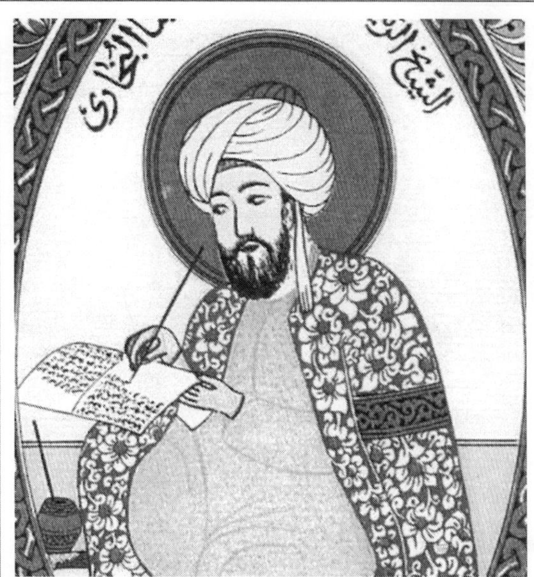

Ibn Sina or Avicenna (980–1037 CE), the most eminent Muslim physician and philosopher of Persia (nowadays Iran) is sometimes described as the father of early modern medicine. His most famous works are *The Book of Healing, The Canon of Medicine*, and a medical encyclopedia.

Unani Medicine

The introduction of the Unani system of medicine, also known as Greco-Arab medicine added further impetus to medical practice of that period. The system was introduced by Arab traders and travelers through the Silk Road and trade routes. Both Ayurvedic and Unani physicians who used herbal remedies for treatment of various respiratory illnesses made substantial contributions. This particular system was practiced by *Hakims* who were brought to India by the foreign invaders during the 10th century AD. The Unani medicine (800–1200 CE), influenced by Ibn Sina adapted Greek knowledge to the Indian context and introduced Arabic medical concepts, including in lung diseases (Ibn Sina's Canon of Medicine, 1030 CE and Al-Razi's Kitab al-Mansuri, 900 CE).

Ibn Sina, often referred to as Avicenna in the West, was a prominent physician and philosopher during the Islamic Golden Age. He is credited with medical works such as *The Book of Healing* and *The Canon of Medicine*. Unani medicine flourished during the Delhi Sultanate (12th–14th centuries) and the Mughal Empire (16th–19th centuries). Unani medicine categorized lung diseases into: *Nafkah* (pneumonia), *Sual* (asthma), *Tansukh* (chronic bronchitis), *Dukhnak* (tuberculosis), and *Riyadh* (pleurisy). The lung diseases were attributed to imbalance of humors (blood, phlegm, yellow bile, and black bile), environmental and dietary factors (climate, air quality, lifestyle, and unhealthy foods), stress, and emotions.

The Unani pharmacy introduced Arabic and Persian herbal medicine to India. The Mughal era in India saw a unique blend of indigenous and Islamic traditions, influencing various aspects of life, including respiratory practices. The Mughal Emperor Akbar (1555–1605) had encouraged the amalgamation of the Unani and the Ayurvedic systems. Both Ayurvedic and Unani systems advocated a holistic approach to treatment with dietary modifications, regular exercise, stress management, and herbal remedies. *Panchakarma* therapies (e.g., steam inhalation and massage were also recommended. There was a revival of Ayurvedic medicine, with a focus on respiratory health. Ayurvedic practitioners developed new treatments for respiratory diseases, using herbal remedies and breathing exercises. *Yogic* and *Tantric* practices continued to evolve with a focus on advanced breathing techniques, such as *Kundalini Yoga* and *Laya Yoga*. These practices aimed to balance the body's energies and access higher states of consciousness. Sufism, a mystical form of Islam, emphasized the importance of breath control (*Habs-e-Dam)* for spiritual growth and self-realization. Sufi practitioners used breathing techniques to quiet the mind and access higher states of consciousness.

India's contributions to lung medicine during this period had a lasting impact on traditional and modern medicine. Ayurvedic and Unani principles continued to influence contemporary respiratory care.

Respiratory Diseases

The common respiratory diseases which were reported during this period included infectious diseases such as tuberculosis (TB), known as "*Rajayakshma*" in Ayurveda, pneumonia described in Unani texts as "*Zat-ul-Janb*" and influenza referred to as "*Mahakasha*" in Ayurveda. Other non-infective respiratory conditions which find a mention are asthma described in Ayurvedic texts as "*Tamaka swasa*", and bronchitis, known as "*Kasa*" in Ayurveda. Epidemics of infections such as cholera and smallpox were common which also affected respiratory systems in some cases. Both Ayurvedic and Unani methods were employed for the treatment.

Contemporary Europe

Meanwhile in the Western world, this period saw significant progress in understanding lung anatomy, classifying respiratory diseases, and developing treatments. These foundational advancements also shaped the course of lung medicine for centuries to come. Galen's works continued to dominate for several centuries. His major contributions to respiratory medicine included the description of lung anatomy and function, diagnosis of pneumonia as a distinct disease and descriptions of various treatments. Galen's first treatise entitled "On the Movements of the Heart and Lung" described the lung as very soft and warm which is kept in constant motion. There was great emphasis on humoral theory in the disease causation put forward by Hippocrates and Galen.

Aretaeus of Cappadocia, a Roman physician, had earlier described chronic respiratory diseases (such as asthma and emphysema) and the importance of environmental factors in lung disease in the 2nd century CE. In the medieval period during 13th and 14th century CE, there were significant advances in the understanding of lung anatomy and function through seminal works of Mondino dei Luzzi (Mundinus) and later Andreas Vesalius (De Humani Corporis Fabrica) as well as on pulmonary circulation by Ibn al-Nafis. Respiratory infections (tuberculosis and pneumonia) were described by physicians such as Guy de Chauliac. The advancements in lung medicine during this period laid the foundation for future discoveries.

Epidemics

Europe was repeatedly ravaged by history's deadliest pandemic of plague, labelled as the Black Death in the 14th century in addition to the prevalence of other infective illnesses such as tuberculosis and pneumonia. Other respiratory illnesses such as bronchitis (chronic cough) and asthma were also common in the medieval Europe. These were generally attributed to various factors similar to what were seen in the rest of the world: Poor sanitation and hygiene; malnutrition; crowding and urbanization; occupational exposures (mining and textile industry); climate and geography (cold and damp environments). The use of purging and bloodletting for treatments was popular in addition to herbal remedies, mineral-based treatments (arsenic), and surgical interventions (thoracentesis). The initial medical responses to the victims of "black death" as well as other illnesses included bloodletting, purging, and quarantine. It was subsequent development of quarantine stations and changes in public health policies during Renaissance, which helped control of different epidemics.

Stagnation of Medical Progress in India

During Renaissance, there was revival of medical learning and of a scientific approach to diseases through improved understanding and increased focus on medicine and science in Europe. But the overall progress in India was rather negligible except for some additions to the indigenous practices discussed earlier. Indian medicine in general lagged behind the global medical practices. This subsequently resulted in increasing the gaps in the knowledge and understanding of diseases as well as the inadequacy of healthcare. Moreover, there occurred a great deficiency of medical researchers and trained health personnel. Numerous factors are likely to be responsible for this slowdown of which the lack of political, academic, and administrative independence due to the foreign rule was the most important.

Introduction of Modern Respiratory Medicine in India

The arrival of European missionaries during the 16th century introduced the modern Western system of medicine and medical practices. From the early 16th century onwards, the Portuguese adopted hospitals as an integrated part of church and treated medical care as a religious practice. Missionaries such as nuns and monks were trained to take care of the sick while the Jesuits introduced basic general medical training program at the hospital. There was initially a conflict with traditional Indian medical systems in particular with the Unani practices. But this exposure also led to a cross-pollination of ideas and amalgamation of practices. The allopathic system of medicine achieved an overall dominance because of its vast scientific foundation and enormity of research base. Allopathic treatments introduced a variety of different remedies for different illnesses. Moreover, they offered early and demonstrable relief from different ailments.

Sources

1. Keele KD. Review of *Glimpses of Health and Medicine in Mauryan Empire* by Reddy DVS. J Hist Med Allied Sci. 1970;25(4):492-94.
2. Sinha P. The Hatha Yoga Pradipika (Translation). Allahabad: Apurva Krishna Bose; 1915.
3. Sastri SS. Yoga Sutras of Patanjali (Translation). Buckingham, Virginia: Integral Yoga Publications; 1963.
4. Naik R, Vekariya S, Acharya RN, Borkar SD. Therapeutic role of vegetables in Respiratory Diseases. A critical review from Ayurvedic classics. https://doi.org/10.21760/jaims.v1i3.4429
5. Feurestein G, The Yoga tradition – Its History, Literatrue, Philosophy and Practice. HOHM Press, Arizona, USA. https://books.google.co.in/books.

6. Magner L. A History of Medicine; 1st edition. CRC Press; 1992.
7. Siraisi NG. Medieval and Early Renaissance Medicine: An Introduction to Knowledge and Practice, University of Chicago Press; 1990. https://books.google.co.in/
8. Porter R. The Cambridge Illustrated History of Medicine; 2006. Wellcome Institute for the History of Medicine, University College London; 2001. https://www.cambridge.org/in/universitypress/subjects/history/history-medicine/
9. Byrne JP. Encyclopaedia of Black Death, 2012. ABC-CLIO LLC, California, USA. https://www.google.co.in/books/
10. Johnston-Saint P. An Outline of the History of Medicine in India. Journal of the Royal Society of Arts. 1929; 77(3999): 843-70.
11. Zaidi SS, Khemchand NS, Akram M, Salman M, Kanaujia P. A comprehensive review of History of Unani Medicine. National Journal of Multidisciplinary Research and Development. 2025;10:31-3.
12. Tiwari SM. Respiratory Diseases in Medieval India. Indian J Hist Med. 2018:63:143-52.
13. Jaggi OP. Medicine in Medieval India: History of Science, Technology and Medicine; Volume 8; 1986.

CHAPTER 5

European Renaissance and Post-Renaissance Period

After a long dark age in history lasting almost around 1,000 years, came the Renaissance period in which Europe went through a cultural and social change during the 15th and 16th centuries, which resulted in a transition from the Middle to the Modern Age. History of any subject, especially if related to science, would now be considered incomplete without going into the developments during this period in Europe. Renaissance not only affected life in Europe but practically throughout the world. This got a major boost for the rediscovery and reinterpretation of ancient texts of different civilizations. Invention of the printing press allowed rapid and wider dissemination of ideas and observations. In due course of time, the Indian practice of medicine got similarly affected. In this chapter, we shall focus on some of the relevant observations related to respiratory medicine.

General Developments

The period of Renaissance was marked by the introduction of newer and frequently revolutionary concepts and beliefs in art, literature, philosophy, and science. There was an increased reliance on observation and reasoning which gave birth to a large number of tumultuous developments and inventions. There was a desire to question the previously held truths and search for new and plausible answers based on empirical and demonstrable evidence, scientific methods, and mathematics.

René Descartes, the 17th century French philosopher and meta-physician was one of the first rationalists in the modern period who believed that questioning and doubt were crucial for finding and discovering true knowledge. Several of these developments were contrary to the previously held beliefs and conventions. Consequently, many of the proponents of new theories, including in medical sciences, had to also face punishments and persecutions. This was also true for medical developments, many of which were also applied to the respiratory system and various respiratory diseases.

There were several other game-changing developments in the health scene including the concepts about cleanliness, invention of toilets, and better understanding of infections. Some of the artists of the period had multifocal interests and contributions, which helped with even greater recognition of their discoveries. Leonardo da Vinci was one such singular example who made extensive contributions to human anatomy through his artistic drawings of dissection. Besides anatomy, he made significant contributions to the study of physics, water flow, movement and aerodynamics, new discoveries in acoustics, botany, geology, and mechanics methods. He is aptly called the "father of modern science".

Human Anatomy

"The substance of the lung is dilatable and extensible like the tinder made from a fungus. But

it is spongy and if you press it, it yields to the force which compresses it, and if the force is removed, it increases again to its original size."

—Leonardo da Vinci, late 15th century

Anatomists during the Renaissance made more precise descriptions of the lungs than medieval medical practitioners. Da Vinci also described the bronchial tree in detail, as well as the phenomenon of bronchial dilatation when the lungs inflate, the residual volume of the lungs, and the interpenetrating networks of lung vasculature. He described the lungs as cooling agents. While Leonardo da Vinci described the feel of lungs, the later 16th century anatomists observed that the lungs had five lobes.

Notable contributions to human anatomy were made by Andreas Vesalius who contradicted many of the old beliefs of Galen who had made observations on animal dissections. Vesalius procured a steady supply of human cadavers for dissection with permission of a judge who was greatly influenced by Vesalius' work and regularly supplied him with cadavers of executed criminals. Vesalius' seven-volume *De humani corporis fabrica* (*On the fabric of the human body*) is a groundbreaking work of human anatomy. He was shipwrecked on an island and died in great debt. It is also believed that he was accused of dissecting a "living" human body.

Respiratory Physiology

Another notable contribution was made by William Harvey during the early 17th century who described the details of the pulmonary circulation in the lungs. He described the role of the lungs as the most eminent in his *Lectures on the Whole of Anatomy* (1653):

"Pre-eminence [of the lung]: nothing is especially so necessary neither sensation nor aliment. Life and respiration are complementary. There is nothing living which does not breathe nor anything which breathing which does not live."

Significant advancements were made in understanding the physical and chemical laws governing the respiratory system. Several of the functions were better explained and understood on the basis of the previously existing laws. Many other observations were explained with newly invented formulae and principles. Robert Boyle's description of the relationship between pressure and volume (Boyle's Law) remains relevant till date. Robert Hooke worked on lung elasticity and lung expansion while the Italian chemist Giambattista della Porta's work on pneumatics was an important contribution. Other key inventors included Santorio Santorio who was a pioneer in pulmonary physiology and measured pulmonary function and respiratory rate. Giovanni Alfonso Borelli applied mechanics to respiratory physiology. Several of these developments were helpful not only for the understanding of physiological principles but also laid the foundations for clinical applications of modern pulmonary and critical care involving oxygen therapy, respiratory gas analysis, anesthesia, and ventilation systems.

Besides the understanding of human anatomy and the discovery of pulmonary circulation, the discovery, or more precisely the isolation of respiratory gases such as oxygen and carbon dioxide helped to define the gaseous exchange in the lungs and formulate the principles of modern human respiratory physiology. Giambattista Porta also discovered oxygen production through heating saltpeter. The discovery of oxygen has been a fascinating story involving several scientists across centuries. Although Leonardo da Vinci had proposed the existence of a vital element in air as early as 1500, it was the English chemist Joseph Priestley who first discovered oxygen over two and a half centuries later, on August 1, 1774, by heating mercuric oxide. He named it "dephlogisticated air" meaning "without flame or combustion". Later, the French chemist Antoine Lavoisier recognized oxygen's significance and renamed it "oxygen" (from Greek "oxys" meaning

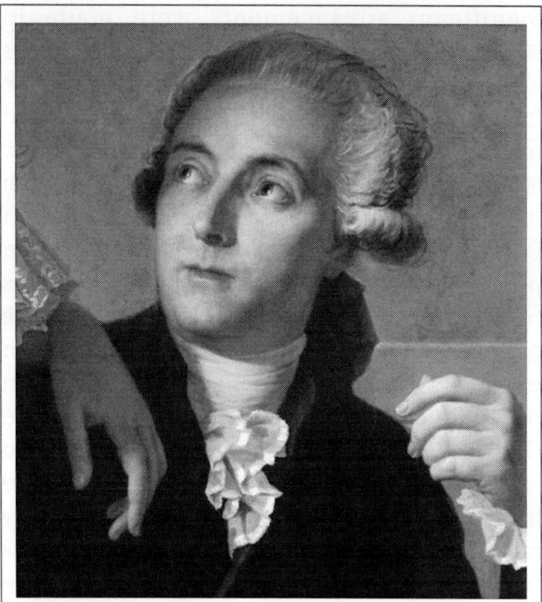

Antoine Lavoisier (1743–1794)—the French chemist known for the discovery of oxygen and its role in combustion.

acid and "genes" meaning generator). He also demonstrated oxygen's role in combustion and respiration. Essentially, oxygen is the "life air" and critical for the survival of each living cell.

Jan Baptist van Helmont discovered a new gas produced due to burning of wood and fermentation. He named it *"gas sylvestre"* or "wild spirit". He was also the first to coin the word "gas", deriving it from the Greek word "chaos". Later Joseph Priestley who had discovered oxygen produced CO_2 (labeled as "fixed air") through heating limestone and used it to produce carbonated water. Antoine Lavoisier recognized CO_2's significance, named it "carbonic acid" (from Latin "carbo" meaning charcoal) and demonstrated CO_2's role in combustion and respiration. In the beginning of 19th century, John Dalton proposed the law of partial pressures, explaining the gas behavior, and Jöns Jakob Berzelius discovered its importance in biological processes. Carbon dioxide's discovery not only revolutionized the developments in basic sciences and medicine but also in the understanding of environmental sciences and climate change research. Carbon dioxide's role extends beyond respiration to photosynthesis, combustion, climate regulation, and industrial processes.

Diseases, Risk Factors, and Treatment Understanding

The most important diseases, which had bothered mankind including Europeans, were tuberculosis, asthma, and lung infections such as pneumonia. It was in the 16th century that contagion theory was proposed for tuberculosis by Girolamo Fracastoro. During the same period, Ambroise Paré had first described pneumothorax and empyema. Pleurisy, i.e., inflammation of the lung lining, often caused by infection and coughing fits presenting with epilepsy-like seizures were also described. Bronchiectasis was first recognized by René Laënnec who also discovered the use of the stethoscope, in the early 19th century. Other frequently devastating respiratory diseases included influenza epidemics which occurred regularly, often with high mortality rates. There were many outbreaks of plague, generally labeled as the Black Death due to a high death rate from plague-pneumonia.

Chronic conditions besides asthma included chronic bronchitis, which was later recognized as a distinct condition by Giovanni Battista Morgagni. Other chronic conditions which posed major health issues included occupational lung diseases, especially among people working in mines. Miner's lung was described in coal workers by Agricola and Silicosis by the Italian physician Bernardino Ramazzini during that period. All these conditions were responsible for high social and economic impact as well as high mortality rates. Some of the diseases such as tuberculosis were also considered as a social stigma.

As discussed in the earlier chapters, the diagnosis of most of these conditions primarily rested on symptoms while the treatments largely included treatments similar to Ayurvedic and Unani remedies. Turmeric, opium, and liquorice root were employed in many conditions. Other measures included diet, isolation, exercises and rest, bloodletting, and purging. Inhalation therapies using herbal remedies and aromatics were used as a treatment for respiratory diseases such as cough, asthma, and bronchitis. Tobacco smoke was also used as an inhalational treatment. Surgical interventions (e.g., thoracocentesis) were rarely employed.

Most of the respiratory diseases could be attributed to multiple causes. Poor sanitation and hygiene; crowding and urbanization; occupational exposures (mining and textile work); malnutrition and weakened immune systems; and climate and environmental factors (cold and dampness) were important risk factors. Detailed pathological autopsies by Giovanni Battista Morgagni shed greater light on respiratory diseases.

The Renaissance period also saw the emergence of new disease-causing risk factors due to increasing industrialization and urbanization. Christopher Columbus introduced tobacco to Europe in 1492 after his return from the voyage to the New World. Previously unknown in Europe, tobacco was first cultivated and used by indigenous peoples in the Americas. The Spanish and Portuguese traders popularized tobacco use in Europe, and it became fashionable, especially among nobility. Smoking, seen as a symbol of wealth, intellectualism, and sophistication, became a social norm. Tobacco houses and smoking clubs widely emerged. Tobacco was initially used for medicinal purposes. Jean Nicot promoted tobacco's medicinal benefits in his *"Traité de la Nicotiane"*. It was during the beginning of 17th century that people started noticing its health concerns when James I of England wrote *"A Counterblaste to Tobacco"* and criticized smoking. The Spain king Philip II prohibited smoking in 1610.

Physical Examination in Diagnosis

The importance of physical examination in making a diagnosis in medicine in India and elsewhere dates back to ancient times. The classical stepwise physical examination of respiratory system today includes inspection (visual examination), palpation (feeling the chest), percussion (tapping the chest), and auscultation (listening to chest sounds). Most of these steps have been used since ancient times. The classic Ayurvedic texts described physical examination techniques. Ebers Papyrus of Egyptian Medicine describes percussion-like techniques for diagnosing abdominal and thoracic conditions. Hippocrates mentioned percussion using terms like "striking" and "tapping". During the medieval period, Hakim Ajmal Khan, a prominent Unani physician, emphasized physical examination. Physicians such as Avicenna and Ibn al-Nafis had also emphasized physical examination.

During modern period, Andreas Vesalius described percussion in his seminal work *"De Humani Corporis Fabrica"*. It was Leopold Auenbrugger who observed that he could determine the presence of fluid or air in the thoracic cavity by tapping on the chest. This technique, known as "percussion," allowed him to make diagnose various respiratory conditions. Auenbrugger published his work, *"Inventum Novum"* (New Invention), in 1761. The book described his percussion techniques and findings. The technique initially met with skepticism due to concerns about the reliability of percussion findings. He was a talented musician and used his musical skills to develop percussion techniques. His work gained recognition later and percussion became a fundamental tool in physical examination. After over half a century, Joseph Skoda, another Austrian physician, refined percussion techniques, introducing the "Skoda's method" in 1819 CE. These contributions to percussion paved the way for modern medical imaging techniques such as ultrasonography.

The technique of listening to the chest sounds (auscultation) also improved later with the use of stethoscope, first introduced by Renne Lennec in 1816 CE.

Treatments and Disease Control

There were few additions to the drug armamentarium. Herbal remedies remained popular. Opium, ipecacuanha, and liquorice root were commonly used to suppress cough and treat asthma. Sarsaparilla and *Guaiacum* were used for respiratory infections and rheumatism. Other treatments included bloodletting (continued from ancient times), poultices and inhalation of herbal vapors and aromatic substances. In particular, inhalation therapy continued to develop and progress with newer introduction of drugs and devices (discussed elsewhere).

More than the disease treatments, several infection control and prevention measures were discovered or developed during this period, which laid the groundwork for modern infection control practices. Handwashing initially recommended by Leonardo Fioravanti and Ambroise Paré, cleanliness emphasized by Giovanni Morgagni and Thomas Sydenham as well as use of personal protective equipment like gloves and masks and greater stress on improved hospital ventilation were able to significantly reduce infection rates. Waste disposal and waste management practices developed in cities such as Venice and London; quarantine stations established in Venice and other Italian cities to isolate plague victims, and lazarettos (isolation hospitals built in Europe to care for patients with infectious diseases) were helpful in the control of tuberculosis and other contagious diseases as well as to prevent recurrent epidemics.

Respiratory Devices, Instruments, and Equipment

Better understanding of disease-causing factors and their impact stimulated the invention of simple devices for prevention and management. Other than for the management of infections such as tuberculosis, steps for prevention of diseases in miners, divers, and other workers exposed to dusty occupations were developed. Respiratory masks used during the 16th century proved to be quite effective for protection of miners and workers from harmful gases at their work places.

Provisions of ventilation shafts enhanced mine airflow while changes in architecture and building ventilation along with chimneys greatly improved indoor air quality during the 15th and 16th century. Pulmonary bellows were developed to improve mine ventilation and served as a precursor to modern ventilators. Diving helmets were initially used at first as diving helmets with air supply for divers. Later, respiratory valves were developed as enhanced diving equipment to regulate air flow. Oxygen supply systems and respiratory valves were introduced for diving and underwater exploration. Naval and maritime ventilation equipment included ship ventilation systems and sail ventilators for enhanced crew comfort.

Devices for pulmonary function measurement developed during this period included pulmonary balance to estimate pulmonary function and respiratory rate. Respiratory gauge was used to measure lung volume and capacity. Some of the clinically applicable devices in respiratory care included early masks for administration of anesthetics and oxygen supply systems for medical use. By mid-17th century, early ventilators came into vogue as experimental devices for respiratory support. Tracheostomy tube was first developed by Antonio Brassavola in the 16th century. Various equipments developed at that time laid the groundwork for occupational safety, understanding of pulmonary function and disease, modern mechanical ventilation, advances in anesthesia, and respiratory therapy.

Post-Renaissance Period

The tumultuous period of the Renaissance had given birth to a relatively fearless era which greatly stimulated the development of a more widespread and scientific approach to new developments and inventions during the 17th century and later. William Stark described several details of lung anatomy and pathology in his studies. Several specific developments in the field of respiratory medicine during the post-Renaissance period in Europe together proved to be game changers in overall medical and respiratory care. Some of these included the discovery of oxygen by Joseph Priestley (1774) and Antoine Lavoisier (1778) and pulmonary function tests by John Hutchinson. The germ theory by Louis and Robert Koch along with a clearer understanding of tuberculosis by Jean-Antoine Villemin and Robert Koch was another critical development which changed the practice of medicine.

There were at least three classical publications during this period which stand out for their impact: "A Treatise on the Diseases of the Chest" by René Laënnec (1819); "The Physiology of Respiration" by John Hutchinson (1846); and "The Germ Theory of Disease" by Louis Pasteur (1861). The period also saw the establishment of some landmark institutions and societies such as the Royal Society of Medicine (1774) in London, Société de Médecine de Paris (1796), and British Thoracic Society (1927) dedicated to respiratory medicine.

Some of the most significant developments which impacted respiratory medicine are described as under.

Pulmonary Stethoscope

Stethoscope, the workhorse of a physician, especially of a pulmonologist, was first invented by René Laënnec in the early 19th century. The word stethoscope includes two Greek words—stethos (chest) and scopos (examination). Before its invention, physicians used to perform auscultation of chest by placing the ear directly on the patient chest. This was rather embarrassing for a shy physician as Laënnec found out in case of a young female patient. Initially, he used an aural tube consisting of a rolled sheet of paper and placing it on patient's chest. He could hear the heart sounds rather clearly. Subsequently, he substituted with a wooden tube and improved with further modifications. Later on, a bi-aural model was made which was further refined by Cammann for commercialization who also wrote a major treatise on diagnosis by auscultation and therefore popularizing its use.

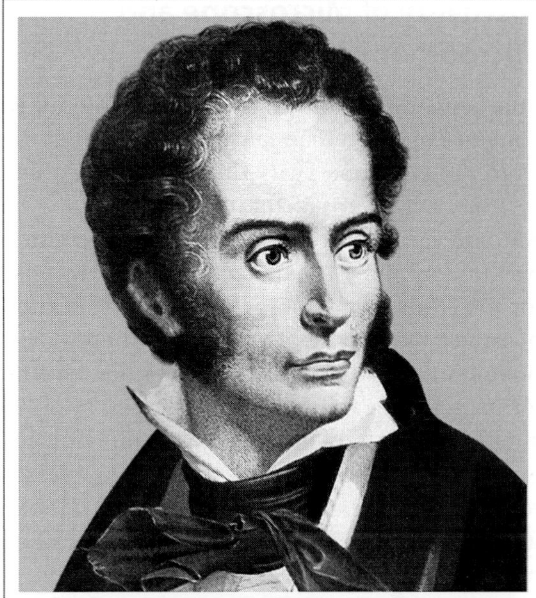
René Laënnec (1781–1826), French physician and inventor of the stethoscope.

Stethoscope acquired an iconic place in medical circles and came to be recognized as a sine qua non for medical practitioners in the eyes of the general public. Several minor changes were made in newer versions to reduce its size, change the appearances and improve the acoustic quality by filtering out external noise. Electronic versions have further improved the quality of auscultation. Even though the essential requirement for a stethoscope for final clinical diagnosis in the modern times has greatly diminished, it remains a useful instrument to perform auscultation and identify specific sounds of the heart, lungs, and the bowels for initial examination and suspecting a diagnosis.

Discovery of Microscope and Microorganisms

In around 1590, Hans and Janssen had created a microscope based on lenses in a tube, but the word "microscope" was first used by Galileo in 1609. Discovery of the light microscope by Antonie van Leeuwenhoek in the 17th century was undoubtedly a new technological wonder for the study of microorganisms and causation of infective diseases including tuberculosis, pneumonia, and others. Leeuwenhoek had no formal scientific training but developed over 500 simple single-lens microscopes following his experience as draper using magnifying glasses to observe threads in cloth. Robert Hooke used a compound microscope and described microscopic appearance of seeds, plants, eye of a fly, and the structure of cork. He mistook the pores inside the cork as "cells". Leeuwenhoek's instruments provided a superior quality of image and were lightweight and portable.

Using a microscope, Leeuwenhoek established that there were live and motile organisms that were not visible to the naked eye. Subsequent observations by Spallanzani and Louis Pasteur proved that the long-held belief that life spontaneously appeared from nonliving substances during the process of spoilage was wrong. Even though there are references in ancient civilizations to the existence of tiny organisms and scholars such as Aristotle and Galen had proposed the existence of microscopic life, there were no visualization tools. Van Leeuwenhoek discovered microorganisms in human mouth and gut and also observed bacteria and yeast. Thereafter, he described microorganisms in letters to the Royal Society. Louis Pasteur was the first to develop germ theory of disease in the year 1861. These observations not only revolutionized the understanding of diseases but also enabled vaccine development and disease prevention. There was significant impact on public health measures and investigations into different epidemics to identify the sources of outbreaks. Microscopic research also led to the discovery of various treatments including antibiotic development. Later development of electron microscopes in the 20th century allowed visualization of viruses, such as Influenza and others.

Mycobacteria and Tuberculosis

Tuberculosis had bothered mankind as a major health illness. The disease was known since antiquity by different names and manifestations and was treated with multiple types of lay therapies. The disease was known to affect and be responsible for deaths of not only the poor in the slums, but also the rich, the celebrities, and the kings and the queens living in palaces. History of Europe is replete with numerous examples of victims of tuberculosis.

Different etiologies had been attributed to tuberculosis in the past. Discovery of the microscope helped in identifying the microbial origin of disease. Several other observations made during the 19th century led to the final discovery about the microbial origin of tuberculosis. Jacob Henle had observed the transmission from cat to human and from humans to rabbits. Later a French doctor, Jean-Antoine Villemin showed that tuberculosis was a transmissible disease among humans and animals. A new staining procedure and use of a solidified, serum-based medium enabled Robert Koch to demonstrate a new organism in tuberculous lesions in 1882. A century later, March 24, the day of demonstration of the mycobacterium in 1882 was designated World TB Day to educate the public about the impact of TB around the world.

Microscopic detection of TB bacteria thus revolutionized the diagnosis and nature of tuberculosis. This proved to be one major milestone which changed the face of respiratory medicine. The disease was no more considered invincible and necessarily fatal. Microbial origin led to the development of a host of therapies directed against the organism. The first antitubercular drug, streptomycin, was discovered 65 years later. This was followed by introduction of several new drugs, vaccination, and disease control programs.

Discovery of X-ray

The German physicist Wilhelm Conrad Röntgen accidentally discovered X-rays on November 8, 1895, when experimenting with cathode rays. *X-radiation* was used to signify an unknown type of radiation. He further discovered the medical use of X-rays when he took a picture of his wife's hand on a photographic plate. The very next year, X-rays were used to radiograph a needle stuck in the hand of an associate by John Hall Edwards who also used it in a surgical operation. Applications of X-rays were made wider with discoveries of Thomas Edison who developed the first X-ray tube and Marie Curie who researched X-ray production.

Otto Walkhoff, another German physician, in 1896 used Röntgen's X-ray technique for the first chest X-ray. Thereafter, its use expanded for diagnosis of pneumonia, tuberculosis, lung cancer, and other diseases. One could more closely and clearly visualize the presence of consolidation, pleural effusion, cavitation, fibrosis, masses, and nodules. Use of X-rays made major impact on disease diagnosis and treatment. The improved diagnostic accuracy also made it possible to start early treatment and improve the patient outcomes.

Other developments on X-rays used in chest medicine happened in due course of time. Some early applications included fluoroscopy enabling real-time imaging and tomography for cross-sectional imaging. In more recent times, the discovery of computed tomography (CT) scans in 1971 has completely revolutionized chest imaging and its applications. Besides its use for medical imaging and diagnosis, X-rays also led to development of radiation therapy for cancer.

Understanding Immunology and Vaccine Development

Intrinsic response to a disease-causing factor in one or the other fashion was recognized since ancient times. Galen had also proposed "intrinsic" in addition to the "extrinsic" factors in response to an infection. There was no clear knowledge

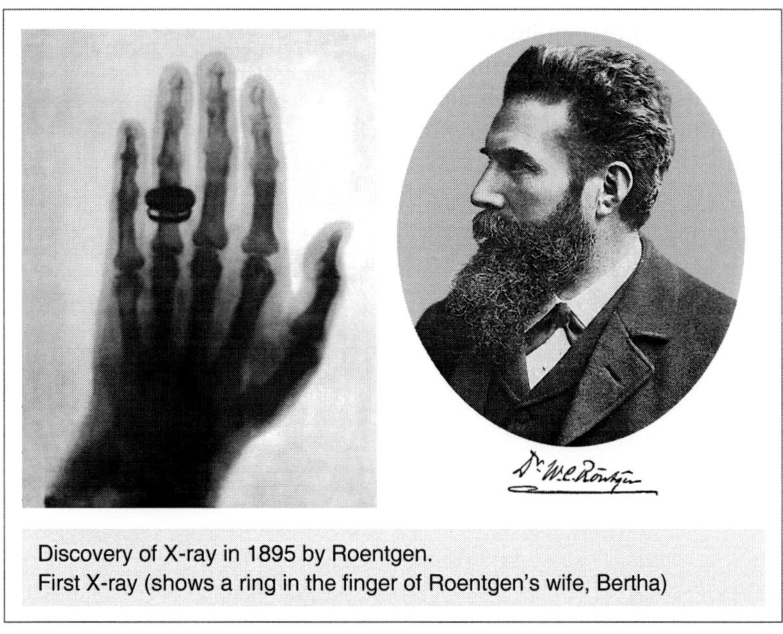

Discovery of X-ray in 1895 by Roentgen.
First X-ray (shows a ring in the finger of Roentgen's wife, Bertha)

about the nature of the intrinsic response. Some of the foundational discoveries during the 18th and 19th centuries, which led to a clear concept about immunological response, included the development of smallpox vaccine by Edward Jenner, germ theory of disease by Louis Pasteur, and the Koch's postulates, which constituted the "gold standard" for microbiological research. It was later that immunology emerged as an important phenomenon of which we are aware today.

Immunology has made a major impact in respiratory medicine and transformed our understanding of diseases and their management. Autoimmune diseases constitute a significant component of medical disorders and respiratory diseases. Immunological mechanisms play an important role in the etiopathogenesis of a large number of both infective and noninfective disorders including asthma, tuberculosis, pneumonias, hypersensitivity disorders, and cancers. Immunological therapies play a significant role in their management.

The other major role of immunology relates to vaccine development. After the first smallpox vaccine in 1796 by Edward Jenner, several new vaccines were developed. Some of the important respiratory disease vaccines include those for diphtheria, measles and mumps, influenza, and pneumococcal pneumonia. Bacillus Calmette-Guérin (BCG) vaccination against tuberculosis has a long history although its efficacy remains debatable.

Sources

1. Wear A, French RK, Lonie IM. The Medical Renaissance of the Sixteenth Century. Cambridge: Cambridge University Press; 1985.
2. Bradley CP. Medical Renaissance in Florence. Eur J Gen Pract. 2006;12(2):51.
3. Siraisi NG. Medieval and Renaissance Medicine: Continuity and Diversity. J Hist Med Allied Sci. 1986;41(4):391-4.
4. Schofield RE. Enlightened Joseph Priestley: A Study of His Life and Work from 1773 to 1804. University Park: Penn State Univ Press; 2009.
5. Roguin A. Rene Theophile Hyacinthe Laënnec (1781-1826): The Man Behind the Stethoscope. Clin Med Res. 2006;4(3):230-5.
6. West JB. History of respiratory mechanics prior to World War II. Compr Physiol. 2012;2(1):609-19.
7. Fitting JW. From breathing to respiration. Respiration. 2015;89(1):82-7.
8. Porter R. The Cambridge Illustrated History of Medicine. Wellcome Institute for the History of Medicine, University College London, 2001. https://www.cambridge.org/in/universitypress/subjects/history/history-medicine/
9. Magner LN, Kim O. A History of Medicine, 3rd Edition, Routledge, 2017. https://www.routledge.com/
10. The Renaissance: the rebirth of medicine, 14th to 17th century. [online] Available from https://www.bbc.co.uk/bitesize/articles/z6hwqfr#z3rpsk7 [Last accessed September, 2025].
11. Murray JF. A thousand years of pulmonary medicine: good news and bad. Eur Resp J. 2001;17(3):558-65.

CHAPTER

6

Modern Allopathic Respiratory Medicine in India

The history of respiratory medicine in India has closely followed the developments elsewhere in the world. This was greatly influenced by the political history ever since the ancient periods. The early period of the dominant *Ayurvedic* medicine got supplemented with *Unani* medicine during the medieval and Mughal eras. During the late 15th and early 16th centuries, European colonialism brought modern (or the Western) systems of medicine in India. Also called *Allopathy,* the Western system of medical practice was based on the evidence and changing concepts about the causes and mechanisms of illnesses, which became available at that time.

Allopathy

The term *"allopathy"* was coined in 1810 by Samuel Hahnemann who also invented *"Homeopathy"* as a preferred alternative. It is derived from the Greek words *"allos"* (meaning "other" or "different") and *"pathos"* (meaning "suffering"). It was considered "heroic medicine" during the 19th century in both Europe and North America because of the extreme measures sometimes employed for treatments. Hahnemann believed that the conventional physicians employed approaches which merely treated symptoms and failed to address the underlying disharmony produced by underlying disease. He considered this "symptomatic" treatment as harmful and harsh equivalent to "opposites treating opposites". It induced symptoms seen as opposite to those of diseases rather than treating their underlying causes.

But the so called "harsh" or modern medicine rapidly spread throughout the world in view of its demonstrable efficacy in treatment of illnesses. Modern medicine continued to expand and absorb many different concepts in its broad spectrum. In 2001, the World Health Organization (WHO) in a study defined *allopathic medicine* as "the broad category of medical practice that is sometimes called Western medicine, biomedicine, evidence-based medicine" or modern medicine as different from the traditional or complementary/alternative medicine practiced in certain areas of the world.

Arrival of Modern Allopathic System in India

The modern allopathic system of medicine arrived in India through various channels from Europe. The Portuguese came in 1500s when the explorer Vasco da Gama landed in Calicut on the Malabar Coast on May 20, 1498. This Portuguese colonialism in India, which started in 1505, lasted until the liberation of Goa in 1961. The explorers were also accompanied by the Christian missionaries who primarily came to spread Christianity and form anti-Islamic alliances with preexisting Christian nations. They also brought Western medicine to India, including respiratory treatments. Francisco de lu Orta, a Portuguese physician, is often credited with the introduction of Western medicine to India. He was also a herbalist and naturalist, who pioneered tropical medicine and pharmacology. He used an experimental approach for the identification and the use of herbal medicines and published a book in 1563 on simple herbs and drugs. It was widely used as a standard reference text on medicinal plants.

The Western medical system spread further with the arrival of the British East India Company. The East India Company which arrived in India in the 1600s also brought some medical officers who served as ship's surgeons in its fleet to take care of sick sailors. But the British stayed and consolidated their rule in the rest of India. They also established allopathic hospitals and medical schools. Moreover, European physicians who visited India off and on shared their knowledge and expertise. The initial medical services in the 18th, 19th, and early 20th centuries were generally sporadic and focused on infectious diseases such as plague, malaria, *kala azar,* and cholera with the primary aim of their prevention. Gradually, there was the introduction of newer trends and systems of medical practice following the newer developments elsewhere in the world.

Introduction of Homeopathy

British and European practitioner also introduced Homeopathy as an off-shoot of Western practices, initially founded by the German physician Samuel Hahnemann. Homeopathy was based on the four key principles: (i) *Law of similars* (a substance that causes symptoms in a healthy person can cure similar symptoms in a person who is ill); (ii) *law of minimum dose* (the smallest dose necessary to stimulate the body's natural healing processes); (iii) *law of individualization* (each person's symptoms and circumstances are unique, requiring a personalized treatment approach); and (iv) *holistic approach* (treat the whole person, not just the symptoms).

Homeopathy soon spread widely in India because of its convincing principles and simplistic treatments. But it evoked criticism from other modern-day practitioners who argued that it exerted merely a placebo effect and that there was lack of any scientific evidence to support its effectiveness. Homeopathy, however, continues to be used by patients for various medical conditions and respiratory diseases, which primarily include common cold, asthma, cough and breathlessness of any cause, bronchitis, and lung infections, including tuberculosis (TB). Even today, a significant number of patients with respiratory disorders keep on switching treatment from one system to the other. Most patients in India do not know about the foreign origins of homeopathy and consider it to be an Indian origin system of medicine. Consequently, India today has the largest number of homeopathic practitioners worldwide.

Impact on Indian Medicine

Western medical practices supplemented and/or replaced traditional Indian methods. Some Indian physicians such as Shivaramakrishnan had also attempted to integrate Western and Ayurvedic medicine during the 19th century. A large number of Ayurvedic physicians continue to use allopathic drugs in one or the other form. Factually, there has been no true integration attributed to different approaches adopted by the two systems.

There were multiple challenges and controversies related to this intermix and integration. Importantly, there was a cultural opposition to Western medicine from traditional practitioners as well as the general public. It was also blamed that European powers exploited India's medical resources. The language barriers between the European and the Indian medical professionals added to the communication challenges.

Almost all the concepts about diseases and their managements came from the Western world.

It cannot be denied that the introduction of Western medicine was responsible for improved healthcare. The various medical advancements included the introduction of the germ theory of disease, which transformed the understanding of infections. Soon, the Western medicine became the dominant system of medical practice in India. There was also increased access to modern medical facilities and training. Adoption of multiple public health programs and systematic sanitation measures, especially in urban areas, helped in reduction of infections such as TB.

Medical Education and Training

The introduction of modern medicine also helped in capacity building, larger collaborations and international cooperation in medical education, training, and research. There was a slow and gradual progress in training and education in medicine in India during the early and mid-19th century. Medical colleges were established in Calcutta (now Kolkata) and Madras (now Chennai) in 1835. The third, Bombay (now Mumbai) Medical College started in 1845. There was a more consistent and faster development after the British government took over control from the East India Company. Establishment of Indian Medical Service was introduced wherein British physicians provided medical education and training. The first training program, Diploma in Public Health, was started in 1890 to address public health concerns. All India Institute of Hygiene and Public Health was started to train students in public health and preventive medicine.

Public Health Initiatives

The pre-Independence era saw the beginning of organized public health initiatives. The Indian government and various health organizations began to recognize the need for comprehensive strategies to combat respiratory diseases. Campaigns aimed at raising awareness about TB and its transmission started to emerge, albeit with limited reach. Significant gaps remained in access to care and public health infrastructure. The legacy of this era would shape the future of respiratory medicine in India, influencing the trajectory of healthcare in the post-Independence period.

Despite these advancements, access to modern medical care remained limited for the majority of the Indian population. Traditional healers continued to play a crucial role in communities, often providing care that combined herbal remedies with practices rooted in indigenous knowledge. The impact of World War II also

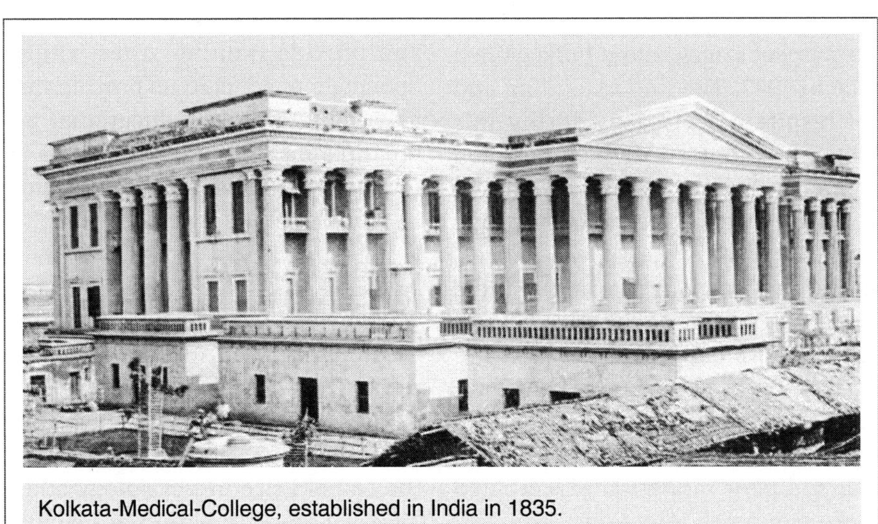

Kolkata-Medical-College, established in India in 1835.

played a role in shaping public health policies. The need to maintain a healthy workforce for the war effort led to increased attention to health issues, including respiratory diseases, and laid the groundwork for post-Independence health reforms.

In spite of the accrued benefits of these activities, there were several challenges and limitations. Most of the education and training programs had limited access and were available only in urban areas at few places. Moreover, there was insufficient funding and infrastructure which hindered growth. British priorities focused on maintaining colonial rule rather than investing in healthcare. But the Indian physicians received training in respiratory medicine, and it laid the groundwork for post-Independence developments.

Status of Respiratory Medicine

The development of modern respiratory medicine in India reflects a journey that integrates colonial influences and independent innovations. Above all, the nation's unique healthcare needs further boosted the efforts, especially in view of the high burden of respiratory diseases. Respiratory diseases, including TB, pneumonia, and chronic obstructive pulmonary disease, were prevalent in India during this time. Respiratory medicine was still in its nascent stages before India gained independence in 1947. The understanding and treatment of respiratory diseases during this period reflected a complex interplay between indigenous medicine and Western medical practices, with significant implications for public health.

Tuberculosis was rampant in colonial India and therefore a major public health concern. Early respiratory care was primarily focused on TB. The disease had deep cultural and social implications, often viewed as a chronic illness associated with poverty and poor living conditions. In urban areas, overcrowding and poor sanitation exacerbated the spread of respiratory infections. The vast socioeconomic disparities meant that healthcare access was highly unequal. Rural populations, in particular, faced immense barriers to receiving appropriate medical care, and respiratory diseases often went untreated.

Additionally, the stigma associated with diseases such as TB hindered early diagnosis and treatment, perpetuating cycles of illness and poverty. The lack of a comprehensive public health infrastructure meant that many respiratory diseases continued to pose serious threats to the population's health. The British administration recognized TB as a significant health issue and began to implement measures for its control, including the establishment of sanatoria. However, these facilities primarily catered to the European population, leaving many Indians without access to adequate care.

Different medical departments existing previously in the presidential system were amalgamated to form Indian Medical Service (IMS), and medical research was also placed on an organized basis. Establishment of IMS and the Indian Council of Medical Research (ICMR) fostered research and education in medicine, including respiratory diseases. Education and training in respiratory medicine during the latter half of the 19th and early 20th centuries made it possible to have an increased accessibility and affordability to respiratory care. Tuberculosis sanatoria were established to treat TB patients and provide training. Chest clinics were also opened in major cities to provide specialized care and training. From educational point of view, the diploma in chest diseases was introduced in 1920s to train physicians in respiratory medicine.

Research Initiatives

There were very few research initiatives in medicine in pre-Independent India. The most recognized achievements included the discovery of the malaria parasite by Sir Ronald Ross, a British-Indian physician who was awarded the Nobel Prize in physiology and medicine in 1902. Dr Upendranath Brahmachari, an Indian physician, developed treatment for *kala-azar* which at that time was a highly significant problem. The Indian Council of Medical Research (ICMR) was established in 1911 with objectives of formulation, coordination, and promotion of biomedical research. ICMR has played a significant role in health research since its inception. The monthly Indian Journal of Medical Research started in 1913 published important research papers and reports. There were other established institutions such as King Institute of Preventive Medicine (Madras, 1903), Pasteur Institute (Kolkata, 1893), and All India Institute of Hygiene and Public Health (Kolkata, 1932).

Research activities in respiratory diseases were rather limited. TB was adopted as a priority area for research largely in the post-Independence period. Madras Chemotherapy Centre (now renamed as National Institute for Research in Tuberculosis) was established specifically to develop the domiciliary treatment with commonly available drugs at that time. ICMR thereafter undertook several research initiatives on epidemiology, diagnosis and management of TB, and Bacillus Calmette-Guérin (BCG) vaccination.

In summary, the developments in modern medicine in India had been significant but slow during the pre-Independence period in India. Both the healthcare and education expanded much faster after India got its freedom from the colonial rule in 1947. There was a wider expansion of medical education, establishment of medical colleges with respiratory medicine departments, and advanced training programs. Research activities were slow to start but picked up soon to catch with the world.

Sources

1. Weatherall MW. Making Medicine Scientific: Empiricism, Rationality, and Quackery in mid-Victorian Britain. Soc Hist Med. 1996;9(2):175-94.
2. Saraf SA. Legal regulations of complementary and alternative medicines in different countries. Pharmacogn Rev. 2012;6(12):154-60.
3. Russell CEB. A History of Medicine in India; 1900.
4. Kumar R. The European Renaissance and Medicine in India; 2015.
5. Arnold D. Medicine and Colonialism in India; 1988.
6. Mushtaq MU. Public health in British India: a brief account of the history of medical services and disease prevention in colonial India. Indian J Community Med. 2009;34(1):6-14.
7. Harrison M. Public Health in British India: Anglo-Indian Preventive Medicine 1859-1914. Cambridge: Cambridge University Press; 1994.
8. Park K. Park's Textbook of Preventive and Social Medicine, 18th edition. Jabalpur: M/s Banarsidas Bhanot Publishers; 2005. pp. 679-80.
9. Medicine-Disease Medical History of British India - National Library of Scotland". https://digital.nls.uk/indiapapers/browse/archive/7446661.
10. Srivastava RK. Reminiscence into history of Medical Research in India with contributions of Indian Council of Medical Research (ICMR) over last hundred years. ICMR Bull. 2011;41(11-12):69-92.
11. Martins P. The history of traditional Indian medicine from beginning to the present day. Int J Adv Res. 2018;6(1):1195-201.
12. India State-Level Disease Burden Initiative CRD Collaborators. The burden of chronic respiratory diseases and their heterogeneity across the states of India: the Global Burden of Disease Study 1990-2016. Lancet Glob Health. 2018;6(12):e1363-74.

CHAPTER 7

Modern Respiratory Medicine—Post-Independence India

There has been a gradual but relatively faster progress of modern medicine after India gained its independence from the British rule in 1947. The indigenous and alternative systems such as Ayurveda, Siddha, and Homeopathy also continue to operate for those who opt for these treatments. The modern system had, however, achieved a dominant position with its demonstrable efficacy, global presence, and dynamic progression. Moreover, there is an immense expansion in the volume of an ever growing medical literature in different spheres. The scope is not just limited to treatment of diseases. Each aspect of health and disease is an endless vista of knowledge, thoughts, and research.

India continued with most of the initiatives started during the colonial era (Pre-1947), for example the establishment of Indian Medical Education Foundations. These were further strengthened while several new activities and programs were introduced. Importantly, independent India incorporated health as one of the Directive Principles of State Policy in Part IV of the Constitution.

Healthcare as a State Policy

The Indian Constitution included and imposed duties on the state related to health. It includes several Articles (such as Article 38, 39e, 41, 42, and 47) which make it incumbent upon State to create a social order that promotes the welfare of the people; to protect the health and strength

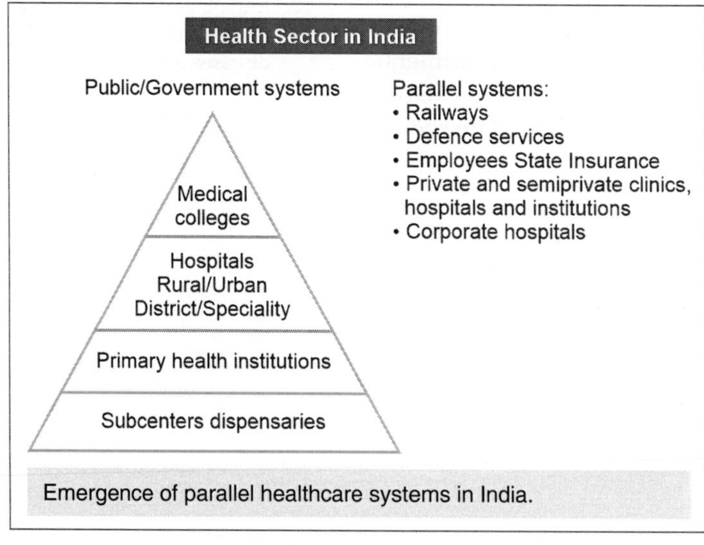

Emergence of parallel healthcare systems in India.

of workers, including children; provide public assistance to the sick, disabled, and elderly; provide reasonable working conditions and maternity leave; improve public health, raise the standard of living, and prohibit the consumption of harmful drugs and alcohol, except for medical purposes. The Article 48A also provides that the state must create a pollution-free environment to promote good health.

Most of the states have adopted a pyramidal model of healthcare with rural and urban health centers at the primary care level, civil hospitals, district hospitals, and medical college hospitals at secondary and tertiary care level. This has resulted in a large expansion of overall healthcare facilities. Army, railway, and many other establishments; a number of private and semiprivate hospitals, charitable institutions, and dispensaries provide healthcare to general public. A large segment of doctors qualified in modern medicine have started with private clinics either individually or in groups.

In addition to the Central and State Health services, the Government of India has introduced different national programs from time to time for control and/or elimination of different diseases. All these programs are now included under the umbrella of unified National Health Mission. Vaccination against different life-threatening childhood infections has been one of the largest health-programs in the world. The Expanded Programme of Immunization (1978) and then Universal Immunization Programme were launched in 1985. One can witness progress in almost all the areas even if it is lacking in research and innovations.

Key Developments in Respiratory Healthcare

Post-Independence, the country witnessed rapid and significant advancements in respiratory healthcare, capacity-building, education, and training of different categories of healthcare personnel. While a large number of private practitioners and hospitals continued to offer service to patients with diseases and disorders of all kinds, there was also an emergence of specialist chest-physicians. Most medical colleges have separate faculty and departments handling lung disease patients. There had been limited diagnostic facilities to start with. But the growth of the available investigations and treatments has been generally smooth and wide-spread. From the standpoint of respiratory medicine, the post-Independence saw two distinct periods—the first four decades and 1990 onward. We believe that the 1990 decade was a watershed period which marked the beginning of somewhat different objectives and approaches.

First Four Decades after Independence

Tuberculosis was rampant in the colonial India. Early respiratory care therefore primarily focused on TB, with sanatoria established by the British in hill stations providing the first structured approach to respiratory diseases. India launched one of the world's largest TB control programs, emphasizing early detection, Bacillus Calmette-Guérin (BCG) vaccination, and streptomycin-based treatment. TB Control Programme which has now converted to National Tuberculosis Elimination Programme (NTEP) has made the most notable impact in reducing the prevalence of tuberculosis. Tuberculosis Association of India (TAI) founded in 1939 became instrumental in promoting TB awareness and management, eventually influencing respiratory medicine.

The Expanded Vaccination Program has been highly successful to significantly reduce the occurrence of several childhood respiratory infections such as diphtheria, measles, pertussis, severe forms of childhood tuberculosis, pneumococcal disease, and influenza (type B). Tobacco Control Program for prevention of tobacco-induced diseases was introduced later. Some other National Programs relevant for respiratory health and disease prevention include the National Programme on Climate Change and Human Health, National Programme for Control of Cancers, and the National Non-Communicable Disease (NCD) Control Programme. Several other similar health-initiatives adopted by the Central and State governments have helped in improving overall respiratory healthcare.

There was a remarkable progress in the general approach to make a clinical diagnosis and treat an illness. The standard approach with history taking and systematic physical examination got largely replaced with an investigative approach. Several new tests and treatments were added in the clinical respiratory medicine. Multiple blood investigations and chest radiography (mostly limited to the plane X-ray film), which were done in the past only in certain specific conditions, came to be routinely performed now. Lung function tests (such as spirometry) were still only occasionally undertaken. In a small survey of respiratory laboratories of 60 Indian Medical Colleges/large hospitals with >500 beds, <25 spirometry tests were performed per week in 1980s. Other pulmonary function tests (PFTs) were only rarely done.

Post-1990 Developments

Clinical Respiratory Medicine

With continued advancements in treating TB, respiratory physicians also began to focus on other respiratory diseases beyond tuberculosis. India in fact now suffered from the dual onslaught of both communicable (or infective) diseases such as tuberculosis and noncommunicable respiratory diseases such as asthma and chronic obstructive pulmonary disease (COPD). An increased economic activity saw greater movement of people responsible for rapid urbanization and unregulated industrialization. Consequently, there was a greater surge in chronic respiratory diseases due to widely prevalent risk factors such as degradation of environment from air pollution due to industrial and traffic exhausts adding to the smokes from biomass fuel use and

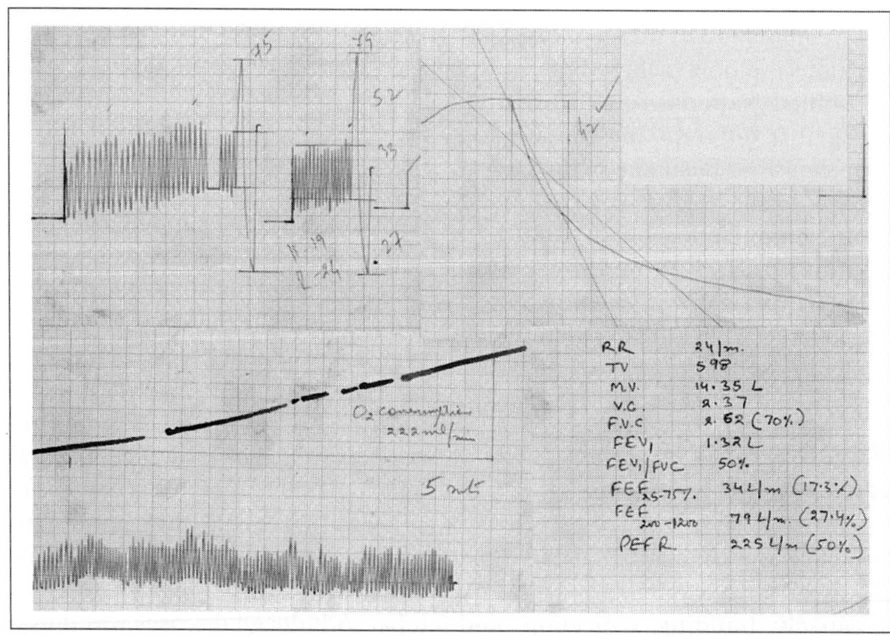

Continued

Continued

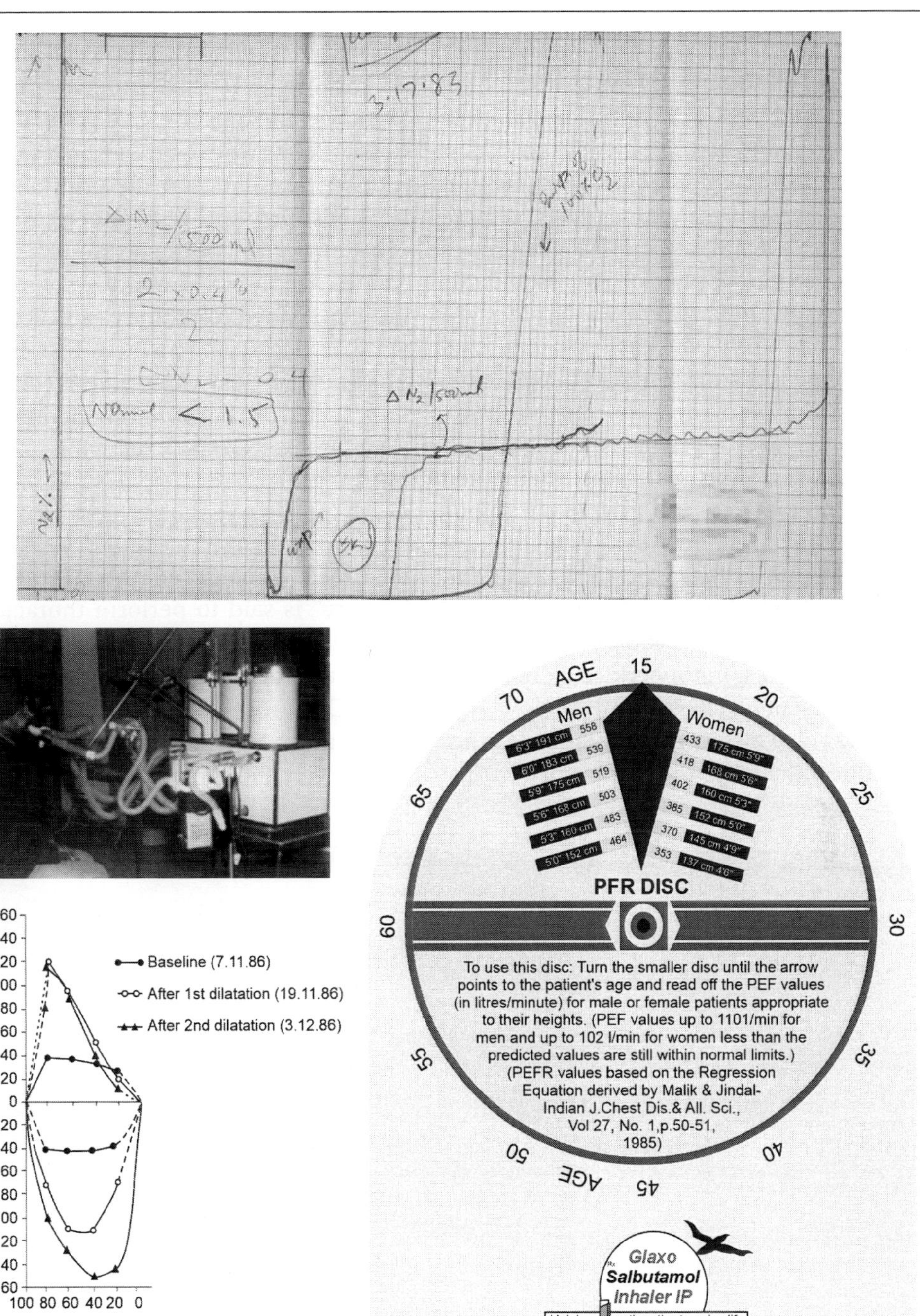

Lung function testing with manual methods during mid-20th century.

Source: Reproduced from Jindal SK. Textbook of Pulmonary & Critical Care Medicine, 3rd edition. New Delhi: Jaypee Brothers Medical Publishers; 2025.

open farm-fires. There was a greater recognition of interstitial lung diseases, environmental and occupational lung diseases, and thoracic cancers.

Respiratory medicine by now had come to occupy a rapidly growing super specialty of medicine. The rising burden of nontubercular lung diseases also augmented the introduction of advanced diagnostic techniques. Entry of large corporate hospitals and commercial companies further facilitated the adoption of global standards and treatments in India. There was greater use of a wider range of PFTs. Chest computerized tomography and pulmonary interventions (such as bronchoscopy and thoracoscopy) became common in diagnostic practices across major hospitals and teaching institutes. Dedicated pulmonary intervention and critical care units were started in larger institutes and private hospitals. Currently, both bronchoscopy and thoracoscopy along with a number of additional advanced procedures are widely available in Indian hospitals. Respiratory critical care is also available in most tier-2 cities.

There was also a slow development of other subspecialties including the respiratory critical care and respiratory sleep disorders. The more recent COVID-19 pandemic from 2020 onward has placed respiratory critical care in the forefront prompting urgent advancements in oxygen therapy, ventilator use, and general critical care. Respiratory critical care also has deep ancient roots with mention of descriptions suggesting tracheostomy and respiratory support. British physicians introduced modern respiratory care techniques and establishment of hospitals which provided respiratory care. Oxygen therapy and ventilatory support was first established in Bombay in1920s while the first intensive care unit (ICU) in the post-Independence era was established at AIIMS, New Delhi.

Thoracic Surgery

Sushruta, considered the "Father of Indian Surgery" is said to perform thoracic surgeries, including rib resections in ancient India. During colonial era, Indian surgeons such as Dr PC Sen (Calcutta) and Dr RN Cooper (Bombay) performed early thoracic surgeries. Surgery was largely done for destroyed lung lobes and

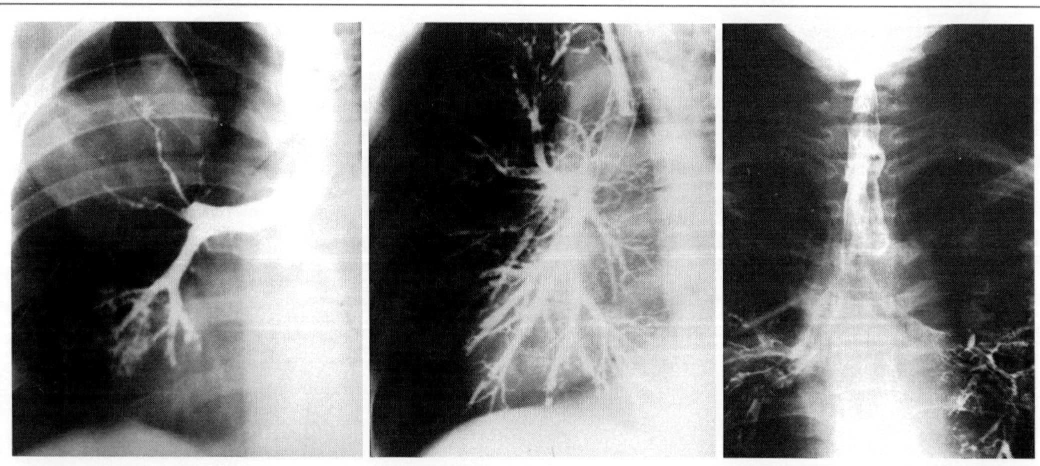

Bronchography—a popular and highly specific method in early and mid-20th century for diagnosis of tracheobronchial lesions.

Source: Reproduced from Jindal SK. Textbook of Pulmonary & Critical Care Medicine, 3rd edition; New Delhi: Jaypee Brothers Medical Publishers; 2025.

other infective conditions such as tuberculosis. Collapse therapy with artificially collapsing the lung to allow healing was commonly practiced. Some old procedures included induction of pneumothorax and/or pneumoperitoneum, phrenic nerve paralysis, and thoracoplasty. Rib resection, lobectomy, and lung decortications were also practiced. Following introduction of effective antitubercular chemotherapy, thoracic surgery went into oblivion. This proved as a great handicap since a significant number of patients such as those of lung cancer or other nontubercular diseases did need surgical interventions for one or the other reason. Thoracic surgery has therefore again gained popularity.

In the modern era, several advancements in techniques have enhanced the scope of thoracic surgery. Minimally invasive surgeries and video-assisted thoracic surgery (VATS) with greater safety have expanded the indications. Robotic thoracic surgery has also become available at a number of centers and is likely to find greater applications with an increase in expertise and affordability. Inspired by global advancements, Indian doctors also began exploring lung transplantation which was first performed for end-stage lung disease in Chennai's Apollo Hospital by KR Balakrishnan in 2013. The facility is now available at a number of hospitals in Chennai, Mumbai, Hyderabad, Bengaluru, Delhi, and other places. There are a number of challenges involved in lung transplantation. Organ shortage, high costs (₹25–50 lakhs), and limited insurance coverage are only a few of the important issues. Inadequate infrastructure and regulatory hurdles also limit the wider availability of the facility.

Training and Education Programs in Respiratory Medicine

Different institutions, organizations, and medical colleges have started with educational programs in respiratory medicine and its subspecialties. These training and education programs aim to enhance the skills and knowledge of healthcare professionals in respiratory medicine, ultimately improving patient care, and outcomes. Unlike most other specialties, educational courses in Respiratory Medicine have generally suffered from the lack of uniformity of a name. Respiratory Medicine has been variously called as Pulmonary Medicine, Pulmonology, Chest Diseases, Thoracic Medicine, and so on. This has sometimes affected the assessment and the quality of different programs.

Diploma in Respiratory Medicine (DRM) was initially started to create a larger manpower especially to handle the large burden of tuberculosis. MD (Respiratory Medicine) which was added thereafter remains the most widely recognized course. Besides MD, the National Board of Examinations offers an equivalent course—Diplomate in Respiratory Medicine (DNB). Since 1989, the postdoctoral (DM) course in Pulmonary and Critical Care Medicine was also started. The Postgraduate Institute of Medical Education and Research, Chandigarh had taken this initiative to broaden the scope of respiratory medicine to a wider spectrum of respiratory syllabus beyond tuberculosis and routine respiratory infections.

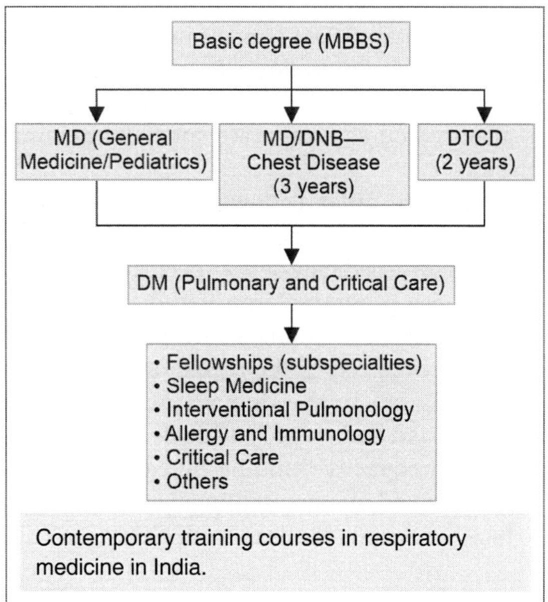

Contemporary training courses in respiratory medicine in India.

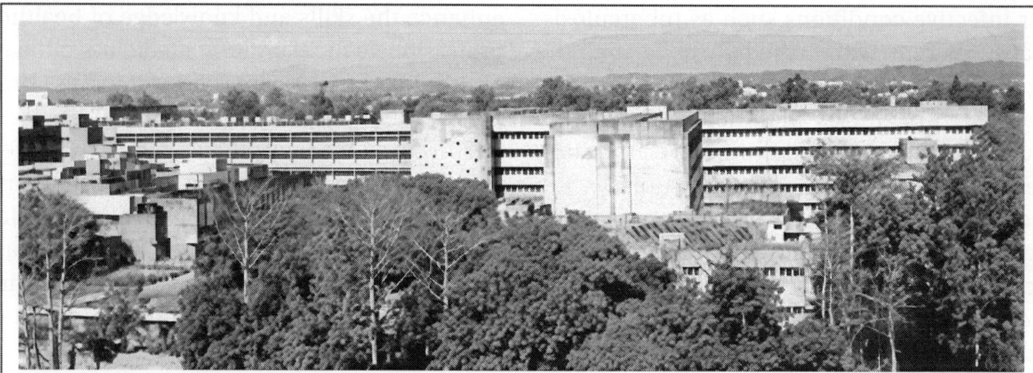

Postgraduate Institute of Medical Education and Research (PGIMER) Chandigarh established in 1960s is one of the pioneer centers in Respiratory Medicine.

Pulmonary interventions, respiratory critical care, sleep medicine, and other subspecialties were included in the course curriculum. This had also enhanced the status of the specialty to that of a super specialty of medicine.

For almost two decades, the Chandigarh institute remained the only place in the country to offer this program in respiratory medicine and critical care. Now, several other institutes in India have also added DM course in Pulmonology/ Pulmonary Medicine. Some institutes have also opted for separate DM courses in Pediatric and/ or Neonatal pulmonology. Pulmonary Critical Care is included in the DM curriculum while it is also treated as a separate specialty at some places.

There are other Fellowship Programs and Certificate Courses either in the broader specialty of respiratory medicine or in a specifically focused area. These programs are offered by different institutions, associations, or hospitals. While a few are recognized by the regulatory provisions, the others fall in the domain of private and unrecognized bodies. Most of these courses have helped in capacity-building by expanding the base of trained manpower. But all cannot be said to have similar standards or credibility.

Educational, Training, and Research Institutes

Tuberculosis was one of the primary focus in the immediate post-Independence period. The Government of India established the Tuberculosis Chemotherapy Centre in Madras (now Chennai) in 1956 which was subsequently renamed as Tuberculosis Research Centre (TRC) in 1978 and then as The National Institute for Research in Tuberculosis. The center has made significant contributions in chemotherapy schedules against tuberculosis, immunology, and molecular biology. The center is now a Supranational Reference Laboratory and a World Health Organization (WHO) Collaborating Center for TB Research and Training. National Tuberculosis Institute (Bangalore) was established in close collaboration with the WHO and UNICEF in 1959 under the Ministry of Health and Family Welfare with specific objective of developing a national TB control program. Other institutes such as National Institute of Tuberculosis and Respiratory Diseases, New Delhi and Rajan Babu Institute of Pulmonary Medicine and Tuberculosis, Delhi were also established primarily for tuberculosis control and research.

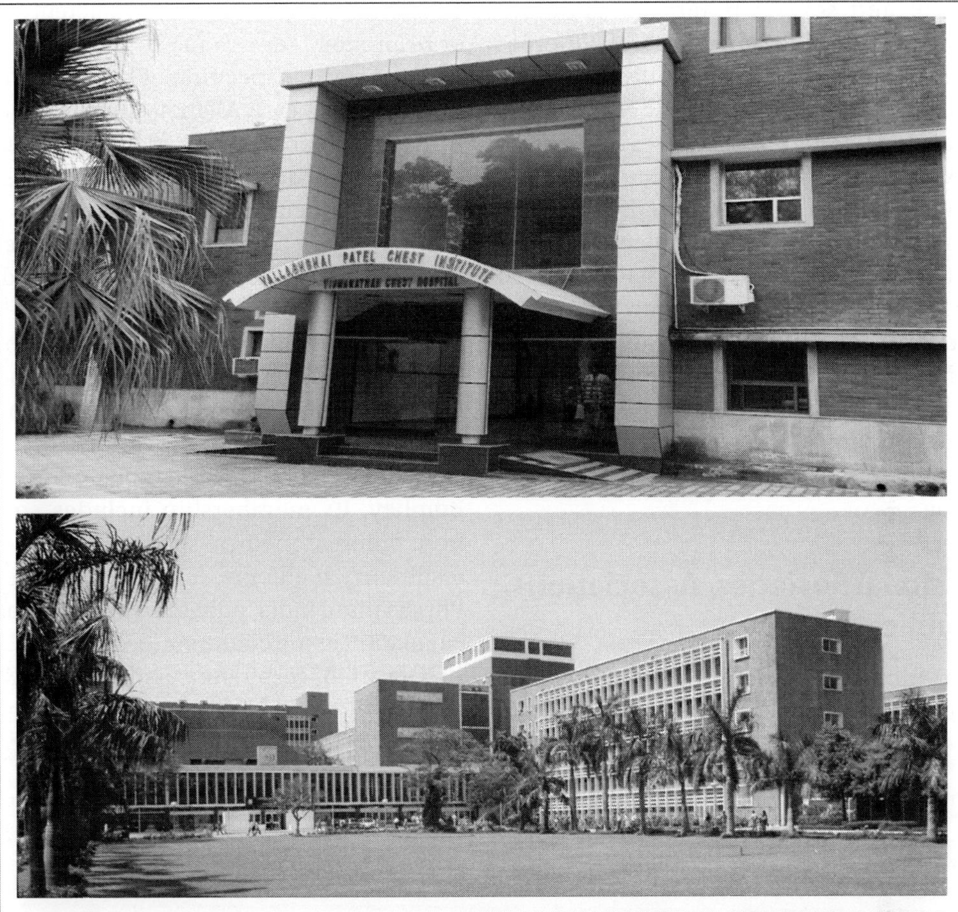

Vallabhbhai Patel Chest Institute (above, Courtesy Dr Ashok Shah) and All India Institute of Medical Sciences (below, Courtesy Dr SK Sharma) are the other primary medical institutes established respectively in 1949 and 1956 in New Delhi.

In the next decade or so, following independence, other government, autonomous, and/ or private institutes also came which offer advanced care for various respiratory diseases. Postgraduate Institute of Medical Education and Research (PGIMER), Chandigarh; All India Institute of Medical Sciences, New Delhi; Christian Medical College (CMC), Vellore; St John's Medical College, Bengaluru; Seth GS Medical College and KEM Hospital, Mumbai; King George Medical University, Lucknow; SGPGI, Lucknow; Kerala Institute of Medical Sciences, Trivandrum; and Nizam's Institute of Medical Sciences, Hyderabad are only some of the examples. The list now is quite exhaustive and includes many other institutes which are engaged in medical as well as respiratory care.

Many other autonomous institutes which contribute with their research work in basic or allied sciences include Indian Institute of Science (IISc), Bengaluru; Tata Memorial Centre (TMC), Mumbai; Institute of Microbial Technology (IMTech), Chandigarh; Jawaharlal Nehru Centre for Advanced Scientific Research (JNCASR),

Bengaluru; and several others. In addition, Governments of India as well as of different states established a wide network of medical colleges and institutes for graduate (MBBS) and postgraduate (MD and DM) courses in different fields. As a result, there was a wide expansion of trained medical and paramedical health personnel. Without any doubt, a large number of private and corporate hospitals have emerged all over the country and significantly contribute to respiratory care and capacity building. Some of the leading corporate chains include the Apollo Hospitals, Fortis Hospitals, Max Super Specialty Hospital, Medanta, Aster, Medicity, Amrita, Metro, and others. The list is huge and keeps on expanding.

Professional Societies, Associations, and Publications

Different professional bodies of doctors and/or other paramedical personnel have played an important role in promoting the different objectives of respiratory care. Some of these associations targeted a wider spectrum of medicine including the respiratory care. All India Medical Association a private, national organization of physicians was established in 1928 and was renamed as Indian Medical Association in 1930. The Association also publishes a monthly *Journal of the Indian Medical Association* (JIMA), is indexed in the Index Medicus. JIMA was founded by Sir Nilratan Sirkar, BC Roy, Kumud Sankar Ray, and others in Calcutta in 1930. Later in 1944, another body was formed with membership restricted to physicians with postgraduate qualifications in different specialties. API was first led by Jivraj N Mehta from Bombay. Its membership includes specialists from different medical specialties including the respiratory medicine. Journal of Association of Physicians of India, published monthly has a wide circulation in the country.

Of various respiratory associations, TAI is one of the oldest and largest voluntary organizations

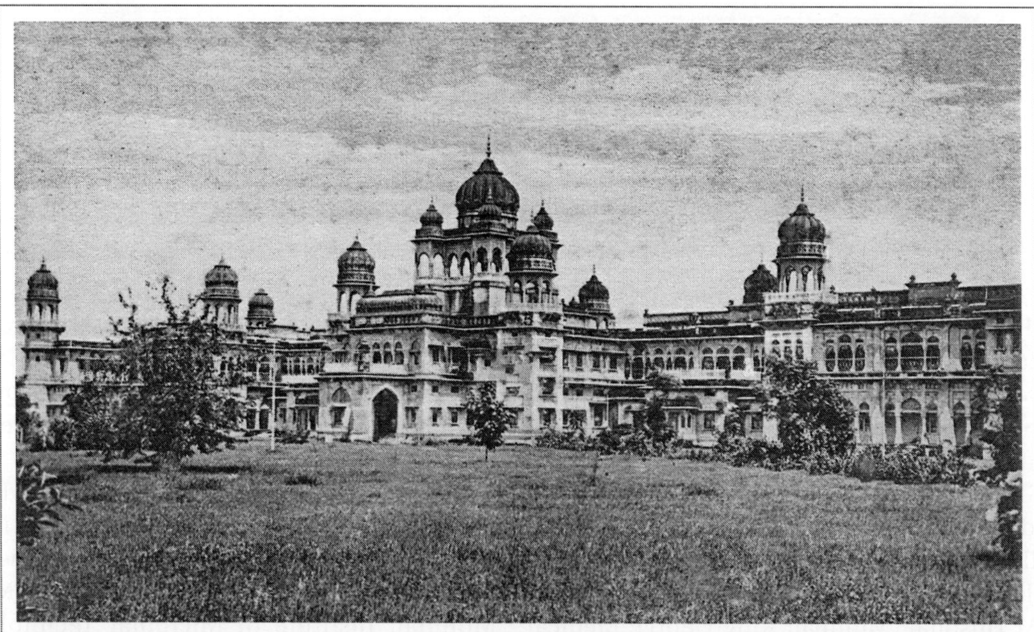

King George's Medical College established in1905 in Lucknow; it was later turned into an University.

having its affiliates all over India. First set up in February 1939, it incorporated the King Emperor's Anti-Tuberculosis Fund and King George Thanks-giving (Anti-Tuberculosis) Fund with the Marchioness of Linlithgow as the first President. Indian Association of Chest Diseases was established in1949 specifically to promote respiratory health by KS Singh, RK Goyal, and SM Tiwari. Later in 1972, it was rechristened as National College of Chest Physicians (NCCP) India. The NCCP brings out a quarterly journal, Indian Journal of Chest Diseases, and Allied Sciences in collaboration with the VP Chest Institute, Delhi.

Indian Chest Society is another organization of Chest Physicians which came into being in 1980. The Society aims to generate and disseminate the knowledge on respiratory medicine and provide a common platform for discussion. The Society holds an annual conference (NAPCON) jointly with the NCCP. From 1982, the Indian Chest Society started publication of a quarterly

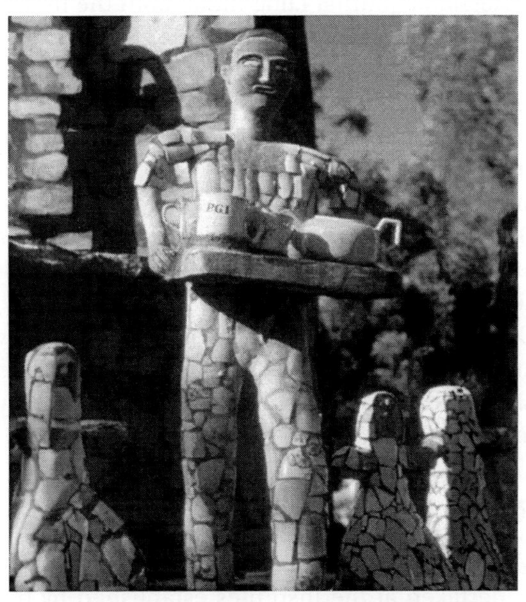

An early creation at Rock Garden of Chandigarh is shown holding an old PGI tea-cup depicted in the hands of a statue.

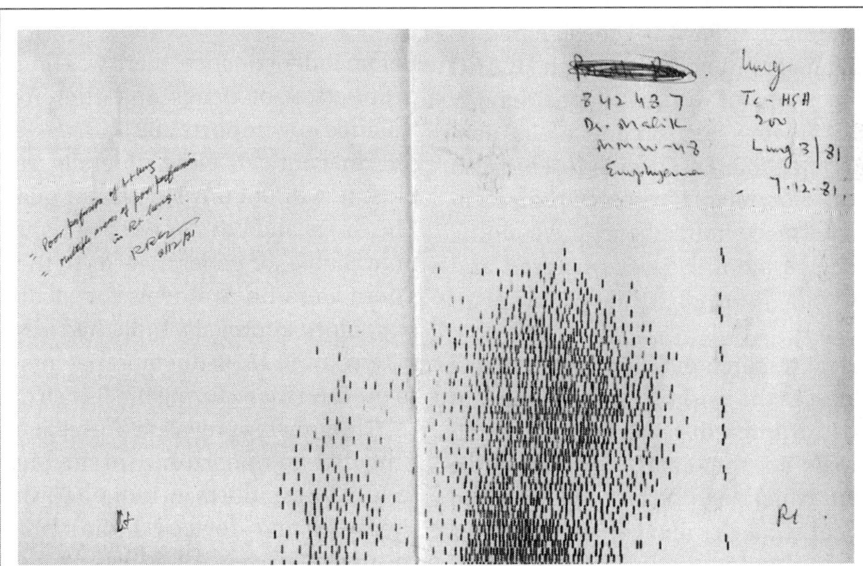

During mid-20th century, ventilation-perfusion scanning was done with help of gamma camera to see structural and functional imaging of lungs; now replaced with CT and PET scanning.

Source: Jindal SK. Reproduced from Textbook of Pulmonary & Critical Care Medicine, 3rd edition. New Delhi: Jaypee Brothers Medical Publishers; 2025.

professional journal Lung India. Both the Indian Journal of Chest Diseases and Allied Sciences and Lung India contain peer-reviewed articles and are indexed by some of the indexing agencies.

There are a few other regional and local groups and/or associations which hold different programs and workshops in respiratory medicine. Different national bodies and associations of other specialties and subspecialties such as of Pediatrics and Pediatric Pulmonology, Critical Care Medicine, Bronchology, Allergy and Immunology, Sleep Medicine, and others also contribute to the discipline of respiratory medicine.

Respiratory Research

Medical research in general was largely undertaken at the Institutes established by the Government of India and its different agencies. Before independence, it had set up the Indian Research Fund Association (IRFA) in 1911 with the specific objective of sponsoring and coordinating medical research in the country. After independence, IRFA was redesignated as the Indian Council of Medical Research (ICMR) in 1949 and its scope of work was considerably expanded. ICMR now has several of its own centers to look after different specified area. It also provides funding for different research projects in subjects of importance from all over the country. ICMR publishes a monthly peer-reviewed and indexed research journal, Indian Journal of Medical Research.

As a medical research organization, ICMR is one of the oldest in the world. It made significant contributions to different aspects of research in tuberculosis in the early decades after independence which significantly contributed to the treatment strategies and control programs of tuberculosis. Demonstration of efficacy of domiciliary and short course antitubercular chemotherapy were some of the key observations made in India which formed the basis of tuberculosis control program in India and elsewhere in several countries. In the later periods, ICMR also sponsored research projects and plans for nontubercular respiratory diseases such as asthma and other lung diseases. Besides ICMR, there are other governmental, semigovernmental, and occasionally private bodies which also sponsor and fund research projects in different scientific subjects including those related to the respiratory medicine. Council for Scientific and Industrial Research (CSIR) and Department of Biotechnology (DBT) are some of such important organizations.

There is no doubt that India has the potential of generating much more original research than that is presently available. It needs to significantly multiply its inputs, investments, and incentives for medical research especially focused on relevant local issues. Some of the important issues of respiratory research from India have been discussed in a separate chapter.

Respiratory Pharmaceutical Industry in India

Before independence, there was limited domestic production of drugs and therefore a greater reliance on imports. Bulk drugs and finished pharmaceuticals were generally imported from outside without any significant quality controls. The drugs and devices were not only costlier but unavailable for general needs of the community. There were no protocols for local streamlined regulatory approvals. India had enacted its own patent law in 1856. But most patents were granted to the foreigners during the British era.

The growing prevalence of respiratory diseases provided an opportunity to the pharmaceutical sector to establish in India and develop novel therapies and devices. India's pharmaceutical industry also started exporting respiratory medications globally. Indigenous production has also eased out a wider availability and affordability of drugs and devices. Bengal Chemicals and Pharmaceutical Works Limited was the first pharmaceutical company in India, which was established in 1901 by Acharya PC Ray. Some other drug companies of the preindependence period included Alembic Chemical Works in 1907 and Bengal Immunity in 1919. Abdul Hamied founded Chemical, Industrial and Pharmaceutical Laboratories (now CIPLA) in 1935 to make India self-sufficient in pharmaceuticals. Cipla assumed leadership in respiratory medicine in India in the 1970s with introduction of salbutamol tablets in 1976 and salbutamol inhalers in 1978.

Several other Indian drug companies which are now contributing to respiratory medicine entered the field in the post-Independence period. Dr Desh Bandhu Gupta founded Lupin in the year 1968 with the initial vision to fight life-threatening infectious diseases and to manufacture drugs of the highest social priority. Other prominent players in the field include Sun Pharmaceutical Industries, Glenmark Pharmaceuticals Limited, Torrent Pharmaceutical, Zydus Cadilla, and multinational companies such as GSK and Astra Zeneca. The list keeps on expanding due to increasing prevalence of respiratory diseases, air pollution, and tobacco usage. Many other regional and national manufacturers and distributors are also engaged with their own brands of inhalers, nebulizers, and oral respiratory medications which dominate the market. Most of these companies offer a wide range of products for respiratory diseases, including asthma, COPD, allergic rhinitis, pulmonary arterial hypertension, lung cancer, and idiopathic pulmonary fibrosis .

India's respiratory pharmaceutical market is currently estimated at ₹17,000 crores (approximately $2.2 billion USD) in 2022. It continues to expand in view of growing demand fueled both by the increase in the disease burden as well as the pressing economic and marketing forces. Inhalation therapy has particularly found a fancy with a number of companies because of their market profitability. The market size of Indian respiratory devices, which includes inhalers, is estimated to be around $one billion in 2024. All kinds of digital inhalation devices and biologics for targeted immunotherapy of asthma are being developed and marketed.

There were a few regulatory acts passed during the colonial era such as the Dangerous Drug Act in 1930 to restrict pharmacy practice; Drug Enquiry Committee in 1930 to investigate the difficulties of the pharmacy profession; and the Drug and Cosmetics Act in 1940 to regulate the import, manufacturing, sale, and distribution of medicines. Now there are regulatory agencies such as the Indian Pharmaceutical Alliance (IPA) and Pharmaceutical Export Promotion Council of India (PHARMEXCIL). The Central Drugs Standard Control Organisation (CDSCO) is the primary apical body under the Government of India with final approval authority.

In addition to the drug industry, there is vast expansion of companies manufacturing and/or supplying diagnostic and monitoring devices such as spirometers, sleep test devices, peak flow meters, pulse oximeters, and capnographs as well as therapeutic devices such as continuous positive airway pressure (CPAP), bilevel positive airway pressure (BiPAP), humidifiers, nebulizers, oxygen concentrators, ventilators, and inhalers. Several different types of disposables such as masks, breathing circuits, and others are also locally manufactured and marketed. The production had multiplied severalfold during the recent COVID-19 pandemic.

It is obvious that India has made rapid strides to cope with its problems and stand along with the developed world in most areas of respiratory medicine. The quality of clinical services as well as of education and training in the subject matches with those available in the advanced Western countries. There is adequate availability of drugs and devices used for disease management. It is true that there are problems of distribution and equity available in the community which are mostly attributed to the economic disparities which are also narrowing with time. There is significant vacuum in the Indian research achievements compared to the international innovations. There are also some lacunae in the uniformity of standards of education. This is not entirely unexpected in a vast country such as India with multiple variations of languages and cultures in different regions. Nonetheless, it is highly desirable that the Indian pulmonary family work harder and make greater investments to cover these gaps.

Sources

1. Garud A, Biswas D, Moitra S, Moitra S. Health promotion in the management of respiratory diseases: an Indian Perspective. Lancet Respir Med. 2024;12(12):e77.
2. World Health Organization. A brief history of tuberculosis control in India. Geneva; World Health Organization; 2010.
3. Jindal SK, Shankar PS, Vijayan VK, Kamat SR, Deivanayagan CN. Down the memory lane: Lung India three decades. Lung India. 2012;29(3):205-11.
4. Malik SK. Developing pulmonary medicine (Pulmonology) in India: A view point. Indian J Chest Dis Allied Sci. 1985;27:254-6.
5. Jain SK. Is teaching and research in respiratory medicine keeping pace with the clinical needs? Indian J Chest Dis Allied Sci. 1988;30:1-4.
6. Jindal SK. Challenges of Training in Pulmonary Medicine in India. Indian J Chest Dis Allied Sci. 2013;55:73-4.
7. Jindal SK. Pulmonary training facilities in medical colleges in India. Indian J Chest Dis Allied Sci. 1989;31:295-8.
8. Editorial. Respiratory medicine: challenging times, hope for the future. Lancet 2012;380:621.
9. Sreedharan JK, Varghese S. (2022). Twenty-Five Years of Excellence; Respiratory Therapy in India - Past, Present, and Future. [online] Available from https://www.ijrc.in/doi/pdf/10.4103/ijrc.ijrc_62_19 [Last accessed September, 2025].
10. Greene W. (2007). The Emergence of India's Pharmaceutical Industry and Implications for the U.S. Generic Drug Market. [online] Available from https://www.usitc.gov/publications/332/EC200705A.pdf [Last accessed September, 2025].
11. PharmaState Academy. (2019). History of Indian Pharma Industry. [online] Available from https://pharmastate.academy/history-of-indian-pharma-industry/ [Last accessed September, 2025].

CHAPTER

8

Tuberculosis

Tuberculosis (TB) which we now know as an infectious disease caused by *Mycobacterium tuberculosis*, has plagued man kind since the very ancient times. In the Indian context, it is also said to have its origin in ancient Hindu mythology. *King Daksha* cursed *Chandra* (the Moon god) to suffer from TB (*Kshayaroga*) after his 27 daughters who were married to *Chandra* complained that *Chandra* ignored them and spent most of his time with Rohini, one of his wives. *Chandra's* brightness immediately disappeared. The curse also affected the medicinal plants and other living beings dependent on *Chandra*'s influence. After pleading by other gods, *Daksha* modified his curse and allowed *Chandra* to be bright or disease-free for half of every month. Subsequently, the disease "descended upon earth to afflict those who overstrained themselves, particularly by sexual excesses". Incidentally, the disease was commonly referred to as the King's Evil and the King fever in the later periods in Europe as well.

21st Century Advances
Vaccines
Preventive strategies improved diagnosis
Adjuvants and vaccines
Newer drugs and combinations
Improved and augmented implementation of treatment and control strategies
TB

Prehistoric Period

History of TB can be traced back to several millennia. Actually, the *Mycobacterium* is believed to exist for over 150 million years long before the origin of man. The molecular evidence was found for the first time in the fossil of an extinct bison about twenty millennia old. In the known historical period, TB was recognized in Egyptian mummies, of around 2400 BC, which had skeletal deformities suggestive of typical Pott's lesions of TB although no such evidence was described in the famous Egyptian papyri. The first written documentation of TB, which is about 3,300 and 2,300 years old, was found from India and China, respectively.

Association of "tubercles" with the pulmonary form of TB was established in the 17th century but the nomenclature of "tuberculosis" was first used by Schönlein in 1839. It was later in 1882 that Robert Koch discovered the bacillus *M. tuberculosis* responsible for human TB.

Archaeological Evidence

The earliest evidence from India is seen in the form of archaeological findings of the Harappan Civilization from skeletal remains showing signs of TB on paleopathological analysis. Of the Harappan Civilization which dates back to

6000 BCE, the two important cities, Mohenjo-daro and Harappa emerged around 2600 BCE in Punjab and Sindh along the Indus River. Both macroscopic and microscopic analyses of some of the 26 remain showed presence of pathological findings of proliferative and lytic lesions and abscess formation associated with reactive bone formation and ankylosis. Specific skeletal features included changes to the spine affecting the vertebral bodies with resulting ankylosis, body collapse, and kyphosis. Single joint ankylosis, specially localized in the hip, knee, and wrist; and new bone formation on the internal surface of the ribs were also seen. There were highly consistent with diagnosis of TB.

Remnants of skeletal TB were also found in Neolithic Mediterranean and Ancient Egyptian mummies. The portraits of hunchbacks pictured by the Egyptian artists on the walls of over 5,000 year old tombs are considered to suggest tubercular vertebral destruction. There is also archaeological evidence dating back to 2400 BC found in Egyptian mummies, as well as the Peruvian mummies from the Andean region. The presence of Pott's deformities of spine due to vertebral *destruction and an associated abscess* suggested the presence of TB disease. It is also said that the queen Nefertiti and her husband, King Akhenaten of ancient Egypt died of TB.

Direct or indirect reference to TB can be found in ancient literature of most of the old civilizations. Interpretation of the old cave-paintings and/or medical records in pictorial writing of over 4,000 years earlier provide indirect evidence of TB. The mention of lung TB can be found in the ancient Chinese, Babylonian, and Indo Aryan literature of 2600–1500 BC, about 1–2 millennia later than the skeletal TB. The code of Hammurabi of Babylon, the Laws of Manu, and the Rigveda of Indo-Aryan period, all of the prebiblical era, do clearly mention about the disease in different descriptions. Body consumption and contagious nature are the two important characteristics which have been pointed out.

Documentation of TB is found in Hebraism in the ancient Hebrew word schachepheth to describe TB. It was used in the Biblical books of *Deuteronomy* and *Leviticus*. In the Indian history, TB is mentioned in the *Rigveda*, one of the four *Vedas* of the ancient *Vedic* civilization written in about 1500 BCE. It provides references to TB as disease *yaksma*. Atharvaveda, which belongs to the later era of around 1200–1000 BCE refers to the disease *balasa* which was similar to TB. TB was also called "*Rajyakshma*" (Royal TB), *Kṣaya* (decay or wasting), and *Sosa* (dryness or wasting). *Atharvaveda* also describes a condition like "scrofula" or lymph-node TB for the first time.

Yaksma (TB) in Ancient Indian Texts

Yaksma is the most commonly used nomenclature at several places in ancient Sanskrit language in the *Vedic* texts, Rigveda and Atharvaveda of 1200–1500 BC. It is often translated as "consumption" or "wasting disease," which could refer to TB. There are also references to a group of diseases called "Sosha" with symptoms of wasting, weight loss, cough, and blood spitting. Though some scholars have argued that *Yaksma* might imply an ailment in general, the characteristics attributed leave little doubt that it referred to what we today understand as "TB". The word "Yakshnā" is mentioned more than 25 times in the *Vedas,* including in a few complete hymns. According to different researchers, symptoms of *Yakshmā* mentioned in *Atharvaveda* include exertion (*Sahasa*), loss of semen (*Sukra*), excessive salivation, fever, cough, bleeding, anorexia, and shortness of breath.

As per some of the most accepted version of the texts, the nature of the disease is explicitly stated in several verses of *Rigveda* (1.102.6, 1.122.6 and 1.123.2):

यक्ष्मा नाश्यति शरीरम् (Yaksmā naśyati śarīram)

यक्ष्मा श्वासो नाश्यति (Yaksmā śvāso naśyati)

क्षयः श्वासः शोष (Kṣayaḥ śvāsaḥ śoṣaḥ)

(The consumptive disease destroys the body; the consumptive disease destroys the life's breath, i.e., the decay/wasting causes dryness/wasting of breath.)

Atharvaveda also described lymph nodal TB in the neck which we now label as scrofula:

अपांगं वृष्णं क्षयाय (Apāṅgaṃ vṛṣṇaṃ kṣayāya)—The swollen gland (Apāṅgaṃ) is destroyed by consumption.

The "*Yajurveda*" advised affected individuals to move to higher altitudes—a belief which persisted up to the 20th century.

Manusmriti, is another ancient Sanskrit text belonging to 2nd century BCE, which prescribes different regulations, doctrines, and principles for the king and the people. It includes the laws, *karma,* and guidelines on proper conduct for the rulers and society based on the principles of *dharma,* the sacraments, and the study of the Vedas. Manusmriti was translated in 1794 by British philologist Sir William Jones into English and later into French, German, Portuguese, and Russian. It was the basis for the legal system established by the British Raj.

The *Manusmriti,* contains descriptions of diseases, including TB, possible for advice on actions for the people. TB is mentioned by same nomenclature uses in the Vedas as *yaksma, kshay, and shosha* in several verses (3.33, 3.34 and 3.36, 3.37, 3.38, 3.39....). It recognized symptoms of cough, fever, weight loss, fatigue, and breathlessness.

Manusmriti also pointed to the communicable character of the disease since it recommended isolation and separation of the sufferer from the family and the society as well as their prohibition from the sacred rituals *(Manusmriti* 3.40, 3.41, and 3.42). It also described the course of disease including the difficulty in recovery and the risk of death (*Manusmriti* 3.43 and 3.44). It also prescribed that persons affected by Yaksma were unclean and that the Brahmins must not marry in those families.

Various treatments were described which included avoidance of excessive physical activity, a balanced diet, avoiding harmful foods, prescriptions of herbal remedies along with rituals and prayers (*Manusmriti* 3.45 to 3.49).

Tuberculosis in Ayurvedic Texts

The reference to *"yaksma"* was generally indirect and contextual in the *Vedas* which were spiritual and philosophical texts. On the other hand, the medical text of the Vedic period, Ayurveda which belonged to 700–800 BC era, contained direct description of "yaksma"—the disease. Both Charaka *Samhita* and *Sushruta Samhita* describe the disease in greater details and provide details of the origin and the symptomatology. It was also stated that "The physician who wants great fame cures a man attacked by consumption". The later Indian manuscript of around 800–1000 CE, *Madhavanidana* and its commentary *Madhukosa* repeatedly refer to "consumption" or *"Rajyakshma"*.

Tuberculosis in Ayurveda was believed to be caused by the defective humoral theory. Of the three known humors (*doshas—vata, pitta, and kapha*), TB was believed to be caused by the defective *kapha* due to accumulation of *ama* (toxins) in the body. Ayurveda prescribed treatment with herbs (turmeric, ginger, and ashwagandha), a balanced diet, and avoidance of excessive physical activity. *Panchakarma* was prescribed as a detoxification procedure to remove toxins from the body.

Tuberculosis was also the most recognized ailment elsewhere in the world during this period. It was recognized as *Phthisis,* i.e., wasting, in ancient Greece by Hippocrates who described the condition as a fatal disease especially for young adults. Galen, in the 2nd century CE described symptoms of such as fever, sweating, cough, and blood stained sputum for which he recommended different empirical treatments with food, fresh air, and others. Galen had also suspected that the disease could be transmitted from one person to another although it was later that this was finally established.

> Atharvaveda authored by a Vedic seer and physician Atharvan is often considered an encyclopedia of medicine and original source of Ayurveda. It incorporates several verses (such as 5.22.5, 6.93.1, and 9.8.2) referring to tuberculosis:
>
> क्षेत्रं क्षयं श्वासम् (Kṣetraṃ kṣayaṃ śvāsaṃ)
>
> यक्ष्मां नाश्यति शरीरम् (Yaksmāṃ naśyati śarīram)
>
> श्वासः शोषः क्षयः (Śvāsaḥ śoṣaḥ kṣayaḥ)
>
> (Consumptive disease causes decay/ wasting of body and life's breath)

Tuberculosis during Medieval Era

Tuberculosis was widespread in Europe after the decline of the Roman Empire. It inflicted and killed not only the poor and the disadvantaged but also the rich and the celebrated. In Europe, TB was also called "consumption" because of extreme wasting. John Keats, the renowned English poet who struggled with TB offer valuable insights into the human experience of living with this illness. He wrote in a letter: *"I am reduced to a state of weakness that makes my life a burden to me. I am dying of a consumption."*

The disease was sometimes referred to as "the white plague" because of extreme paleness of patients. Sometimes, the terminology "white death" was used for TB to differentiate from "black death" or the plague which had caused devastating epidemics in that period. In the 14th century, the first plague epidemic was described first in vivid terms: "... *and so many died that all believed it was the end of the world"* (The Plague in Siena: An Italian Chronicle). Similarly, TB was believed as the *"Captain of all these men of death".*

It also continued to be an issue of significant health and social concerns in India during this period. TB patients often faced social exclusion not just because of its contagious nature but due to an associated social stigmatization. It seriously impacted daily life and incomes of not only the patients but the entire family. Sometimes, it was considered as a divine punishment by the gods and a curse for the religious and social misdoings and acts. It also posed a great economic burden and adversely affected the trade and commerce.

Several different forms of TB were described. Scrofula, i.e., lymph node TB, known since the time of *Atharvaveda* in India and Aristotle in Greece, was described as a new clinical form in Europe. The disease was known as "king's evil" since it was commonly believed that the disease could be treated with the "royal touch". It was also believed by many physicians such as Rene Laennec there were multiple clinical presentations of the same disease characterized with coughing, fever, and night sweats. Miliary TB, described by Thomas Willis was also a common presentation. It was also believed that miliary TB was more prevalent at that time than seen in the modern era.

From the 14th century onward, the period is referred to as the Renaissance or the Age of Discovery. There were many discoveries which also helped in making significant advances with reference to TB. Benjamin Marten had hypothesized that consumption could be caused by minute living creatures which were similar to those seen earlier by Leeuwenhoek. But he could not demonstrate any such creatures. Description of the microscopic structure of the lungs by Malpighi, demonstration of the presence of tubercles in different organs by Bayle as well as of lesions described by Hyacinthe Laennec made it possible to further understand TB. It was Johann Lukas Schönlein who gave the terminology "tuberculosis" in 1839. Discovery of X-rays and of the stethoscope also advanced the knowledge about TB.

It was still not clear how the disease was caused. It was believed to be hereditary by Hippocrates

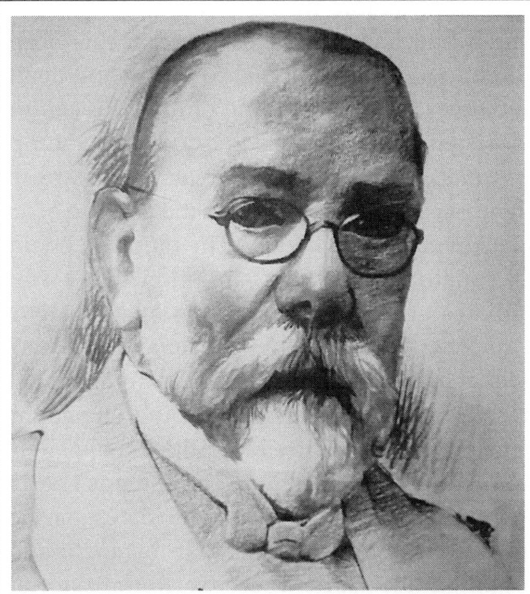

Robert Koch—the discoverer of *Mycobacterium tuberculosis* was a German physician and microbiologist. He had first announced the discovery on March 24, 1882, at the Berlin Physiological Society.
(*Tissue dissections from guinea pigs infected with tuberculous material from lungs of infected apes, brains, and lungs of humans who had died from blood-borne tuberculosis, from the cheesy masses in lungs of chronically infected patients and from the abdominal cavities of cattle infected with TB. In all cases, the disease which had developed in the experimentally infected guinea pigs was the same, and the cultures of bacteria taken from the infected guinea pigs were identical.*)
"I hold that evening to be the most important experience of my scientific life"—Paul Ehrlich (Nobel Laureate in 1908).

while Galen was the first who suspected that the disease could be transmitted. The contagious nature of TB was described in the 16th century by an Italian physician, Girolamo Fracastoro, who showed that some diseases could be transmitted between humans through breathing of "particles".

The *Mycobacterium* causing the disease was discovered much later by Robert Koch, in 1882. On March 24, he announced the discovery of the microorganisms to the Berlin Society of Physiology as "*Thin, whose length is half-a-quarter of the diameter of a red blood cell, very similar to the lepers' bacillus, but sharper*". Subsequently, the microorganisms were labeled as *M. tuberculosis*. It was later proposed by Virchow that a number of other factors such as poverty, malnourishment, and poor hygiene were also important in the development of the disease.

Koch's observations also laid the foundation of Koch's postulates which were relevant to all infectious diseases. In essence, the Koch's postulates implied that the causative agent, i.e., the microorganism should be present in every case of the disease and not in healthy subjects; the microorganism should be isolated from a diseased patient and grown in pure culture, and should cause the same disease when introduced into a healthy subject. Later in 1905, Smith added the fourth postulate that the microorganism should be reisolated from the new host and identified as being identical to the original microorganism. Koch's postulates, however, do not apply to all microbes and different variations have been developed for different types of diseases. The revised postulates propose the replacement of organism with the molecular and DNA copies, and so on.

Tuberculosis was a significant public health concern in India during this era although there is very little documented information available about the disease. TB was, however, mentioned in court records and literature of the Mughal Empire. The disease had been referred to in different terminologies in some Ayurvedic and Unani texts of medicine. Kitab al-Saydalah' of Al-Biruni belonging to the 11th century described TB symptoms and treatments while Ibn Sina's "The Canon of Medicine" of the same period also referred to the disease in Unani medicine. Later, the Ayurvedic text, Bhavaprakasha of the 16th century described ayurvedic treatments and other details. Both Unani medicine and Ayurveda employed herbal preparations, dietary regimens, minerals, and yoga. Sometimes, surgical interventions were also employed by skilled physicians.

Discoveries related to the disease during European Renaissance rapidly traveled to India as well. A greater understanding was therefore possible, which helped in taking gradual steps for disease control.

Tuberculosis during the Colonial Era in India

In India, TB became an issue of larger public health due to a number of social and economic factors. There was great poverty, malnutrition, and poor living conditions which all promoted and exacerbated TB. Other factors such as increasing urbanization and industrialization, migration, and labor movements helped increased TB transmission and spread. TB, however, also affected the people in higher echelons. Muhammad Ali Jinnah, the founder of Pakistan, suffered from this illness for several years before his death in 1948.

India, however, was quick in applying the treatment and prevention measures which had become available due to the new discoveries which had happened elsewhere in the world. The initial British Colonial response and health initiatives in the beginning of the 20th century consisted of the establishment of TB sanatoria for isolation and rest-based treatment as was the common practice in Europe in the absence of any specific pharmacotherapy. The rationale behind TB sanatoria was the assumption that certain climates prevented TB and that open-air living would heal the disease. The sanatoria, usually built at high attitude, provided environment with fresh air and nutritious food for the TB patients. Sanatoria were also used for isolation of patients from the family and the local community. The first such open air sanatorium in India was established in 1906 in Tilonia in Rajasthan by a Christian organization while the first nonmissionary sanatorium was built near Shimla in 1909. Several sanatoria were subsequently started in different parts of India.

TB clinics and hospitals were also established for early diagnosis and treatment. The government also adopted legislative measures and policies such as making TB a *"notifiable disease"*

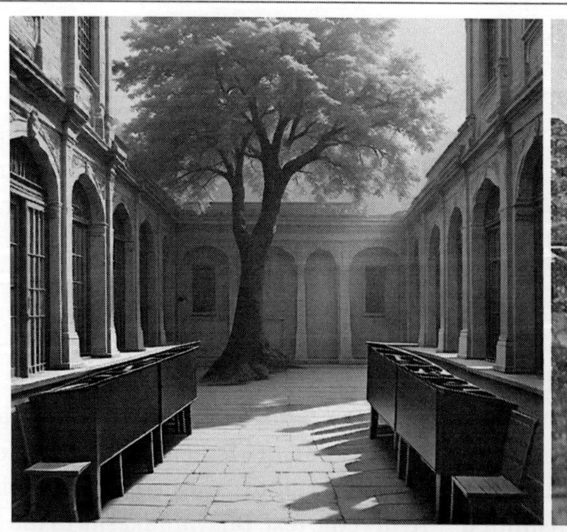

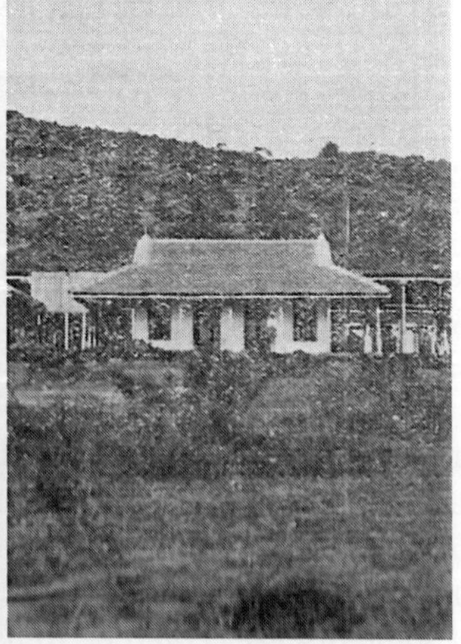

TB Sanatoria in the 19th and early 20th century: (L) Conceptual; (R) Tambaram sanatorium, Chennai.
Courtesy: DJ Christopher

under the Indian Lunacy Act (1912). The Public Health Act (1897) enabled local authorities to establish TB clinics. The country also adopted the Bacillus Calmette-Guérin (BCG) Vaccination programs in1920s after the discovery and development of the vaccine by Albert Calmette and Camille Guérin at the French Institut Pasteur between 1908 and 1921. The vaccine was made from a weakened strain of *Mycobacterium bovis*, and found effective after the initial administration to an infant whose mother had died of TB. Mass production of the BCG vaccine was taken up in 1924. The BCG vaccine prevented child mortality as well as the occurrence of TB in about 20% of children.

Without a doubt, the colonial era laid the groundwork for later TB control efforts in India, despite the several challenges which persisted. The cultural and social stigma associated with TB in the Indian community hindered TB diagnosis and treatment. Funding constraints and the colonial focus on European health concerns rather than that of Indians were major challenges at the governmental level. TB control activities were also taken up by voluntary and semigovernment agencies and individuals. A British physician, Sir Robert Philip strongly advocated for TB control measures while an Indian physician, Dr M Kesava Pai led TB control efforts in the Madras Presidency. Another important step included the establishment of Tuberculosis Association of India in 1920 which promoted TB awareness and control activities with strong support of the government.

Tuberculosis in the Post-Independence Period

The discovery of mycobacterial origin of TB led to intensified efforts for drug treatment. Till then, treatment in Western Europe and America largely consisted of isolation of patients in Tb Sanatoria meant for this purpose. Surgical treatment including artificial pneumothorax, lobectomy, and pneumonectomy were quite widely used. Chemotherapy with mercury, iodine and creosote, etc., was also employed. Robert Koch in 1890 discovered tuberculin which was tried for treatment of TB but proved to be futile. Sulfanilamide which could inhibit the growth of mycobacteria in guinea pigs was also unsuccessful in humans. The most significant step consisted of the discovery of streptomycin in 1943 by Waksman and colleagues which marked a big step forward in the treatment of TB. Streptomycin was administered for the first time in 1944 and was almost immediately effective. Subsequently, isoniazid was discovered in 1951, which marked the beginning of the modern era of TB treatment. Other drugs such as ethambutol in 1961 and rifampin in 1966 were able to increase the efficacy. Additional of pyrazinamide further helped to reduce the length of TB treatment from the earlier 9–12 months to 6-month, leading to the term "short course chemotherapy".

TB control efforts significantly expanded after independence in 1947. Diploma in TB after the MBBS undergraduate degree was started as a capacity-building measure to increase TB specialists. Later, the diploma was upgraded to a 2-year postgraduate MD which was further expanded to include nontubercular lung diseases in its ambit.

A large public health campaign of mass BCG vaccination was undertaken which included health education to reach the rural areas. National Sample Survey on TB served the useful purpose of assessment of national prevalence and distribution in different populations of the country. National Tuberculosis Institute was established in 1959 in Bangalore with the help of the World Health Organization (WHO) to develop a national TB control program (NTP) which was soon thereafter launched by the government of India in 1962. The Program designed to provide free TB treatment to all integrated TB control into the government's health services.

NTP in India had shown good success in the beginning but did not achieve the objectives of TB control which were laid out earlier. This also led to some truly warning comments by the WHO at the international level. In 1993, the then Director General, H Nakajima had commented on the TB problem as a *global emergency* while the earlier DG, *H Mahler* was quoted to have said that *"All countries benefit from the fruits of Indian research—all countries except India".*

The NTP failure was mostly attributed to lacunae such as poor rates of diagnosis and inadequacy of treatment on assessment. Different scientific studies and investigations reported the use of erratic and irregular drug-regimens at multiple levels as well as poor compliance by the patients as most significant factors responsible for the continued rise in prevalence of TB. All these factors also added to an increase in the number of cases with drug-resistance. The Government of India therefore launched the Revised National TB Control Programme (RNTCP) in 1997. This program incorporated political commitment and Directly Observed Treatment, Short-course (DOTS) strategy as an essential component. RNTCP was gradually expanded to cover the entire country in the next few years. Since human immunodeficiency virus (HIV) infection was an important risk factor for TB, integrated TB-HIV services were also added. Many other initiatives were also taken which included *Nikshay,* i.e., National TB surveillance system and a community-led initiative—TB-Free India Campaign.

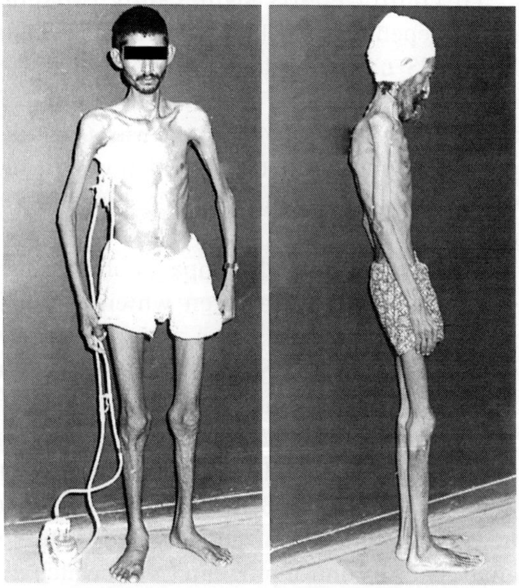

Tuberculosis patients—mid-20th century (*Source*: Reproduced from Jindal Sk. Textbook of Pulmonary and Critical Care Medicine, 3rd edition. New Delhi: Jaypee Brothers Medical Publishers; 2025.)

Indian Research in Tuberculosis

India had produced some excellent outcomes of its long-term field research in TB, particularly related to treatment strategies. Most of this research was undertaken at NTI, Bangalore and the Tuberculosis Chemotherapy Centre, Madras. The Tuberculosis Chemotherapy Centre was set up in 1956 in collaboration with British Medical Research Council, WHO, ICMR and the Madras Government. The primary objective was to study the feasibility of domiciliary treatment on a larger scale.

ICMR in 1961 had made several recommendations for the district TB Program including domiciliary treatment. It was convincingly shown that hospitalization was not essential and that domiciliary treatment was all that was essential. Bacteriological demonstration was considered of supreme importance in diagnosis and control of TB. It was also found that intermittent therapy was as good as daily treatment if compliance was ensured. Several of these findings formed the basis of the DOTS strategy recommended in RNTCP which was launched in 1997. The revised program included "bacteriological demonstration" as essential for diagnosis of active disease. "Intermittent" and "direct observation of administration of drugs" were other principles of therapy.

A field study on efficacy of BCG vaccination against bacillary forms of pulmonary TB was undertaken by the Indian Council of Medical Research in Chingleput district of South India in a large population. The findings at 15 years showed that BCG did not offer any protection against adult forms of bacillary pulmonary TB. The reporting of the study caused a global hue and cry. Subsequent analyses of the results revealed that the vaccination was successful only in preventing the severer forms of TB such as military TB and tubercular meningitis in children.

Current Indian Scene

The millennia-old disease continues to pose challenges related to treatment failure and multidrug resistance. Several factors such as variable quality of care, delayed diagnosis, disparities in access to care, persistent social stigma, and limited public awareness contribute to this.

Mr Narendra Modi, the Prime Minister of India, demonstrated his firm resolve to eradicate the disease by 2025 at the national level. The Government of India decided to restructure the previous program as "National TB Elimination Programme (NTEP)" to frame the national commitment. TB elimination, defined as an incidence of <20 cases per 100,000 population, was determined to be the goal. NTEP had four important components as part of the National Strategic Plan, i.e., detect, treat, prevent, and build. NTEP also included the strategy of "active case finding" among key populations, i.e., high-risk populations and preventing the development of active TB in people with latent TB. Programmatic Management of Drug Resistant TB (PMDT) was another thrust area of NTEP.

India has moved forward in TB control and achieved significant results. According to TB-India 2024 Report, there was a 16% decline in 2024 in incidence of new cases emerging each year compared to the 2015 figures. Mortality rates had also reduced by 18% during the same period. There was an improvement of up to 65% of treatment success rate among notified drug-resistant TB patients. The report also highlighted the continued challenges of multidrug-resistant TB, TB-HIV co-infection, and socioeconomic barriers to TB care.

In addition to the launch of NTEP, the government had implemented several other initiatives to address these challenges. *Pradhan Mantri TB Mukt Bharat Abhiyan* provides additional patient support while Corporate Social Responsibility activities are undertaken to augment community involvement. *Nikshay Poshan Yojana* was designed to provide financial incentive for TB patients registered on the *Nikshay* Portal. NTEP intends to engage the private sector as well as plug the "leak", i.e., loss of patients from the care-cascade.

The United Nations Sustainable Development Goals aim to end the epidemics of TB along with some other communicable diseases as public health challenges by 2030. It is expected that India can move closer to achieve its ambitious goal of becoming TB-free by 2025 by addressing various challenges and building on existing initiatives, 5 years earlier than the global goals. Political commitment, availability of adequate administrative, and funding support should help achieve this aim.

Sources

1. Bühler G. Manu Smriti. Oxford: Clarendon Press; 1886.
2. Ganganatha Jha. Manusmriti with the Commentary of Medhatithi, 1920 https://www.wisdomlib.org/hinduism/book/manusmriti-with-the-commentary-of-medhatithi.
3. Manusmriti: Origins, Influence, and Legacy. https://medium.com/part-of-the-cuture/manusmriti.
4. Max Mueller's Edition of Rig Veda with Sayana's Commentary . Muller, F. Max, Rig-Veda-Samhita, the Sacred Hymns of the Brhmans together with the Commentary of Sayanacharya, 4 volumes (Varanasi: Krishnada Academy, 1983. https://www.peterffreund.com/Dissertation/Freund_Dissertation_Vedic_Library.pdf

5. Griffith, Ralph TH, The Hymns of the Rigveda, translated with a popular Commentary, (Delhi: Motilal Banarsidass, 1973). https://www.peterffreund.com/Dissertation/Freund_Dissertation_Vedic_Library.pdf
6. Atharvaveda, edited by William Dwight Whitney (1905); Delhi: Motilal Banarsidass, https://www.scribd.com/document/660540859/
7. Maji L. (2021). Tuberculosis (Yakṣmā or Rājayakṣmā) in the Atharvaveda. In Atharvaveda and Charaka Samhita. [online[https://www.wisdomlib.org/hinduism/essay/atharvaveda-and-charaka-samhita/doc1210492.html [Last accessed September, 2025).
8. Samal J. Ayurvedic management of pulmonary tuberculosis: A systematic review. J Intercult Ethnopharmacol. 2015;5(1):86-91.
9. Mohan A, Sharma SK. History. In Tuberculosis (2nd Ed). Jaypee Brothers Medical Publishers, New Delhi, 2009: pp 7-15.
10. Robbins Schug G, Blevins KE, Cox B, Gray K, Mushrif-Tripathy V. Infection, disease, and biosocial processes at the end of the Indus Civilization. PLoS One. 2013;8(12):e84814.
11. Meulenbeld GJ. A history of Indian medical literature. Groningen Oriental studies. Groningen: Egbert Forsten; 1999.
12. Prasad PV. General medicine in Atharvaveda with special reference to Yaksma (consumption/tuberculosis). Bull Indian Inst Hist Med Hyderabad. 2002;32(1):1-14.
13. Barberis I, Bragazzi NL, Galluzzo L, Martini M. The history of tuberculosis: from the first historical records to the isolation of Koch's bacillus. J Prev Med Hyg. 2017;58(1):E9-E12.
14. Aufderheide AC, Rodríguez-Martín C, Langsjoen O. The Cambridge encyclopedia of human paleopathology. Cambridge, UK: Cambridge University Press; 1998. pp. 126-7.
15. Riccardi N, Canetti D, Martini M, Diaw MM, DI Biagio A, Codecasa L, et al. The evolution of a neglected disease: tuberculosis discoveries in the centuries. J Prev Med Hyg. 2020;61(1 Suppl 1): E9-E12.
16. Cambau E, Drancourt M. Steps towards the discovery of *Mycobacterium tuberculosis* by Robert Koch, 1882. Clin Microbiol Infect. 2014;20(3):196-201.
17. World Health Organization. A brief history of tuberculosis control in India. Geneva: World Health Organization; 2010.
18. Radhakrishna S. Tuberculosis chemotherapy centre–The beginning. Indian J Tuberculosis. 2020;67:S3-S6.
19. Murray JF, Schraufnagel DE, Hopewell PC. Treatment of Tuberculosis. A Historical Perspective. Ann Am Thorac Soc. 2015;12(12):1749-59.
20. Mahadev B, Kumar P. History of tuberculosis control in India. J Indian Med Assoc. 2003;101(3): 142-3.
21. Fifteen year follow up of trial of BCG vaccines in south India for tuberculosis prevention. Tuberculosis Research Centre (ICMR), Chennai. Indian J Med Res. 1999;110:56-69.
22. National Tuberculosis Elimination Programme. (2024). TB India Report 2024. [online] Available from https://tbcindia.mohfw.gov.in/2024/10/11/india-tb-report-2024/ [Last accessed September, 2025].
23. National Tuberculosis Elimination Programme, Central Tuberculosis Division. (2025). Home. [online] Available from https://tbcindia.mohfw.gov.in [Last accessed September, 2025].
24. NTEP. (2025). Evolution of TB-Elimination Program in India. [online] Avaiable from https://ntep.in/node/116/CP-evolution-tb-elimination-programme-india [Last accessed September, 2025].
25. Frith J. History of Tuberculosis. Part 2 - the Sanatoria and the Discoveries of the Tubercle Bacillus. J Milit Veteran Health. 2014;22(2).

CHAPTER

9

Bronchial Asthma and Allergy

Bronchial asthma affects people of all ages but is more common in children and young adults. Although primarily an allergic disorder, non-allergic asthma is almost equally common. Allergic diseases are caused by a complex interplay of genetic and environmental factors. Allergies and airway diseases like asthma together can be considered as "*the epidemic of the twenty-first century*." In the first half of the 20th century, asthma was known as one of the "holy seven" psychosomatic illnesses. The burden caused by these non-communicable diseases is rather enormous all over the world and is responsible for a huge drain of economic resources in spite of several treatment options which have now become available. While asthma has a long history dating back to over 5,000 years, the evidence for the presence of allergies in the ancient times is scarce.

History of Allergy

There is only meagre evidence to trace the history of allergy to ancient times although there is some mention of suggestive symptoms in the ancient texts of the Egyptian, Chinese, and Greco-Roman civilizations. A Pharaoh, King Menses of Egypt, was reported to have died after a wasp sting which could be attributed possibly due to an anaphylactic shock. Another ancient report of allergy from Europe is that of Brittanicus, the son of the Roman Emperor Claudius who used to develop rashes on exposure to horses. In the medieval period, King Henry III of England was reported to develop acute urticaria when he ate some strawberries. He reportedly blamed Lord William Hastings who had met him before that event and ordered his beheading for the curse.

The first convincing description of hay fever was in 1828 by John Bostock, who described his own symptoms. It was however in the 20th century when the term 'allergy' was first defined. This was also the time when it was postulated that asthma is also an allergic disease. After about a decade, Francis Rackemann described that asthma could be caused by both allergic and non-allergic factors.

Indian History of Allergy

Desensitization or immunotherapy now practised for treatment of allergies, can perhaps be traced to the concept of '*Vish-kanyas*' *(poison-girls)* mentioned in Chanakya's *Arthashastra,* associated with the Maurya Emperor, Chandragupta I. Some suggest that *Vish-kanyas*, used as assassins and spies, were given minute but increasing doses of poison from childhood, making them immune to toxins while allowing them to poison others. Similarly, native American Indians were known to chew poison ivy to prevent severe skin rash or anaphylaxis.

Both the *Charaka Samhita* and *Sushruta Samhita* described conditions similar to allergies, such as "*shvasa*" (breathing difficulties) and "*kasa*" (coughing) and the concept of "*virudha*" as a condition where the body reacts adversely to certain substances. *Atreya Punarvasu,* an ancient Indian physician, described a condition characterized by nasal congestion, sneezing, and runny nose. These symptoms are similar to those experienced by people with allergic rhinitis. *Vagbhata,* another ancient Indian physician, described a condition characterized by skin rashes, itching, and redness. These symptoms are similar to those experienced by people with skin allergies.

Unani medical texts, such as the "*Qanun*" by Ibn Sina described conditions similar to allergies, including skin rashes and respiratory issues. *Ayurvedic and Unani* doctors used *neem* and turmeric as herbal remedies to treat allergic conditions. Neem and turmeric respectively have been shown to possess anti-inflammatory properties anti-allergic properties. Later when the Western medical system got introduced to India with the arrival of the Europeans, concepts with reference to allergic disorders were similarly adopted. Later during the British rule, allergy was recognized as a separate medical condition in differential diagnosis of various diseases. Anti-allergic drugs and de-sensitization treatments also began to be used rather frequently in medical practice.

Allergy clinics were established in major Indian cities with recognition of allergy as an important cause of overall-all health care burden. Allergy also became a part of teaching curricula of for medical students of Respiratory medicine, Dermatology, Oto-rhino-laryngology and other medical specialities. Indian researchers have also contributed significantly to the understanding of allergies, and awareness campaigns have been launched to educate the public about allergy prevention and management.

History of Asthma

History of asthma has been excellently described by Mark Jackson in a fascinating book which explores asthma from ancient to modern times in a fascinating manner. He has also cited autobiographical commentaries from patients including Marcel Proust, the French author who was confined to his bedroom from ailments, chiefly asthma. Another celebrated example was that of the US President Theodore Roosevelt who used to suffer from recurring and terrifying night time asthma attacks during his youth.

Ancient History of Asthma

History of asthma dates back several millennia in the past. Asthma was mentioned differently in different languages in ancient literature such as the Egyptian, Indian, Chinese and Greco-Roman medical manuscripts of that period. Ebers Papyrus (1550 BC) of ancient Egypt refers probably to asthma which was treated by clysters (enemas), animal excreta and herbs. The early Chinese writing Neu Ching of the third millenium BCE mentioned the plant Ma Huang which is used to extract asthma drug (ephedrine) in modern times. The disease was considered to be caused by an imbalance of *yin and yang* principles. Acupuncture and moxibustion were recommended for treatment. The Japanese also used these methods in their *kampo* system of medicine.

The term 'asthma' is derived from the Greek word '*aazein*' which implies exhaling through an open mouth. It was first used by Homer in his classic the *Iliad* for panting or distressed breathing. It was in the 1st- 2nd century CE when Aretaeus of Cappadocia mentioned asthma as a disease rather than merely a symptom. He provided one of the more clear description of asthma in ancient times.

Indian History of Asthma

Asthma was referred to as '*Tamaka Swasa*' in Sanskrit in ancient Vedic scripts (*Rigveda* and *Atharvaveda*). *Rigveda* describes *Tamaka Swasa* as an ailment characterized by difficulty breathing, wheezing, and coughing while

Atharvaveda called the same as *Swasa Roga* with symptoms like wheezing, coughing, and difficulty breathing—'*Tamaka*' is translated as 'wheezing' and '*Swasa*' as 'breathing'. Detailed descriptions of clinical symptoms, causes, and treatments which were commonly prescribed were also included. In later period, the same expressions were used in the original *Ayurvedic* manuscripts (*Charaka Samhita and Sushruta Samhita*) and other texts for further definitions and descriptive understanding. Later texts such as '*Ashtanga Hridayam*' which also describes asthma as "*Tamaka Shvasa*" provides information on its diagnosis, prognosis, and treatment. The concept of "*Pratishyaya,*" also refers to the same- a respiratory disorder with symptoms like wheezing, coughing, and difficulty breathing.

तमकश्वासो नाम वातपित्तप्रकोपजः (*Charaka Samhita, Chikitsasthana,* 17.3)

(*Tamaka Swasa* is a disease caused by the aggravation of *Vata* and *Pitta doshas*)

श्वासकासं च वै पिपासां चैव हिक्कां च (*Charaka Samhita, Chikitsasthana,* 17.4)

(Symptoms of *Tamaka Swasa* include difficulty breathing, coughing, thirst, and hiccups)

श्वासरोगः कफपित्तप्रकोपजः (*Sushruta Samhita, Nidanasthana,* 6.3)

(*Swasa Roga* is a disease caused by the aggravation of *Kapha and Pitta doshas*).

श्वासकासं च वै पिपासां चैव हिक्कां च (*Sushruta Samhita, Nidanasthana,* 6.4)

(Symptoms of *Swasa Roga* include difficulty breathing, coughing, thirst, and hiccups)

तमकश्वासो नाम वातपित्तप्रकोपजः (*Ashtanga Hridayam, Chikitsasthana,* 12.3)

(*Tamaka Swasa"* is a disease caused by the aggravation of *Vata* and *Pitta doshas).*

श्वासकासं च वै पिपासां चैव हिक्कां च (*Ashtanga Hridayam, Chikitsasthana,* 12.4)

(Symptoms of *Tamaka Swasa* include difficult breathing, coughing, thirst, and hiccups)

The disease was believed to be caused by an imbalance of the three *doshas or humors (Vata, Pitta, Kapha)* similar to what was also believed in ancient Greek medicine. Traditional treatment methods primarily focussed on herbal remedies, *Yoga* and breathing exercises (like *Pranayama*). Herbs like Turmeric, Ginger, and *Ashwagandha* were used both orally and as herbal *vapours*. Patients were advised to follow a balanced diet and avoid excessive physical activity. *Panchakarma,* a detoxification procedure to remove toxins from the body was also employed.

The same beliefs and treatments continued during the Mauryan Era in India. Archaeological evidence in form of inscriptions on Mauryan-era monuments, such as the Ashokan Pillars, provides evidence of the existence of asthma during this period. Ancient Ayurvedic manuscripts, such as the *Charaka Samhita and Sushruta Samhita* of the Vedic age continued to provide valuable insights into the understanding and treatment of asthma during the Mauryan era. There were remarkable similarities of concepts about the cause of asthma, diagnosis and treatment with Greco-roman and Egyptian beliefs.

Post-Mauryan Era

There were significant anecdotal developments related to asthma in the contemporary Arabia and Europe during this period. Avicenna of Arabia recommended alchemy and astrology in his medical practice although some physicians continued to adhere to Hippocratic concepts. The Jewish theologian and philosopher, Moses Maimonides wrote his Treatise on asthma which was the first work composed specifically on the subject, in the 12th century. Maimonides had fled to Egypt for fear of persecution in Spain and was appointed as the physician to Almalik Alafdal, the asthmatic son of Sultan Saladin. Although his advice helped the Prince, his theories on asthma were rather orthodox. Later during the period of European Renaissance, a ***Swiss physician, who changed his name from v***on Hohenheim

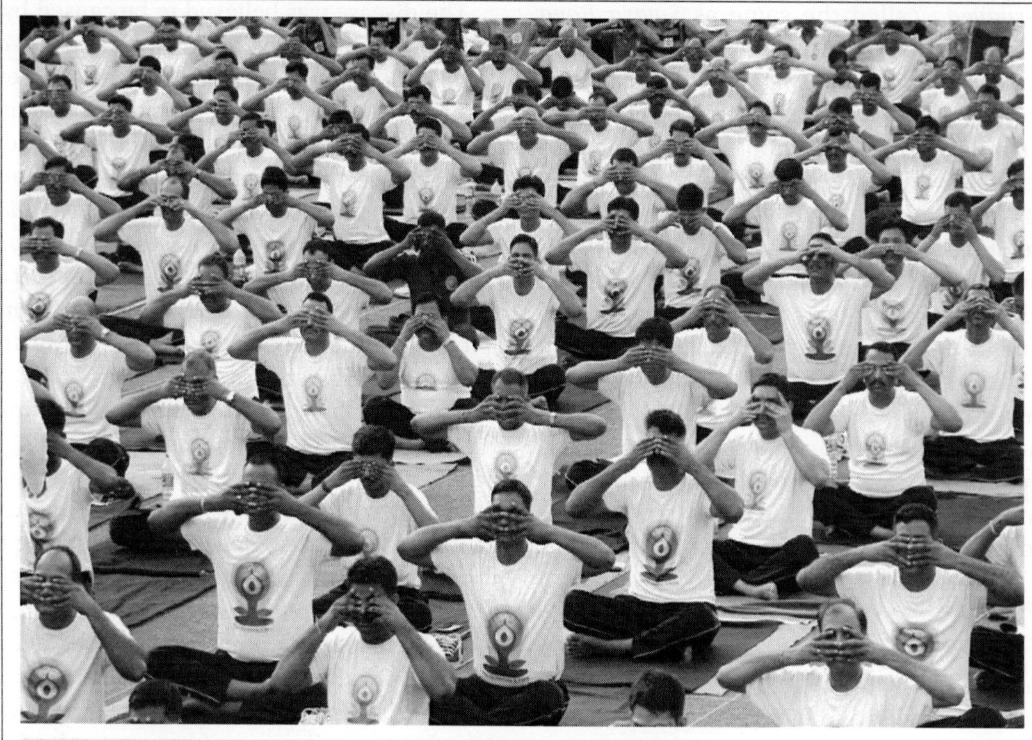

Yoga—Pranayama practice in a group for healthy lungs and body.

to Paracelsus, ('equal to Celsus') rejected earlier theories pronounced by Galen, Celsus and others that health and disease were controlled by the four humours, as redundant. In a symbolic gesture, he burned the old works of Galen and Avicenna and told students and colleagues to study nature and develop personal experience through experiment.

In India, during the post-Mauryan period up to about 500 CE, asthma continued to be described in various Ayurvedic medical texts of that time. Post-Mauryan monuments, such as the Satavahana-era inscriptions, provide evidence of the existence of asthma during this period. *'Ashtanga Hridayam'* written by *Vagbhata* in around 7th century CE described asthma as *'Tamaka Shvasa'* while *'Kashyapa Samhita'* attributed to Kashyapa, described asthma as *'Shvasa Roga'*. Both the texts provided detailed descriptions of its symptoms and treatment. Medical physicians continued to be influenced by Ayurvedic principles, including the concept of the three *doshas* (*Vata, Pitta, Kapha*) and their importance in the balance and harmony in the body. Treatments were prescribed with use of herbal remedies.

Medieval and Mughal India

There was no major development during medieval India (500 CE–1500 CE) but for the introduction of additional Unani system of medicine which originated in Greece. There is archaeological evidence in form of inscriptions found on medieval Indian monuments of the Delhi Sultanate-era and the Mughal-era monuments, such as the Taj Mahal. Some of these inscriptions provide evidence of the existence of a respiratory disease like asthma during that period. The Taj Mahal inscription written by Amir Khusro, the court-poet of Mughal Emperor Shah Jahan mentions the emperor's struggles. The main inscription on the gate reads: *O soul, you are at rest. Return to the Lord in peace with him, and he at peace with you.*

His autobiography Shahjahan Nama also mentions that he suffered from a severe respiratory illness, "dyspnea" or "breathlessness", which could be either asthma or 'chronic obstructive pulmonary disease'.

Asthma continued to be described in various Ayurvedic and Unani medical texts. Ayurvedic texts such as *Bhavaprakasha* written by *Bhavamishra* and *'Madhava Nidanam'* by Madhava respectively described asthma as *'Tamaka Shvasa'* and *'Shvasa Roga'*. The texts also provided detailed descriptions of symptoms, diagnosis and treatment. Unani texts which were new additions included *'Al-Qanun fi al-Tibb'* by *Ibn Sina* (Avicenna) and *'Kitab al-Manzari'* by *Ali ibn al-Abbas al-Majusi,* which described asthma as *'Rabw'* and provided detailed information on its symptoms, diagnosis, prognosis and treatment.

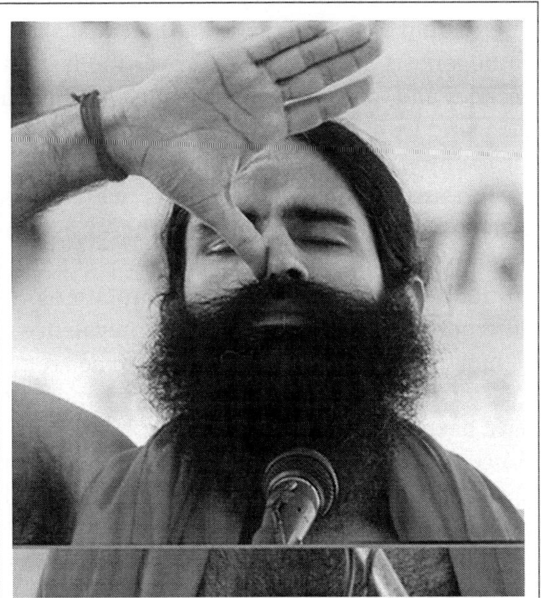

Yoga Guru, Ramdev demonstrating *'Patanjali'* yoga.

Asthma symptoms described during medieval India included difficulty breathing, wheezing, coughing, and chest tightness. Unani physicians also described asthma as "*Nazzla*" or "*Zeq-ul-Nafas*", emphasizing its respiratory symptoms. Various treatments for asthma were essentially the same herbal remedies, as well as dietary changes and yoga practices. In addition to herbal drug, Unani treatments also included modalities like bloodletting and purging which were not used earlier. During Mughal period, Hakim Ajmal Khan's text *'Tibb-e-Nabawi' and Al-Shifa by Hakim Muhammad Sharif Khan* described asthma as "*Rabw*" and provided detailed descriptions.

Impact of European Renaissance

Meanwhile contemporary developments in the European continent during fourteenth to seventeenth centuries, i.e., the Renaissance and after had greatly transformed Western concepts about asthma and provided a fresh impetus to medical thoughts in Europe. This was an indication of a break with the past. With reference to asthma, an Italian physician Savonarola provided a detailed description of asthma symptoms while Sydenham, an English physician, provided a comprehensive clinical description. Sydenham differentiated asthma from other diseases, such as tuberculosis and pneumonia.

Schneider in Germany and Richard Lower in England discarded the ancient Greek concept of catarrh having its origin in the brain. Lower also conducted experimental studies on asthma, including the use of animal models to study the disease and described the presence of bronchial constriction that occurs during an asthma attack. By the end of the seventeenth century, Sir John Floyer who himself an asthmatic, wrote a treatise of asthma which tended to differentiate the condition from other types of dyspnoea. That was the first monograph on the subject in the English language. He developed a method to measure lung function which helped to better understand asthma, and was also the first to appreciate the importance of the expiratory component of breathing. Floyer described asthma as a chronic disease, rather than an acute condition. Rene Laennec who invented the stethoscope in 1816 was also an asthmatic in addition to suffering from phthisis (tuberculosis). He described the importance of physical examination using the stethoscope for the nature and diagnosis of asthma.

These discoveries during the Renaissance laid the foundation for our modern understanding of asthma and its management. The ideas and developments slowly permeated the medical practice elsewhere in the world including in India. Arrival of Europeans and other foreigners which also included physicians who were sometime invited by the Royalty facilitated frequent exchange of ideas and expertise. There was a faster transmission and adoption of newer methods of diagnosis and treatments.

British Colonial Era

During the colonial British rule in India (1858 CE–1947 CE), asthma was described in various medical texts, including those written by British physicians and Indian practitioners of traditional medicine. British Administration showed greater interest in developing an overall health-system for multiple purposes. It vigorously promoted the establishment of the European modern system of medical practice and established hospitals for management of diseases even though the facilities were rather limited for the general populace. The British also established medical institutions such as the Calcutta Medical College, to train Indian physicians in Western system of medicine as well as promoted the dissemination through different medical publications such as the Indian Medical Gazette by the British Medical Association.

Medical records from colonial-era hospitals and dispensaries provide evidence of the significant existence of asthma during this period. Similarly, advertisements for asthma medications, such as inhalers and powders, provide evidence of the availability of Western medical treatments. Journals like the Indian Medical Gazette and Transactions of the Medical and Physical Society of Bombay contained articles on asthma, including its symptoms, diagnosis, and treatment. This period saw the introduction of Western medical treatments like use of opium and belladonna, and the use of inhalers and other medications.

Post-Independence India

Asthma continued to remain a significant public health concern. Its prevalence continued to increase and involve people from all sections of population including the rich, the politicians, the elite and the celebrities. Many eminent sports persons, artists and writers continue to suffer from the illness. But the suffering and distress caused by asthma have significantly diminished because of the availability of newer treatments.. The global concepts about its causes and pathogenesis greatly changed over the last few decades and new discoveries made anywhere in the world were adopted within a short period in the country.

Indian medical researchers were more actively engaged in understanding of asthma and undertook studies on causes, genetics, epidemiology, and treatment outcomes. In different epidemiological studies, prevalence of asthma in India has been estimated to be around 2–5% of the population. Rates of asthma mortality have been declining over the years, but remain a concern. Most of the current forms of treatments have become widely available and are commonly used to treat asthma.

Pulmonary medical services have expanded in India, with many hospitals and clinics offering specialized care for asthma patients. There are some important challenges which continue to concern the overall health sector. There is a continued need to increase awareness and education about asthma among the general public, healthcare providers, and policymakers. Several populations particularly in rural, hilly and remote areas lack access to healthcare services, including asthma care. Air pollution is a significant concern in India, and efforts are needed to reduce exposure to pollutants that can exacerbate asthma. While the National Health Mission has been working to strengthen healthcare services the Indian government has also implemented various measures to control air pollution, including the National Clean Air Programme.

Asthma Management

In the past, bizarre treatments such as animal excrement, especially the dung of stallions and *Lohoch e Pulmone Vulpis* (linctus of fox's lung) were also recommended as popular therapies. Astrology was also employed sometimes with a strong belief that: *'A physician without astrology is like a lamp without oil.'* Some other recommendations included 'sleeping on a chair for nocturnal asthma which was attributed to 'the heat of the bed'. Use of antispasmodics such as spirit of hart shorn, sedatives, powder of shells, millipedes, heavy waters, spirit and volatile salts were sometimes prescribed.

Some of these therapies remain popular in certain sections even now. In Hyderabad in India, the Bathini Goud family administers a "miracle" remedy called "*fish prasadam*" (a live fish, with a herbal paste) which is believed to cure asthma. This is inserted directly into the mouth of a patient to swallow on a particular day. Annually, there are huge crowds on that day in spite of the lack of any proven evidence.

In medical parlance, episodic airways-obstruction was thought to occur due to contraction of the airway-smooth muscles (or bronchospasm) in response to an allergic response. The concept had prevailed for almost around a century. Therefore, bronchodilators and expectorants were most commonly used for treatment which was the practice since ancient times when herbs such as '*dhatura*' and '*ephedra*' used for relief of cough and breathlessness contained bronchodilator ingredients. *Dhatura* was used in multiple ways- leaves were smoked or made into tea; seeds were powdered and mixed with honey while the root decoction was used for bronchitis and asthma.

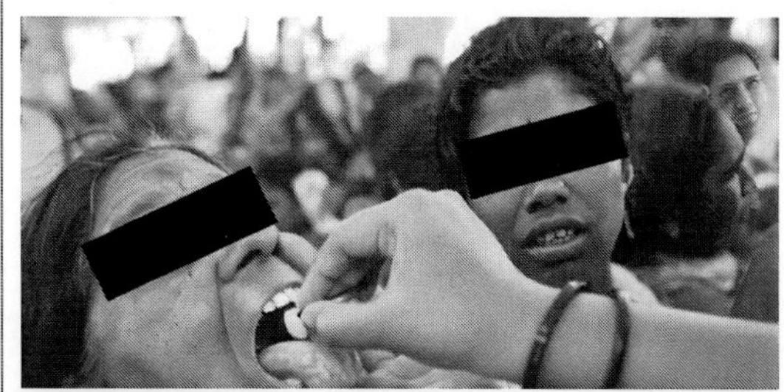

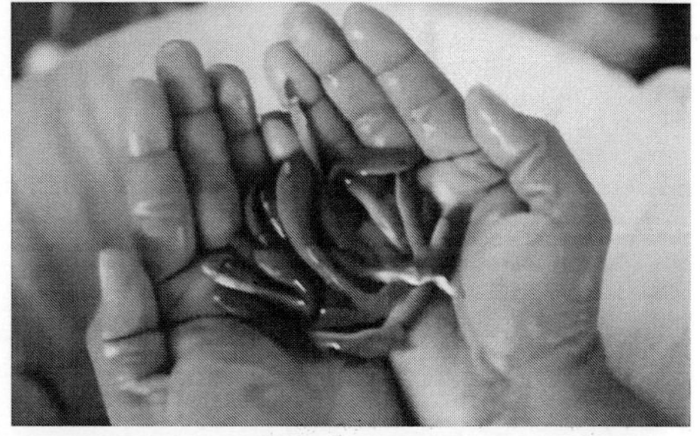

"Fish prasadam" (a live fish, with a herbal paste) being administered directly into the mouth of a patient of asthma in Hyderabad, India
Courtesy: Dr Vikram Jaggi, New Delhi.

There was introduction of new herbal remedies such as the dried root of the Brazilian shrub *ipecacuanha* following the discovery of America by Christopher Columbus in the 15th century. Tobacco was also used for its medicinal properties for respiratory ailments. It was only around the 19th century that bronchodilator drugs (atropine and ephedrine compounds) were identified from these herbs. *Dhatura* contained key alkaloids such as scopolamine (with antispasmodic and

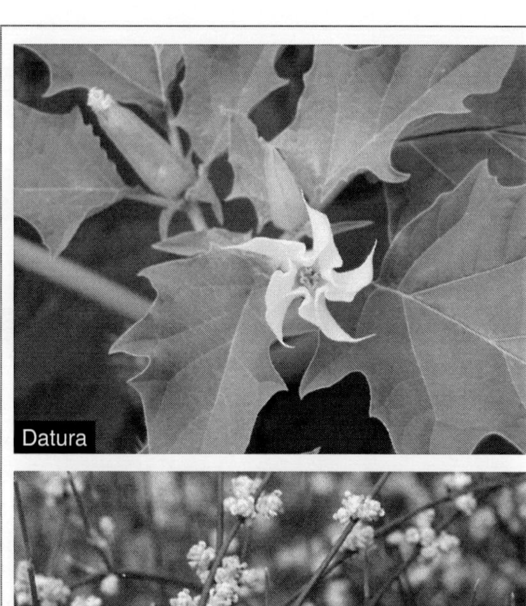

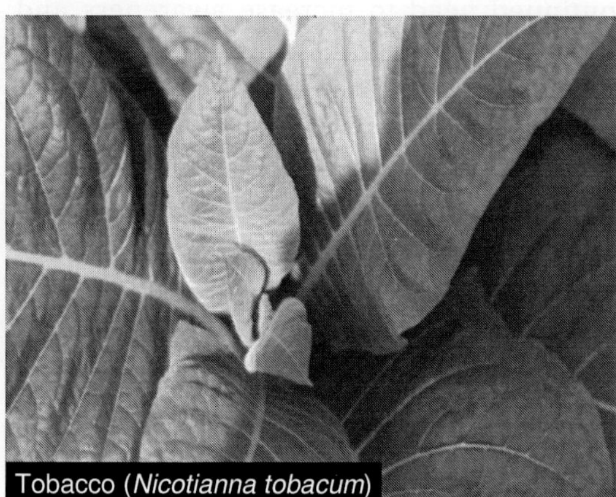

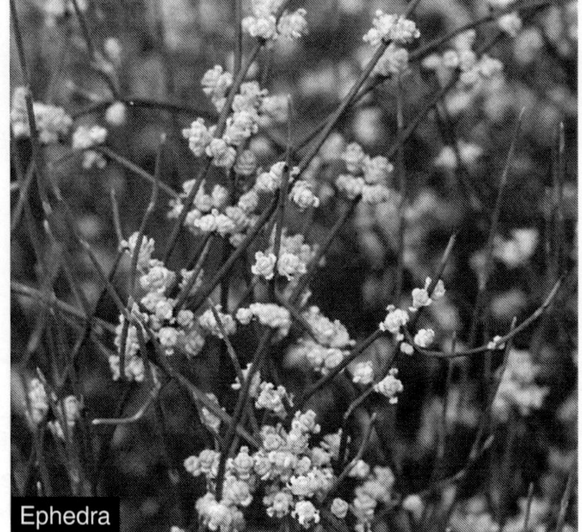

Herbs which were commonly used for management of cough and phlegm; *Datura* and *ephedra* constitute the natural sources of modern day bronchodilators (anticholinergic alkaloid atropine and sympathomimetic ephedrine respectively). Tobacco leaves are used in various forms by smokers to induce cough and expectorate.

antitussive properties) and hyoscyamine (with anticholinergic and bronchodilatory effects). While intravenous pilocarpine was tried in the late 19th century, epinephrine was first used for treatment of asthma in 1905. Therapy with bronchodilator drugs constituted the main-stay of treatment of asthma till the 1980s and 1990s.

Towards the end of the 20th century, it was established through different studies that airway inflammation following stimulation by different triggers such as inhalation of an allergen was the primary pathological mechanism of asthma. Respiratory tract infection, exercise, cold air and other stresses also precipitate the complex inflammatory cascade which causes airway-narrowing and air-flow obstruction responsible for clinical symptoms and signs of asthma. Recognition of airway-inflammation was the game-changer for management of asthma. The focus of treatment changed from oral bronchodilators to the inhaled bronchodilators and anti-inflammatory agents. While oral corticosteroids for asthma were first used in 1950, the management strategies were completely revamped with introduction of inhaled corticosteroids and selective short acting beta agonist in the 1960s. Today, the inhaled modality remains the most effective and widely available form of therapy.

Inhalation Therapy

Inhalation of vapors of different intoxicants and medicinal herbs has a long history in respiratory medicine. As per the ancient Hindu epic, Ramayana, it was the inhalation of the miraculous herb *(Sanjeevni booti)* which revived *Lakshmana,* the brother of *Lord Rama,* after he fell unconscious in the war. In Greek mythology, the priestess *Pythia* of the Temple of Apollo at Delphi would inhale the vapors from clefts in the slopes of Mount Parnassus where the temple was located. In a delirious state due to effects of those vapors, she used to deliver prophecies about the future.

Fumes of different herbs had been also used several centuries before the common era in India, China, Egypt and Greece. The Greek and Roman Physicians like Hippocrates and Galen used inhalation therapy to treat respiratory conditions. Indians used fumes of stramonium and hemp while the Egyptian produced vapours of black henbane by heating the weed on hot bricks. *Dhatura* continued to be smoked for its cough relieving properties practically throughout the past five millennia in most of the ancient cultures in the world.

In known medical history, inhalation of vapours of different herbal drugs produced by heating had been practised for respiratory ailments since the ancient times. In Ayurvedic tradition, both Sushrata and Charaka had recommended herbal vapours as *Dhupana*. In medieval era, the Unani medicine introduced Arabic inhalation technique, *Tariqat-al-Bukhār.* Inhalational administration of different drugs had become a more popular method for not only the treatment of cough and breathlessness but also for relief of anxiety, stress and pain. Inhalational route was also extensively employed for induction of anesthesia for different surgical treatments. Smoking of stramonium, a thorn-apple derivative was known for its relaxation properties. It was used for management of asthma, a practice which continued to be practiced by the British army in India during the early colonial era.

Inhalation treatment has made a steady progress in the last two hundred years or so. Several different kinds of inhalers varying from earthen and metal pots to the sophisticated form of metered dose devices had been developed and used. Technological advances of the modern era have made inhalation a popular and effective route for administration of drugs in medicine. For anesthesia, the initial inhalational anesthetic gases have been replaced with more efficient intravenous drugs. On the other hand, the treatment for respiratory diseases such as asthma and airways obstruction is now more effectively done with inhalational drugs.

The first inhaler was created in the late 18th century by John Mudge, an English physician and astronomer. The inhaler facilitated people with catarrh and mucus production to breathe opium vapour from a cylindrical metal cup with a handle. The initial metal cup laid the foundation for development of subsequent inhaler designs like different kinds of ceramic inhalers and atomizers. The journey to the modern design was long but continuous. Nebulizers were developed on the pattern of inhaling hot water vapours at spas which was a popular fashion in France. The first modern metered-dose inhaler (MDI) produced by Riker Laboratories (now 3 M Drug Delivery Systems) in 1956, can be considered as a milestone in the development of inhalation therapy of asthma.

Inhalers have come to occupy the centre-stage for asthma management in spite of the difficulties associated with their use. Inhalation route is also employed for other airway diseases and for administration of some antibiotics for respiratory infections. Inhalational devices now also include the Dry Powder Inhalers, nebulizers, soft-mist inhalers, breath-actuated inhalers and others. In India, the British Colonial Era saw the introduction of Western inhalation therapy. Cipla Ltd which had produced the bronchodilatory salbutamol tablets in 1976, also introduced the first salbutamol inhaler in 1978 in India. This was followed by the development of indigenous inhalation devices in 1980s with a large number of multi-national and Indian companies producing asthma inhalers in a highly competitive market.

Current and Future Scene

Asthma is a highly dynamic disease characterized with rapid and fast moving changes in concepts of causation and management strategies. Asthma is now considered as a systemic syndrome with different allergic and non-allergic phenotypic clusters defined by different inflammatory responses identified on the basis of biomarkers. The treatment trend also seems to be moving towards personalized therapy with biological agents (such as the mono-clonal antibodies) based on individual phenotype. This is rather a costlier form of treatment which very few in India afford for the present. Inhalational and other medical therapy therefore remains the most commonly available option.

In India, the disease burden due to asthma continues to be huge. Besides genetic factors, the presence of high levels of environmental air-pollution and smoke act as important triggers and risk factors for asthma, allergies and other airway diseases. Without a doubt, better treatments and control options are now widely available. In the near future, it is likely to persist as a chronic disease but possibly with diminished morbidity and mortality.

Sources

1. KC Bergmann . History of Allergy; Karger AG. 2014. https://doi.org/10.1159/isbn.
2. Platts-Mills TA. The allergy epidemics: 1870-2010. J Allergy Clin Immunol. 2015;136(1):3-13.
3. Sharma PV. Charaka Samhita Text With English Tanslation. digitallibraryindia; JaiGyan. https://archive.org
4. Patel V, Patel M, Desai V. Asthma Therapy in Ayurveda: An Ancient Scientific Approach. 2013; 1:57.
5. Singhal GD, Tripathi SN, Sharma KR. Madhava-Nidhan (Rogaviniscaya) Ayurveda Clinical Diagnosis. https://www.exoticindiaart.com/
6. Murthy KRS. Vagbhatta Astanga Hrdayam Vol. 1. Chowkhamba Krishnadas Academy, Varanasi; 2019. https://www.amazon.in/Vagbhatta-Astanga-Hrdayam-Vol-1-Srikanth/dp/B08SHCNP3T
7. Tiwari RV. Kasyapa Samhita (English). Chaukhamba Bharati Academi, Varanasi. 2013. https://www.chaukhambabooks.co.in/product/Kasyapa-Samhita-English-aXLBt
8. Kulkarni PH. Bronchial Asthma Care in Ayurveda and Holistic Systems (Indian medical science series). 2001. https://www.amazon.in/Bronchial-Ayurveda-Holistic-Systems-medical/dp/8170307139/
9. Singhal GD, Shukla, Sharma KR, Mitra J. Susruta Samhita (Ancient Indian Surgery). Chaukhamba Sanskrit Pratishthan. 2015; 1-3 https://www.exoticindiaart.com/
10. Murthy KRS. Bhavaprakasa of Bhavamisra (Two Volumes), Chowkhamba Krishnadas Academy, Varanasi. 2019. https://www.exoticindiaart.com/book/
11. Panda AK, Doddanagali SR. Clinical efficacy of herbal Padmapatradi yoga in bronchial asthma (Tamaka Swasa). J Ayurveda Integr Med. 2011;2(2):85-90.
12. Ayurveda for Bronchial Asthma. https://health.vikaspedia.in/viewcontent/health/ayush/ayurveda-1/ayurveda-for-common-disease-conditions/ayurveda-for-bronchial-asthma?
13. Masic I. Thousand-year anniversary of the historical book: "Kitab al-Qanun fit-Tibb"- The Canon of Medicine, written by Abdullah ibn Sina. J Res Med Sci. 2012;17(11):993-1000.
14. Saunders C. (2021). From Romance to Vision: The Life of Breath in Medieval Literary Texts. In: Fuller D, Saunders C, Macnaughton J. (Eds) The Life of Breath in Literature, Culture and Medicine. Palgrave Studies in Literature, Science and Medicine. Palgrave Macmillan. Cham. https://doi.org/10.1007/978-3-030-74443-4_5

15. Cserháti E. The history of bronchial asthma from the ancient times till the Middle Ages. Acta Physica Hungarica A) Heavy Ion Physics.2004 91(3-4): 243-61.
16. Kapri A, Pant S, Gupta N, Paliwal S, Nain S. Asthma History, Current Situation, an Overview of Its Control History, Challenges, and Ongoing Management Programs: An Updated Review. Proc Natl Acad Sci India Sect B Biol Sci. 2022: 1-13.
17. Unani System of Medicine Ministry of Ayurveda, Yoga & Naturopathy, Unani, Siddha and Homoeopathy (AYUSH). Government of India. 2016, https://ccrum.res.in/writereaddata/
18. Reddy DVS. The Outline of the History of the Unani Medical Literature *Part-ll, 1970. Lippincott https://journals.lww.com › oaks.journals.
19. Kadam SD, Chavhan SA, Shinde, PN. Sapkal. Pharmacognostic Review on Datura. Res. J. Pharmacology & Pharmacodynamics. 2018;10(4): 171-8.
20. The Social History of Health and Medicine in Colonial India, Edited By Biswamoy Pati, Mark Harrison, 2011. Routledge. https://www.routledge.com/
21. Holgate ST. A brief history of asthma and its mechanisms to modern concepts of disease pathogenesis. Allergy Asthma Immunol Res. 2010;2(3):165-71.
22. Cserháti E. The history of bronchial asthma from the Renaissance till the beginning of the twentieth century. Acta Physiol Hung. 2005;92(2):181-92.
23. Arnold, David. The rise of western medicine in India. The Lancet. 1996;348:1075-78.
24. Jackson M. Asthma: The Biography (Biographies of Disease), Oxford: Oxford University Press, 2009. https://academic.oup.com/shm/article-abstract/24/3/859/1646066.
25. Patel HH. Asthma History. https://www.news-medical.net/health/Asthma-History.aspx
26. Sakula A. A History of Asthma. Journal of the Royal College of Physicians of London,1988;22:36 - 44. https://api.semanticscholar.org/CorpusID:30832025.
27. The History of Therapeutic Aerosols: A Chronological Review. National Institutes of Health (gov.) http://www.ncbi.nlm.nih.gov>articles>PMC5278812
28. Jindal SK, Aggarwal AN, Gupta D, Agarwal R et al. Indian study on epidemiology of asthma, respiratory symptoms and chronic bronchitis in adults (INSEARCH). Int J Tuberc Lung Dis. 2012;16(9):1270-7.
29. Jindal SK. Do we care asthma? Indian J Med Res. 2012;135(2):157-9.
30. Singh S, Salvi S, Mangal DK, Singh M et al. Prevalence, time trends and treatment practices of asthma in India: the Global Asthma Network study. ERJ Open Res. 2022;8(2):00528-2021.
31. Gupta BM, Bala Adarsh. Mapping of asthma research in India: A scientometric analysis of publications output during 1999-2008. Lung India. 2011;28(4):239-46.
32. Jindal SK. Bronchial asthma: the Indian scene. Current Opinion in Pulmonary Medicine. 2007; 13(1): 8-12.

CHAPTER 10

Tobacco Smoking and Respiratory Disease

Tobacco is an important cause of multiple respiratory and other diseases such as cancers, heart, cerebrovascular and obstructive lung diseases. These effects are attributed to a large number (over 4,000 in numbers) of chemical substances in tobacco, many of which are metabolically active and/or carcinogenic in nature with nicotine as the most addicting alkaloid. It is extensively consumed all over the world including in India. Tobacco products currently generate revenue of almost a trillion US dollars worldwide with China topping the list while the Indian revenue was estimated at about 13.3 billion US dollars in 2024. These staggering figures account for the financial compulsions and other difficulties associated with its control.

Tobacco is commonly produced from the fresh leaves of plants of genus *Nicotiana* which are dried and cured to allow the slow oxidation to produce some aromatic and habituating compounds. The tobacco, thus, obtained is mixed with other additives to make it more palatable and/or addicting before final packaging. Subsequently, tobacco is used in different forms both by inhalational and oral routes.

Tobacco Consumption in India

According to the Global Adult Tobacco Survey (GATS) 2016–2017, around 30% of adults in India use tobacco in some form. In terms of number of tobacco users, India is estimated as second globally and first in the South-East Asia Region. Smoking involves the practice of burning of tobacco in a cigarette, *bidi,* pipe, cigar, or cigarillo, and inhaling the resulting smoke. Smoking from a *hookah* or handheld *hookli* is also practiced in certain populations in India. *Chhutta* smoking is another peculiar form of smoking along the Eastern coasts of Orissa and Andhra Pradesh in which the burning end is kept inside the mouth *(Reverse smoking).* Tobacco is also used in several nonsmoking forms for chewing, snuffing, and eating in India and some other South-Eastern Asian countries.

History of Smoking

There is good archaeological evidence indicating that humans used tobacco in the Americas for over 10 millennia, 1,000s of years earlier than previously believed. Smoking history can be traced back to 5000–3000 BCE since when tobacco was grown as an agricultural product in ancient Mesopotamia and South America. Inhalation of tobacco smoke might have followed due to either incidental or accidental burning of the plant which subsequently was adopted as ritualistic and/or a pleasure habit. It got introduced in Europe in the late 17th century after Columbus traveled to South America. Soon thereafter, the trade in tobacco expanded between Europe and Americas. It was often adopted as a fashionable and sophisticated habit by the rich and the royalty. Also, it was used as a cure for coughs, cold, and pains as well as for management of asthma and tuberculosis.

The term *smoking* was used in the late 18th century and replaced the earlier description of the practice such as *drinking smoke*. Smoking was the most common method of consuming tobacco which remains the most common substance smoked. The agricultural product was often mixed with other additives before consumption. Tobacco smoking attracted criticism from various sections of the society, clergymen and religious leaders who considered the habit as immoral or outright blasphemous. In spite of severe opposition to tobacco use, it rapidly grew in most countries in Europe, USA, and Asia.

But, there were increasing concerns about harmful effects of smoking. In the early 19th century, German scientists identified a link between smoking and lung cancer. This led to a widespread antismoking campaign which got subdued during the world war period. Subsequently, British researchers demonstrated a clear relationship between smoking and cancer. New evidence continued to emerge from all over the world which linked smoking with several diseases which made it compelling for different countries to take political action against smoking.

Indian History of Smoking

Like other ancient civilizations, smoking in India has a long history that spans 1,000s of years. According to the texts, the use of smoking substances was popular for medicinal and recreational purposes in Ancient India (2000 BCE–500 CE). Cannabis smoking was first mentioned in the "Atharvaveda" of that period. Besides cannabis, various plants and medicinal concoctions were recommended to promote general health. Smoking of tobacco is not mentioned as such but other substances such as *Datura stramonium* (*Ganja) and Cannabis sativa* (*Bhang,* i.e., a preparation made from cannabis leaves and flowers) were smoked or consumed as a beverage for their psychoactive properties. Herbs like *Tulsi* (*Ocimum sanctum*; Holy basil), *ajwain* (carom seeds), and *dhatura* (jimsonweed) were smoked for their perceived medicinal properties. It was a common practice to use fumigation with burning of incense sticks *(dhupa), dhumrapana* (meaning "drinking smoke") and fire offerings *(homa)* to Gods for religious and medical purposes.

Medieval and Mughal India

In more recent history, tobacco is first mentioned in Indian texts in the *"Ain-i-Akbari"*, a Persian manuscript written by Abu'l-Fazl ibn Mubarak, which describes the use of tobacco in India during the Mughal Empire. It was introduced to India by the Portuguese in the 17th century during the reign of Jahangir, soon after it came to Europe. In India, it came to be referred as *Tamaku* (तामाकू) in Sanskrit and Hindi languages and as *Tamakhu* (तमाखु) in Urdu and Persian texts. Ayurvedic texts, such as the *"Bhavaprakasha"* and *"Rajnighantu"*, as well as the Unani texts, such as the *"Qanun"* by Ibn Sina, began to mention tobacco as a medicinal herb during the 17th century. Tobacco became an integral part of Indian culture, with hookah smoking becoming a symbol of luxury and sophistication.

In the following decades, tobacco became widely available in the coastal regions, as the Portuguese established trade routes. The use of tobacco for smoking in the "hookah" became more widespread as it began to be seen as a luxury and a status symbol. It quickly gained popularity among the Mughal nobility and upper classes. The *hookah*, a waterpipe used for smoking tobacco, became a popular pastime among the Mughal elite. *Hookah* smoking was often considered as a social activity, with friends and family gathering to smoke and converse.

Hookah Smoking

"Hookah" smoking, also known as *"hukka"* or waterpipe smoking is believed to have originated in India and Persia (modern-day Iran) in the 16th century. The word "hookah" is derived from the Persian word *"huqqa"*, which means *"waterpipe"*. It gained popularity in the Mughal Empire in India, where it was patronized by the Royal Court. Emperor Akbar was initially skeptical about tobacco, but eventually became curious about its properties, experimented with tobacco, and eventually adopted it as a habit, using it for medicinal and recreational purposes. Emperor Jahangir was known to have enjoyed tobacco smoking and even wrote about it in his memoirs.

Shah Jahan was a known tobacco-smoker. He had got elaborate and expensive hookahs made for his court. But, there was criticism from Islamic scholars who considered smoking as a sinful and unhealthy habit. Some Mughal physicians and scholars warned about the health risks associated with tobacco smoking. Emperor Aurangzeb, the son of Shah Jahan, was a critic of tobacco smoking and banned it in his court, citing Islamic principles and health concerns.

From India and Persia, hookah smoking spread to the Middle East, Turkey, and eventually Europe. The Ottoman Empire played a significant role in popularizing hookah smoking in the Middle East and Europe. Over time, the design of the hookah evolved, with various materials and shapes being used. The modern hookah, with its characteristic water chamber and hose, emerged in the 19th century. Today, hookah smoking remains a popular pastime in India, with various flavors and styles available. It was often used as a symbol of hospitality, relaxation, and social bonding especially in rural India.

Tobacco smoking was frequently depicted in Mughal art, including miniature paintings and decorative arts reflecting their cultural and social aspirations. Tobacco had become an integral part of Indian culture, with hookah smoking becoming a symbol of luxury and sophistication. However, it also raised health concerns and criticisms from some Islamic scholars. Akbar's physician, Hakim Humam is said to have warned him about the potential health risks associated with tobacco smoking. But, Akbar believed that tobacco had medicinal properties and could be used to treat diseases. He also enjoyed tobacco for recreational purposes, using it to relax and socialize.

British India: Introduction of Cigarettes

The British introduced cigarettes as the most popular tobacco product which was widely consumed in Europe in the late 19th century. The British East India Company commercialized tobacco production in India, leading to widespread cultivation and trade. Soon, tobacco became a major profitable industry in the country with big companies such as Imperial Tobacco Company of India and the Indian Tobacco Company entering the business of production and trading of tobacco products.

Tobacco cultivation rapidly expanded in various regions, including the Indo-Gangetic plain and the Deccan plateau. Besides cigarettes, pipes and *"hookah"*, people also started smoking tobacco in other forms such as *"bidis"*, *"chillum"*, *"chhutta"*, and *"hukkli"*. Nonsmoking forms such as chewing or snuffing crude tobacco or other different products became equally or even more popular among the women in some Northern and Western regions.

Quit Smoking
Why and How
Surinder K Jindal
Why did the issue of quitting arise?
• Recognition of health hazards – killing risks
• Economic burden
• Environmental risks
– Deforestation
– Loss of biodiversity
– Indoor pollution–ETS
• Fire hazards

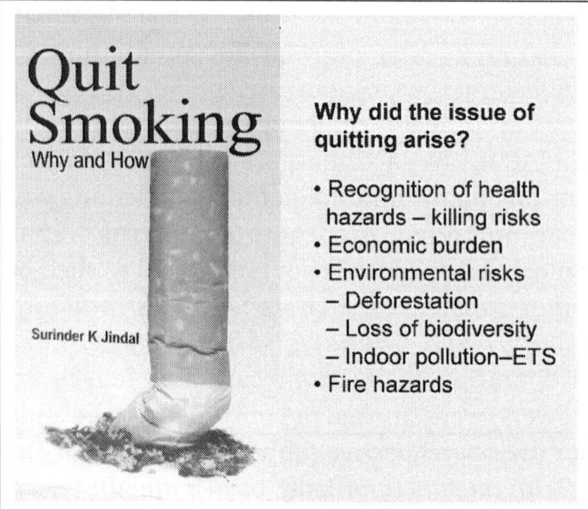

Bidi smoking, the indigenous product of cottage industry which involved handrolled tobacco leaves, became a popular and affordable alternative to cigarettes for the rural and urban poor. The word "*bidi*" is derived from the Sanskrit word *"vidi"* which means *"leaf".* Bidis are made from dried *tendu* leaves, which are wrapped around tobacco and secured with a thread. Today, *bidis* are widely used in India, with millions of people employed in the *bidi* manufacturing business.

Cigarette companies aggressively marketed and advertised their products, targeting the Indian elite and middle classes. Cigarettes became more widely available and smoking became increasingly popular among Indians, particularly among the urban population. Overall, smoking became a widespread habit in India during British rule, with the growth of the tobacco industry, popularization of cigarettes, and continued use of traditional forms of tobacco.

Post-Independence India

The trend continued in post-Independence India with an increase in tobacco-trade and growth of domestic tobacco companies such as ITC Limited and Godfrey Phillips India which expanded their operations and increased tobacco production. Tobacco companies also launched aggressive marketing campaigns to promote their products among the growing middle class to attract nonsmoking populations. Youth and women were specially targeted employing celebrities, sportspersons, and popular icons. Cigarette smoking had now become a symbol of status for men, bravery for the youth and of equality and freedom for women.

Electronic cigarette, also called a vaporizer, was promoted as an alternative to smoking traditional cigarettes. It consists of a device used to sublimate the active ingredients of plant material in a partial vacuum rather than burning the tobacco which produces potentially toxic substances. More recent literature, however, suggests that the vaporizer is equally addicting and harmful as are other forms of smoking.

Health Concerns

Tobacco has remained a popular personal and social habit for *centuries. But now* it tops the list of causes of death and disability. The last 50 years have seen some decline of smoking in the developed countries of the West which had continuously shown a rising graph in the preceding 500 years. But, there is rather an increasing trend in some of the developing countries. It is feared that the unsold tobacco products of the West are being dumped in these countries for commercial purposes and profits.

Smoking today is recognized as the single most significant factor responsible for a large number of noncommunicable diseases. It is also an important contributory factor for several infectious diseases including tuberculosis. The WHO Director General, Dr Gro Brundtland had summarized the adversities in his statement: *"A cigarette is the only consumer product which when used as directed kills its consumer."* Anne Edwards of Philip Morris, the major multinational tobacco company had even more explicitly expressed: *"What I think is clear is if someone came to us with a cigarette today and said, hey, here is a new product, I'm going to bring it to market. Would it be allowed in the market anywhere? No, it would not. It is a very harmful product" (Sex, Lies, and Cigarettes)".*

From time to time ever since the introduction of tobacco, there had been religious, social, and health concerns which were raised in Europe as well as in India. There was no firm or proven scientific evidence in favor of the harmful effects of tobacco. In the first quarter of the 20th century, almost 300 years after its introduction, the antismoking groups in Germany first published an advocacy against the consumption of tobacco in the journal *Der Tabakgegner* (The Tobacco Opponent). A paper on statistical evidence linking smoking with lung cancer was also published by Fritz Lickint and the German dictator, Adolf Hitler termed his earlier smoking habit as a waste of money. Germans also viewed women who smoked as not fit as wives or mothers. But, the end of World War II saw the end of antismoking initiatives in Germany with the entry of American cigarette manufacturers, illegal smuggling of tobacco as well as shipment of free tobacco to Germany.

Lung Cancer

Ancient texts of most civilizations do not specifically mention lung cancer, although there is occasional description of lung conditions that may have included symptoms related to lung cancer. The understanding and diagnosis of lung cancer as we know it today did not exist in the ancient world. The first case can be attributed to the Italian physician Giovanni Battista Morgagni who in 1761 described a patient of lung cancer. In 1800s, pathologists like Matthew Baillie and Samuel Soemmering studied lung cancer cases on autopsies providing more insight into the disease. The link of smoking with lung cancer was finally proven in the British Doctors Study by Richard Doll in England while the United States Surgeon General Report suggested the same relationship. With mounting evidence, the four largest US tobacco companies and the attorneys general of 46 states entered into a *Master Settlement Agreement* for their contributory negligence, restricted certain types of tobacco advertisement and made huge payments for health compensation.

Simultaneously, there appeared many social campaigns to discourage smoking in different countries. Since then, smoking in the United States and most Western countries has significantly declined to almost half or less. Advances in diagnostic imaging, radiation, chemotherapeutic drugs, and immunotherapy have now tremendously improved the diagnosis, staging, and management of lung cancer.

Cancer is a general term for a large number of different diseases with similar relentless progression leading to early death. Lung cancer in India is a leading cause of cancer-related deaths in India. Cancers of lung, blood, and brain caused by smoking have different rates of progression than cancers of mouth attributed largely to chewing of tobacco. Several studies from different parts of the country have pointed to a strong link of the problem with tobacco smoking of different kinds, including the *bidis* and the *hookah.* Exposure to secondhand smoke especially at home, is also a causative factor. Other risk factors include different occupational exposure and domestic indoor air pollution.

Undoubtedly, tobacco is the strongest cancer producing consumer product. Cancer Registry Reports from India have clearly shown a significant relationship of cancers with both cigarettes and *bidis*. A 2008 Report "*Bidi Smoking and Public Health*" published by the Ministry of Health and Family welfare, Government of India had summarized the Indian evidence linking *bidi* smoking with cancers.

Tobacco-use in India

I. Tobacco smoking

Bidis	Cigarettes
Cigars	Cheroots
Chutta (Reverse)	Dhumti
Hookahs and Hukklis	Pipe and Chillums

II. Nonsmoking tobacco consumption

(Oral use and applications)

Gudhaku (Paste)	Creamy snuff
Tobacco water (Tuibur and Hidakphu)	
Paan masaala	
Mainpuri	Mawa
Khaini	
Snus, mishri, gul, bajjar, and betel quid	

Noncancer Diseases

Tobacco is also responsible for a large number of noncancer diseases of which respiratory problems are described for several centuries. Chronic obstructive pulmonary disease which includes conditions such as chronic bronchitis and emphysema is the most important and disabling condition associated with smoking.

Chronic obstructive pulmonary disease: Although physicians like Thomas Sydenham and John Floyer had described lung diseases that were likely related to smoking, it was only by the 19th century that Samuel Green and Charles-Édouard Brown-Séquard recognized the harmful effects of tobacco on the lungs. It was in the late 1940 and 1950s after the end of World War II that chronic bronchitis and emphysema were linked with tobacco smoking. The relationship was more clearly demonstrated by Hammond in 1958. Around that time, COPD emerged as a collective term for chronic bronchitis and emphysema bearing a strong association with smoking. Strong evidence linking tobacco with smoking appeared from large-scale epidemiological studies like the Framingham Heart Study (1960s–1970s) and the Lung Health Study (1980s–1990s). Clinical and experimental studies further elucidated the mechanisms underlying the relationship between smoking and COPD, including inflammation, oxidative stress, and airway remodeling.

Throughout the 20th century, the evidence linking smoking to COPD has grown stronger, and our understanding of the pathophysiological mechanisms has deepened. Fletcher and Peto's pioneering work established the role of smoking in impaired lung function and the importance of smoking cessation. From 1964 onwards, the US Surgeon General's annual reports consistently highlighted the link between smoking and COPD. In 1984, the Surgeon General cited cigarette smoking as the major cause of COPD and other respiratory diseases. Smoking damages the lungs by causing diffuse changes to the lining of the airways, epithelium, and bronchioles. Cigarette smoke contains 1,000s of chemicals, including oxidants and free radicals, which can overwhelm the body's antioxidant defenses.

Chronic obstructive pulmonary disease is now recognized as a major public health burden, with smoking being the primary risk factor. Moreover, quitting smoking is considered the most effective way to prevent and manage the disease. Rates of smoking in the United States have significantly declined from 42 to 20.8%. Similar trend was observed in many other industrialized nations where smoking rates have either leveled-off or declined. In particular, the professional and affluent men have quit. It is also likely that those who continued to smoke started consuming lighter cigarettes. It is rather ironical that tobacco consumption continued to rise in the developing countries. Today, Russia leads as the top consumer of tobacco followed mostly by other Eastern countries.

Passive Smoking

Smoking also endangers the health of nonsmokers who live in the company of smokers. Exposure to secondhand smoke (Passive or sidestream smoking) can also increase the risk of COPD-associated mortality. Passive smoking has been shown to be directly related to cancers and other diseases. Such a relationship was first shown among nonsmoker wives of smokers from Japan. Studies from Greece and the United States have also demonstrated an increased risk of diseases such as lung cancer and angina pectoris among people who did not smoke themselves but got passively exposed to others' smoke. Such an exposure, often referred to as passive or secondhand smoking was common in India. Passive smoking was commonly observed in homes of smokers where nonsmoking women and children were exposed to their smoke. Evidence of an increased risk of COPD and lung cancer was also shown in some Indian studies.

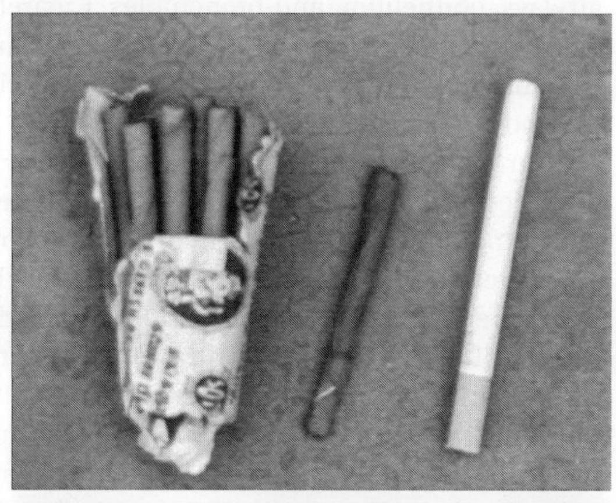

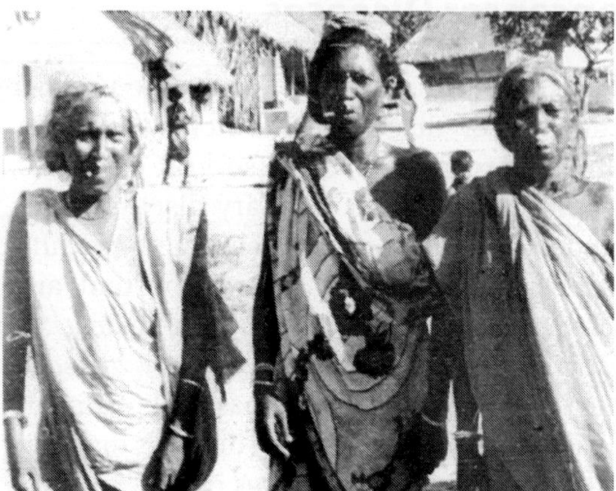

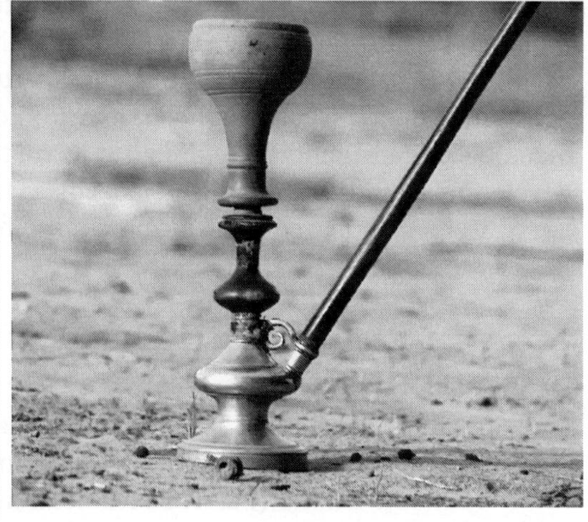

Some common smoking products in India—cigarettes, *bidis, hukkah*, and "*chhutta*". *Chhutta* (Reverse smoking with the lighted end inside the mouth) is restricted to the coastal regions of Eastern states of Andhra Pradesh and Orissa.

Bronchial asthma and other respiratory diseases: Although tobacco smoking is not directly responsible as a cause for these diseases, it is an important factor for promotion and aggravation of problems such as nonspecific cough, upper-respiratory catarrh, bronchial asthma, and interstitial and occupational lung diseases. Other medical and surgical disorders such as a majority of heart attacks, strokes, general ill health, atherosclerotic narrowing of vessels of the legs, eyes and other organs leading to serious disorders have been recognized in the last 200 years. In women of child-bearing age, tobacco is responsible for infertility, prematurity, and low birth weight of newborn babies, and abortions.

Tobacco Control in India

Tobacco use remained a significant public health concern in post-Independence India, with the growth of the tobacco industry, increased availability and marketing of tobacco products, and continued use of various forms of tobacco. Mahatma Gandhi, the Father of Indian Nation, was a vocal critic of smoking and tobacco use, viewing it as a corrupting influence on Indian society. After independence, the Indian government and health organizations have implemented various measures to control tobacco use and promote public health. In 1955, the Indian government nationalized the tobacco industry, leading to increased government control over tobacco production and trade.

The World Health Organization had initiated several measures for tobacco control programs and adoption of the Framework Convention on Tobacco Control (FCTC) at the World Health Assembly. India was one of the first few countries which had ratified the convention. Several important legislative measures have since been implemented to reduce tobacco consumption in the country like taxation, advertising restrictions, and public awareness campaigns. As the health risks associated with smoking became more widely known, the Indian government strengthened its tobacco control efforts with the implementation of the Regulation of Production, Supply and Distribution Act, 1975.

Antitobacco campaigns and awareness programs were launched to educate the public about the health risks associated with tobacco use. Antismoking efforts received a major boost with the landmark judgment of the Supreme Court of India in 2001 in a lawsuit, Murli S Deora vs. Union of India and Ors. The Court recognized the harmful effects of smoking in public places on nonsmokers in the indoor public places such as the auditoria, cinema halls, hospitals, and educational institutions. This type of exposure was also common even in the indoor microenvironments during travel in the public transport buses and the railways.

There was no statutory provision at that time to prohibit smoking in public places. The Court observed:

"Tobacco is universally regarded as one of the major public health hazards and is responsible directly or indirectly for an estimated eight lakh deaths annually in the country. It has also been found that treatment of tobacco-related diseases and the loss of productivity caused therein cost the country almost Rs. 13,500 crores annually, which more than offsets all the benefits accruing in the form of revenue and employment generated by tobacco industry".

(Supreme Court of India, Murli S Deora vs. Union of India And Ors on 2nd November, 2001)

Thereafter, smoking in public places was prohibited nationwide from 22nd October, 2002. There was a growing awareness of health risks associated with tobacco. As the public awareness increased, antitobacco campaigns also became stronger and started gaining popularity. India enacted the cigarettes and Other Tobacco Products (Prohibition of Advertisement and Regulation of Trade and Commerce, Production, Supply and Distribution) Act, 2003, which banned tobacco advertising and promotion. A warning against smoking was also required to be displayed on the screen in all smoking scenes of a movie. Another major initiative, National Tobacco Control Program (NTCP) was launched in 2007–2008. The government introduced graphic health warnings on tobacco product packaging in 2009.

The NTCP primarily aimed to reduce tobacco use and promote tobacco control measures. The "Program" was scaled up in the 12th 5-Year Plan with a goal to reduce the prevalence of tobacco use by 5% by the end of the 12th Plan. The primary objectives of NTCP were to: (1) create awareness about the harmful effects of tobacco consumption, (2) reduce the production and supply of tobacco products, (3) ensure effective implementation of the provisions under "The Cigarettes and Other Tobacco Products (Prohibition of Advertisement and Regulation of Trade and Commerce, Production, Supply and Distribution) Act, 2003" (COTPA); (4) help the people to quit tobacco use, and (5) facilitate implementation of strategies for prevention and control of tobacco advocated by WHO Framework Convention of Tobacco Control.

NTCP provisions included establishment of Tobacco Cessation Centers (TCCs) in district hospitals for free counseling and pharmacotherapy services. A toll-free number (*Quitline*) and mobile SMS service (*mCessation*) were started to provide counseling in all languages. Steps taken by the Indian Government under the "Program" have been fairly successful in overall implementation. It will, however, take longer time to evaluate the health impacts of various measures. A retrospective analysis aimed to quantify the implementation of MPOWER tobacco control policies in India has shown that the status is still far from the ideal situation and that there is considerable room for improvement.

Sources

1. Duke D, Wohlgemuth E, Adams KR, Armstrong-Ingram A, Rice SK, Young DC. Earliest evidence for human use of tobacco in Pleistocene Americas. Nat Hum Behav. 2021;6(2):183-92.
2. Rammanohar Puthiyedath. Smoking and Ayurvedic Medicine in India January 2004, In book: Smoke A Global History of Smoking. Publisher: Reaktion Books. Editors: Sander L Gilman, Zhou Xun Amrita Vishwa Vidyapeetham. https://www.researchgate.net/publication/215533875
3. Dey P. Culture of Tobacco Smoking in Mughal India: A Historical Analysis. Karatoya: NBU J Hist. 2013;6:20-4.
4. Mishra S, Mishra MB. Tobacco: Its historical, cultural, oral, and periodontal health association. J Int Soc Prev Community Dent. 2013;3(1):12-8.
5. United States. Public Health Service. Office of the Surgeon General. Center for Chronic Disease Prevention and Health Promotion (U.S.). Office on Smoking and Health Centers for Disease Control (U.S.). Reducing the Health Consequences of Smoking—25 years of Progress. A report of the Surgeon General: Executive Summary. USA: US Department of Health and Human Services; 1989.
6. Reddy KS, Gupta PC. Report on Tobacco Control in India. Government of India: Ministry of Health and Family Welfare; 2004.
7. The Health Consequences of Smoking. A Report of the Surgeon General, Department of Health and Human Services, USA. 2004.
8. Doll R, Peto R, Boreham J, Sutherland I. Mortality in relation to smoking: 50 years' observation on male British doctors. BMJ (Clin Res Ed.). 2004;328(7455):1519.
9. Doll R. Uncovering the effects of smoking: historical perspective. Stat Methods Med Res. 1998;7(2):87-117.
10. Rani M, Bonu S, Jha P, Nguyen SN, Jamjoum L. Tobacco use in India: prevalence and predictors of smoking and chewing in a national cross sectional household survey. Tobacco Control. 2003;12:e4.
11. Rapiti E, Jindal SK, Gupta D, Boffetta P. Passive smoking and lung cancer in Chandigarh, India. Lung Cancer. 1999;23:183-9.
12. Parikh PM, Ranade AA, Govind B, Ghadyalpatil N, Singh R, Bharath R, et al. Lung cancer in India: Current status and promising strategies. South Asian J Cancer. 2016;5(3):93-5.
13. Watson A, Pride NB. Early History of Chronic Obstructive Pulmonary Disease 1808–1980. COPD. 2016;13(2):262-73.
14. Verma A, Gudi N, Yadav UN, Roy MP, Mahmood A, Nagaraja R, et al. Prevalence of COPD among population above 30 years in India: A systematic review and meta-analysis. J Glob Health. 2021;11:04038.
15. Jindal SK, Aggarwal AN, Jindal A, Talwar D, Dhar R, Singh N, et al. COPD exacerbation rates are higher in non-smoker patients in India. Int J Tuberc Lung Dis. 2020;24(12):1272-8.
16. Jindal SK, Aggarwal AN, Chaudhry K, Chhabra SK, D'Souza GA, Gupta D, et al. A Multicentric Study on Epidemiology of Chronic Obstructive Pulmonary Disease and its Relationship with Tobacco Smoking and Environmental Tobacco Smoke Exposure. Indian J Chest Dis Allied Sci. 2006;48:23-9.
17. National Tobacco Control Programme (NTCP). (2017). National Health Mission. [online] Available from http://nhm.gov.in [Last accessed Sept., 2025].
18. Jindal SK, Gupta D, Singh A. Indices of morbidity and control of asthma in adult patients exposed to environmental tobacco smoke. Chest. 1994;106:746-9.
19. Jindal SK, Sapru RP, Aggarwal AN, Chaudhry K. Excess morbidity and expenditure on healthcare in families with smokers: A community study. Nat Med Jr India. 2005;18:123-6.
20. Malhi R, Gupta R, Basavaraj P, Singla A, Vashishtha V, Pandita V, et al. Tobacco Control in India: A Myth or Reality—Five Year Retrospective Analysis Using WHO MPOWER for Tobacco Control. J Clin Diagn Res. 2015;9(11):ZE06-9.
21. Jindal SK. Quit Smoking: Why and How? New Delhi: Vitasta Publications; 2008.

CHAPTER

11

Occupational Respiratory Diseases

The respiratory system bears the primary brunt of environmental dusts produced due to different occupational activities. There exists a wide spectrum of disorders caused due to environmental exposures, which extend from deposition of dust particles in the lungs to allergic manifestations, lung fibrosis, and carcinogenesis. The current burden of occupational respiratory disease in India is substantial. According to the Global Burden of Disease Study 2016, there were over half a million deaths from chronic respiratory disease due to occupational airborne risk factors. Around 4% of total deaths were attributable to exposure to pneumoconiotic dusts.

Occupational Lung Diseases

Pneumoconioses due to deposition of inhaled dusts in the lungs constitute the most serious form of occupational lung diseases of which silicosis is the prototype pneumoconiosis. Silica is present in abundance in the earth's crust, which is disturbed during heavy mining, tunneling, and foundry activities. Cumulative exposure to silica dust over the years results in silicosis. There are about 3 million workers exposed to silica dust in India, whilst 8.5 million more work in construction with similar exposures. Prevalence rates of silicosis range from about 5% to over 50% among miners. Similarly, *Anthracosis* occurs in coal miners and workers exposed to coal dusts in factories and foundries. Asbestosis is another important condition seen in workers engaged in asbestos mining, manufacturing, construction, and shipbuilding. The prevalence varies from 2.5 to 14.5% among asbestos-exposed workers. Asbestos exposure is important in the etiology of pulmonary fibrosis and respiratory cancers.

Hypersensitivity pneumonias as a result of recurrent exposure to organic and toxic dusts constitute another important group of occupational lung diseases. It includes diseases such as *byssinosis* in textile workers, *bagassosis* in workers engaged in sugar-cane processing, *farmer's lung,* and several others. A large number of hypersensitivity pneumonia are now recognized, which besides causing respiratory and systemic symptoms may frequently lead to lung fibrosis, chronic respiratory disability, and premature death.

Ancient History

The history of occupational respiratory diseases, primarily the pneumoconioses, is as long as the history of human labor. Since times immemorial, occupation and environment were recognized as an important factor in the causation of the respiratory symptoms of cough, phlegm, and breathlessness, although the definite relationship with specific diseases was described in only the modern period. Ancient medical texts of Egyptian, Greek, and Roman civilizations describe occupational diseases, including those affecting miners and stonecutters. Physicians like Hippocrates and Galen described occupational diseases, including lead poisoning and respiratory problems.

References to respiratory diseases caused by occupational exposures to dust, smoke, and other pollutants are also found in ancient Ayurvedic texts.

These ancient texts demonstrate a clear understanding of the relationship between occupational exposure and respiratory diseases, highlighting the importance of preventive measures and treatment. Ancient Indians were skilled miners and metalworkers. Ancient Indian civilization is known for its sophisticated mining and metallurgy techniques. Workers in these industries likely suffered from respiratory diseases caused by inhaling dust and fumes.

Dust inhalation was also associated with *Kshaya* (tuberculosis) described as a wasting or consumption of the body.

Inhalation of dust and other pollutants was related to *Tamaka Shwasa* (like asthma), characterized by coughing, difficulty breathing, and chest pain in *Charaka Samhita*:

"Tamaka shwasa nam vataja vyadhihi, kshataja, pittaja, kaphaja cha" (Charaka Samhita, Chikitsa Sthana, 17.13).

This verse describes a respiratory disease (*Tamaka Shwasa*) caused by occupational exposure to dust, which leads to an imbalance of the three *doshas (Vata, Pitta, and Kapha)*.

"Mrityormukham prapya, dhumenaiva yujyate, tamaka shwasa nam vataja vyadhihi" (Charaka Samhita, Chikitsa Sthana, 17.14).

This verse describes a respiratory disease caused by inhaling dust, which can lead to severe symptoms and even death.

Sushruta Samhita also describes the respiratory disease in miners and textile workers:

"Khani-gara-karma-kara, tamaka shwasa nam vataja vyadhihi" (Sushruta Samhita, Uttara Tantra, 40.13).

This verse describes a respiratory disease (*Tamaka Shwasa)* affecting miners, caused by occupational exposure to dust.

"Tantuvaya-karma-kara, tamaka shwasa nam vataja vyadhihi" (Sushruta Samhita, Uttara Tantra, 40.14). This verse describes *Tamaka Shwasa*, affecting textile workers, caused by occupational exposure to dust and fibers.

Later Ayurvedic texts in the current era (such as *Ashtanga Hridayam* and *Bhavaprakasha*) also described *Tamaka Shwasa* caused by occupational exposures.

Occupational exposure among ancient agriculture and textile industry, particularly the weaving and dyeing sectors, also exposed workers to respiratory hazards of inhalation of particulate fiber and agricultural products, cotton dust, dye fumes, and other chemicals.

Middle and Modern Ages

Temple building, stonecutting, and carving was extensively practiced since the Mauryan period in India. Hindu rock-cut temples as well

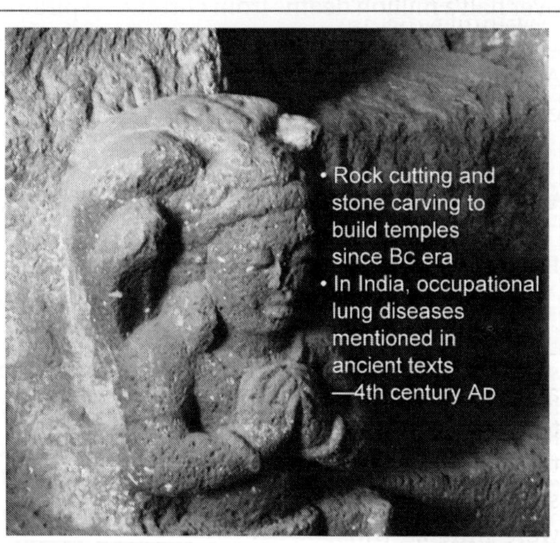

• Rock cutting and stone carving to build temples since BC era
• In India, occupational lung diseases mentioned in ancient texts —4th century AD

Rock cutting and stone carving to build temples and sculptures were highly developed arts in ancient India.
Stone carvings from Ajanta caves, Maharashtra, built in two periods—first around the second century BCE to first century CE, and the second from the fifth to sixth centuries CE.

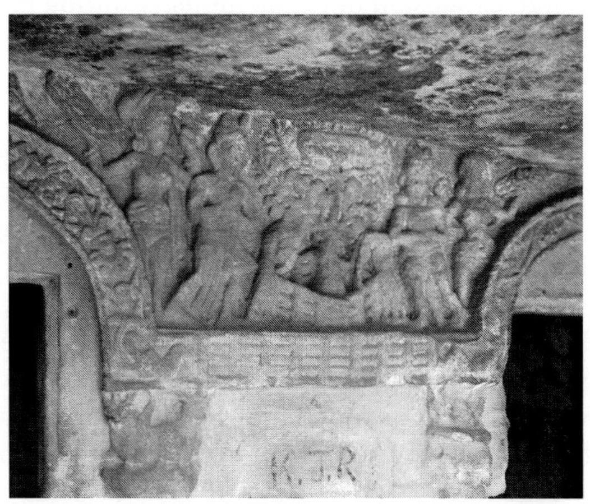

Carving from Sun Temple, Konark, Orisssa built in the 13th century, around 1250 CE.

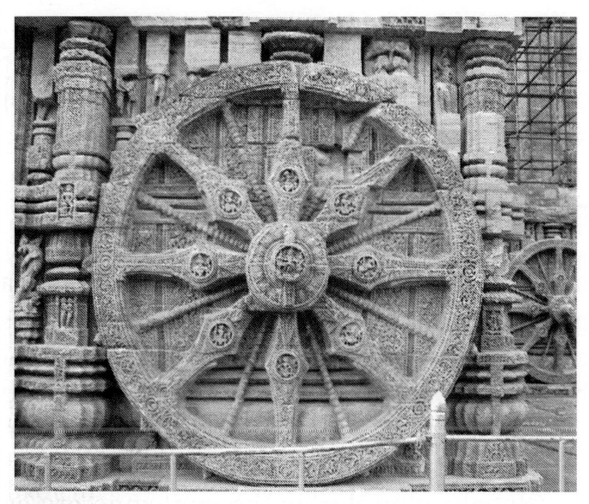

as the Buddhist Pagodas built during third to seventh centuries bear a strong testimony to these activities all of which involved exposure to silica dust and other particulate matter, which were inhaled by the workers engaged in these occupations. Silappatikaram (second century CE) described a worker who died due to exhaustion while working in a quarry: "The worker's body was worn out, his hands were bruised, and his feet were swollen. He died, exhausted by his labour." Similar case examples were cited by others—Manimekalai (second century CE) and Tirukkural (third century BCE).

The hymns and poetry related to the building of stone monuments in Mahabalipuram on the Eastern sea coast of Tamil Nadu, built during the Pallava Dynasty of the seventh century CE, provide some evidence of increased physical disability of workers engaged in these occupations. In all probabilities, they suffered from silica deposition in the lungs and died of premature deaths.

Manikkavachakar, a renowned Tamil poet and saint, highlighted the physical and emotional toll of manual labor:

"I am worn out by the labour of stone quarrying,

My body is weakened by the dust of the red stone,

I am exhausted by the hard work of sculpting the white stone,

My life is consumed by the suffering of my craft, the black stone."

Similarly, Tevaram Hymn by Appar, a renowned Tamil poet and saint, highlighted the pangs of stone carving.

From India, there is limited evidence of the occupational lung diseases during the Mughal and colonial periods. Medieval Indian texts, such as the "*Ain-i-Akbari*" and "*Bhavaprakasha*" of 16th century CE describe respiratory diseases, including those likely caused by mining and quarrying activities. The construction of monumental buildings, such as the Taj Mahal (1632 CE), would have required large numbers of stonecutters and construction workers, who would have been exposed to silica dust. The Persian manuscript "*Insha-i-Mahru*" by Muhammad Arif Qandhari mentions the challenging working conditions of a large number of workers involved in masoning, stonecutting, and laboring activities. The memoir of the Mughal emperor Jahangir, "*Tuzk-i-Jahangiri*" by Nur-ud-din Muhammad Salim describes the emperor's concerns about the welfare of the workers involved in construction of the Taj Mahal. A recent research article "The Construction of the Taj Mahal: A Study of the Labor Force' by Ebba Koch (2006) provides a detailed study of the labor force involved in the construction of the monument and describes the harsh and challenging conditions and that the workers may have been at risk of various health problems.

Similar description of the sufferings of textile workers in the 16th century are found in the *Ain-i-Akbari*, 1590 CE: "*The weavers work day and night, their bodies bent and their eyes strained... They are paid very little, and their work is not valued.*"

Global Developments

Meanwhile, occupational problems attracted greater attention in the European continent. Respiratory problems due to inhalation of dusts in miners were reported by Agricola in the 16th century. It was more than a century later when significant focus was laid on health effects of various occupations. Bernardino Ramazzini, an Italian physician, often considered the "Father of Occupational Medicine" in Europe published his book "*De Morbis Artificum Diatriba*" (Diseases of Workers). He described the respiratory problems faced by miners and textile workers as well as conditions such as metal poisoning and health effects of agricultural work including respiratory problems and skin conditions. He also described respiratory problems associated with baking, and what is now known as extrinsic allergic alveolitis. He recognized the link between specific occupations and health problems and suggested ways to prevent occupational diseases by improving ventilation and using protective equipment. He emphasized the importance of protecting workers' health and well-being. Ramazzini's work laid the foundation for modern occupational medicine and continues to influence the field today.

The Industrial Revolution saw a significant increase in coal mining, leading to a rise in pneumoconiosis cases among coal miners. As mining activities increased during this period, silicosis became a significant occupational hazard for miners. Asbestos was used in shipbuilding and sailing, exposing workers to asbestos fibers and increasing the risk of asbestosis. There was a large expansion of textile industry during this period. Therefore, byssinosis became a major occupational hazard for textile workers due to their exposure to cotton, wool, and other fibers. Workers in industries like metalworking, woodworking, and chemical manufacturing were exposed to various respiratory irritants, leading to occupational asthma.

In view of an expanding list of occupational diseases, Governments in European countries began to enact regulations and laws to protect workers. The occupational health movement gained momentum, with the establishment of organizations like the International Labour Organization (ILO) and the American Conference of Governmental Industrial Hygienists (ACGIH). Governments began to establish regulations and standards for occupational health and safety. The late 20th century saw the expansion of occupational health services to cover more industries and workers. Research on occupational health led to a better understanding of occupational diseases and the development of new treatments.

Employers were required to implement better ventilation systems and provide personal protective equipment to reduce workers' exposure to respiratory hazards. Researchers and healthcare professionals raised awareness about occupational lung disorders and studies were conducted to better understand these conditions.

Globalization during the contemporary era has led to new occupational health challenges, including the spread of diseases across borders. New occupational health issues continue to emerge, including musculoskeletal disorders, occupational cancer, mental health, and others. There is a growing recognition of the importance of occupational health and safety, with increased efforts to prevent occupational diseases and promote healthy workplaces. New industries and technologies have introduced new respiratory hazards, such as nanoparticles and biologic agents, which require continued research and attention.

Modern Period in India

There was little respite from the harsh working conditions during the colonial period. Indian workers were employed in mining, quarrying, and stone-cutting industries, leading to silicosis. Miners working in coal mines and in the Kolar Gold Fields were similarly exposed to dusts containing silica, coal, and other minerals. The British physician WH Wills in 1865 described a lung disease among Indian stonecutters in Calcutta. The Report of the Indian Mining Commission, 1891 CE described their sufferings: "The miners work in dark and damp conditions, their bodies worn out and their lungs affected... Many miners die due to accidents and diseases."

There were several other factors which contributed to the prevalence of occupational lung diseases among workers in various industries during British colonialism in India. Presence of poor working conditions, inadequate ventilation, poor lighting, and unsanitary conditions further augmented the risks. There were inadequate laws and regulations governing workplace safety and health. Moreover, workers had limited access to medical care. Workers were often exploited, with long working hours, low wages, and limited social protections.

Recognizing the significance of the problem, the British government enacted the Factory Acts (1883, 1911, and 1922) to regulate working conditions and protect workers' health. The colonial government also established occupational health services, including medical inspections and health records. Most of the occupational problems, however, continued to pose concerns because of the inadequate enforcement.

The post-Independence period witnessed exaggerated industrial growth, which led to increased mining and quarrying activities. The Indian Government introduced the Factories Act (1948) and the Mines Act (1952) to regulate working conditions. It also established the Central Labour Institute (CLI) in Mumbai (1966) to undertake research in occupational health. Silicosis was recognized as a major occupational health concern and regulations were introduced to set silica exposure limits and use respiratory protection measures. Later, National Institute of Occupational Health (NIOH) was established in Ahmedabad in 1980 to undertake studies on silicosis prevalence and prevention measures.

The Indian government formulated policies such as the National Policy on Occupational Health (2003) and the National Occupational Health Programme (2013). Occupational health services expanded to cover more industries, including construction and agriculture services. Research on occupational health began to gain momentum with studies on occupational diseases such as silicosis and asbestosis. Research on occupational health continues to grow, with a widened focus on other emerging issues such as occupational cancers and mental health.

Silicosis

Although the first recorded mention of silicosis-like symptoms in India dates back to the late 18th century when the British physician Francis Buchanan-Hamilton described a disease among

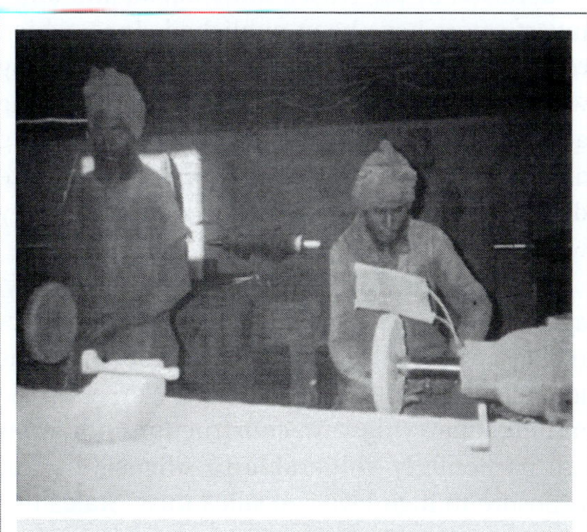

Grinding work producing extensive dust in a close environment in contemporary India.

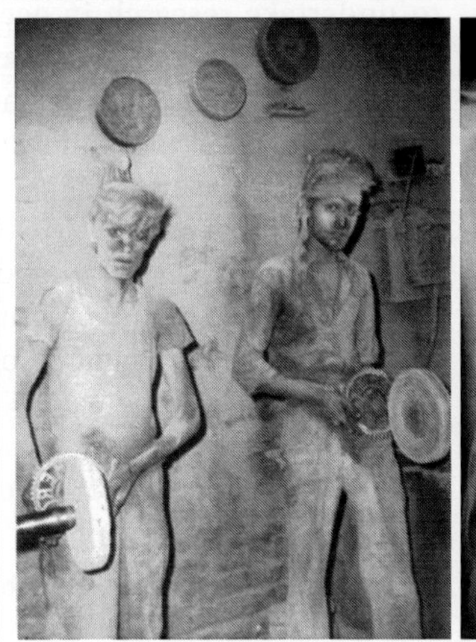
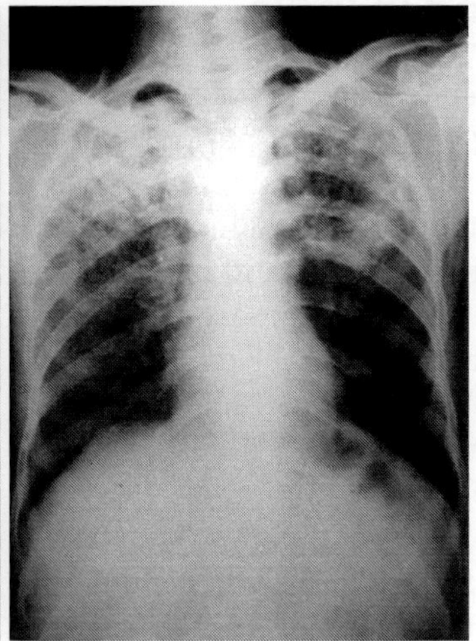

Prevalence of silicosis varies widely among various industries; lowest in iron and steel and ordnance factories (2–3.5%) and highest in agate, slate pencil, lead, zinc and mica mining, and stone cutting/quartz grinding (>30%).

Indian stonecutters, documented reports became available only in the late 19th and early 20th century. The problems of pneumoconiosis in the Kolar Gold mines in Karnataka were described in 1933, and the first case of silicosis was reported in 1947. Several reports of medical surveys undertaken by the NIOH, Ahmedabad and other investigators have been published since, which reported a high prevalence of silicosis among workers engaged in construction, sand blasting and crushing, drilling, masonry, tunnelling and grinding; mining, sand stone, and granite drilling; and slate pencil work and foundry work.

Manufacturing of ceramic and clay pottery, agate cutting and polishing, and glass manufacturing are some other important occupations identified to predispose to silicosis. Workers in the mining, quarrying, and construction industries are particularly vulnerable to silicosis due to exposure to high levels of silica dust. States like Madhya Pradesh, Chhattisgarh, and Rajasthan have been identified as high-risk areas for silicosis due to the presence of significant mining and quarrying activities.

Despite the risks, many Indian workers are not aware of the dangers of silicosis, and regulatory measures to prevent exposure are often inadequate. The Indian government has launched initiatives to prevent silicosis, including the National Policy on Occupational Health (2006) and the National Programme for Prevention and Control of Occupational Diseases (2013).

Indian research on silicosis has highlighted the significant occupational health risks faced by workers in various industries. According to recent studies, more than 10 million workers in India are exposed to silica particles, putting them at risk of developing silicosis. Researchers are also exploring new diagnostic techniques and treatment options including the use of biomarkers and antifibrotic therapies. Overall, Indian research on silicosis highlights the need for greater awareness, regulation, and research to prevent and control this significant occupational health risk.

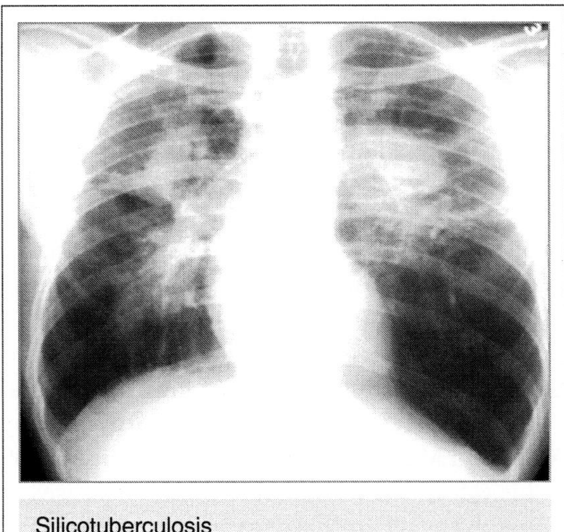

Silicotuberculosis

Silicosis was officially recognized as an occupational disease in India in 1948, with the enactment of the Employees' State Insurance Act. This act provided medical benefits and compensation to workers suffering from occupational diseases, including silicosis. Recognizing the significant burden of silicosis and disability of workers in a Public Interest writ petition filed by the People's Rights and Social Research Centre, the Supreme Court of India made important observations and asked the National Human Rights Commission (NHRC) to take up steps with the States for relief to patients with silicosis. The NHRC of India organized a national conference on silicosis in 2011. A special report was also prepared and submitted to the Ministry of Home Affairs for laying before Parliament. The report highlighted the inhumane conditions faced by those with silicosis and also suggested various preventive, management, compensation, and rehabilitative measures. It remains a national health challenge and requires the active participation of stakeholders including the industry management, labor-unions, regulatory authorities, state governments, civil society organizations, national institutions, and central government ministries.

Asbestosis

Asbestosis, a lung disease caused by inhaling asbestos fibers, has been a significant occupational health concern in India for several decades. Asbestos exposure is linked to progressively fatal lung disease such as pulmonary fibrosis, lung cancer, and malignant tumors of the pleura.

While asbestos was known and used in ancient civilizations, including ancient India, there is limited evidence of asbestosis being recognized as a distinct medical condition. There is indirect mention in ancient Indian texts, such as the "Rigveda" and the "Mahabharata". It was used in medieval Indian architecture, particularly in the construction of temples, mosques, and other buildings. But the medieval Indian medical texts, such as the "*Bhavaprakasha*" and the "*Madhava Nidanam*" do not contain direct references to asbestosis although they do describe various respiratory diseases, including those caused by dust and fiber inhalation.

During the British colonial period, India was a significant exporter of asbestos with major asbestos mines in the states of Andhra Pradesh, Bihar, and Rajasthan. It was widely used during this period for construction, insulation, and manufacturing purposes, including in the production of asbestos cement products. The asbestos cement industry emerged in India in the early 20th century, with the establishment of companies like the Associated Cement Companies (ACC) and the Hyderabad Industries Limited (HIL). Asbestosis was likely present among Indian workers exposed to asbestos in mines, construction sites, and manufacturing facilities.

One of the earliest documented cases of asbestosis in Europe was that of Nellie Kershaw, a British textile worker who died in 1924 at the age of 33 years. It led to increased awareness of the health risks associated with asbestos exposure. The case was investigated by the British government, and it resulted in changes to workplace safety regulations and improved protection for workers handling asbestos. From India, cases of asbestosis and other asbestos-related diseases were likely underreported due to limited medical awareness and inadequate diagnostic facilities. The first reported case in India was published in 1957, in the Indian Journal of Medical Research, about a worker who had been exposed to asbestos for 20 years in a textile mill. There were subsequent reports of asbestos-related diseases, including asbestosis and mesothelioma, in Indian literature in the 1990s and early 2000s. These reports demonstrated the importance of occupational health surveillance and the need for continued research, awareness, and regulation to prevent asbestos-related diseases in India.

The asbestos industry expanded rapidly after independence, with the government encouraging the growth of the industry. But there were no effective regulations to protect workers from asbestos exposure, leading to widespread occupational health hazards. Asbestosis was officially recognized as an occupational disease in 1983, with the enactment of the Factories Act. The Indian Factory Acts of 1883 and 1911 had provided some basic protections for workers, but they did not specifically address asbestos exposure. The 1983 Act mandated the use of asbestos substitutes and provided guidelines for the safe handling and disposal of asbestos. In 1986, the Indian government established the Asbestos Rules, which regulated the use of asbestos in various industries, including construction, manufacturing, and mining. In 2011, the Indian government banned the use of asbestos in the country, citing its hazardous effects on human health and the environment.

Debates about banning asbestos in India began in the 1990s, with some countries like the United States and European nations already having banned or restricted its use. The Indian government developed a national asbestos profile in 2011, which highlighted the extent of asbestos use and the need for better regulations. In 2011, the Indian government banned the use of asbestos in the manufacture of asbestos-cement corrugated sheets. Despite these efforts, India still struggles with asbestos-related diseases, including asbestosis, due to ongoing exposure and inadequate regulations.

Coal Workers Pneumoconiosis

Coal Workers Pneumoconiosis (CWP), also known as black lung disease, has been a significant occupational health concern in the coal mining industry. Viscount Charles Montague, a British physician, had first described a condition called "coal miner's asthma" in 1713. However, the first comprehensive description was provided by Archibald Makellar, a Scottish physician in 1839 in his work, titled "A Treatise on the Diseases of Miners." The term "coal worker pneumoconiosis" was officially adopted in the 1940s to describe this occupational lung disease.

Coal mining in India was started in the mid-19th century, with the establishment of the first coal mine in Raniganj, West Bengal. There were anecdotal reports of respiratory problems among coal miners, but these were not formally documented or recognized as an occupational disease. The first recognition of coal worker pneumoconiosis in India is attributed to AK Sen, a renowned physician, who reported a series of cases of CWP among coal miners in the Jharia coalfields of Bihar (now Jharkhand) in 1936. Dr Sen's work, published in the Indian Medical Gazette, highlighted the occupational health hazards faced by coal miners in India and emphasized the need for better working conditions, dust control measures, and medical surveillance. Dr Sen's pioneering work laid the foundation for future research and studies on CWP in India, which ultimately led to the development of policies and regulations to protect the health and safety of coal miners in the country.

Coal Workers Pneumoconiosis became a major concern with increased reporting of cases and growing awareness among workers, employers, and healthcare professionals. CWP was formally recognized as an occupational disease in India in the 1950s, with the publication of studies documenting the respiratory problems faced by coal miners. The Indian government introduced regulatory measures, such as the Mines Act (1952), to control dust exposure as well as established schemes to provide compensation and rehabilitation to the affected workers by CWP.

Despite efforts to control, the disease remains a significant occupational health concern in India's coal mining industry.

Byssinosis

Byssinosis, also known as "brown lung disease," caused by inhaling cotton dust, is commonly seen in workers in the textile industry. The ancient texts described *"shwasa rog"* or breathing disorder caused by dust inhalation. Archaeological findings suggest that textile production was a significant industry in ancient India, with evidence of cotton production dating back to the Indus Valley Civilization. It is likely that ancient Indian textile workers were exposed to cotton dust, which could have led to respiratory problems similar to byssinosis.

The first recognition of byssinosis, a respiratory disease caused by inhaling cotton dust, is attributed to Bernardino Ramazzini, an Italian physician, who described a condition called "*mal de los hilanderos*" (disease of the spinners) in his book "*De Morbis Artificum Diatriba*" (Diseases of Workers) in 1700. However, the term "byssinosis" was not used until 1936, when the disease was formally recognized and named by the American physician, David H Brown. The medieval Indian Unani text, "*Tibb-e-Nabawi*" (14th century), written by Ibn-e-Hajr, describes a condition called "*Zukam-e-Nassaji,*" which translates to "disease of the weavers".

India's textile industry experienced rapid growth during the British colonial period, with the establishment of numerous cotton mills and textile factories. There were anecdotal reports of respiratory problems among textile workers, but these were not formally documented or recognized as an occupational disease. The first recognition of byssinosis in India is attributed to NSN Rao, who reported a series of cases of byssinosis among textile workers in Bombay in 1928. Dr Rao's work, published in the Indian Medical Gazette, highlighted the occupational health hazards faced by textile workers in India and emphasized the need for better working conditions, dust control measures, and medical surveillance.

Byssinosis was formally recognized as an occupational disease in the 1960s when it gained the attention of the Indian Council of Medical Research and other organizations. The Indian Government introduced regulatory measures such as the Factory Act (1948) to control dust exposure. The Government also established compensation and rehabilitation schemes for the affected workers. Despite efforts to control the disease, it remains a significant occupational health concern in India's textile industry. Researchers and industry stakeholders are exploring new technologies and innovations to reduce the incidence in the future.

Miscellaneous Occupational Lung Diseases

There is a long list of occupational respiratory diseases of multiple etiologies and different patterns, which are now recognized. Changing industrial technology and the growth of the healthcare sector has led to new patterns of work-related lung diseases that can be caused, aggravated, or exacerbated by workplace exposures. Occupational exposure to different organic and inorganic dusts, allergens, smokes, and chemicals are also listed as important causes of asthma, chronic obstructive pulmonary disease, and interstitial lung diseases. As an example, occupational asthma and hypersensitivity pneumonias can be caused by over 200 known occupational agents. Occupational asthma and occupational COPD are now recognized as distinct entities.

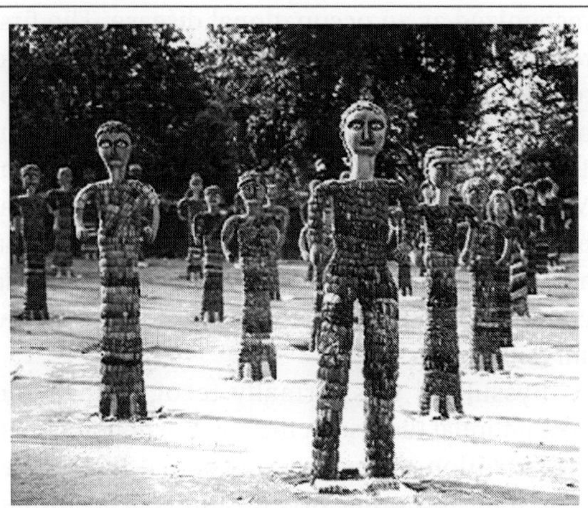

A large collection of statues made from broken glass-bangles (product of extensive glass industry in India) in the famous Rock-garden of Chandigarh created mostly from old and broken material.

Domestic exposure of women to household smoke from solid fuels due to cooking is also categorized as an occupational risk factor for chronic lung diseases. A rare condition granulomatous lung disease is reported in workers exposed to glass particles, characterized by the formation of granulomas in the lungs. Exposure to pesticides and other toxicants has been linked to various respiratory problems. Prolonged exposure to loud noises can cause not only hearing loss but also respiratory issues, such as asthma and COPD.

Modern Shift in Disease Pattern

There is a marked shift in the types of work and occupational exposures in the modern world. Incidence of some of the ancient diseases such as coal workers' pneumoconiosis, asbestosis, and even silicosis has significantly declined. The elimination of beryllium from fluorescent light bulbs has led to a decline in chronic beryllium disease although beryllium sensitization and the disease are being increasingly reported in workers exposed in defense and aerospace industries.

Several new lung diseases, especially of the hypersensitivity phenotypes, are being recorded in the last few decades. Some such examples include the indium lung disease in workers exposed to indium, a rare earth metal used in flat-panel displays and other electronics; hard metal disease caused by exposure to hard metals, such as tungsten carbide and cobalt, used in machining and manufacturing; diacetyl-induced lung disease caused by exposure to diacetyl, a chemical used in food flavorings, and Flock Worker's Lung caused by exposure to nylon flock, a material used in textile manufacturing. Exposure to vapors of pharmaceutical and personnel care products as well as to nanoparticles, such as carbon nanotubes and metal oxides, has been linked to lung inflammation and damage. Recently, 3D printing-related lung disease caused by exposure to emissions from 3D printing, which can include particulate matter, volatile organic compounds, and other hazardous substances has been reported.

These reports of new exposures and newer health problems highlight the continuity of history of occupational lung diseases. They also point out the need for continued research, surveillance, and prevention efforts to protect the health of the workers and all other exposed personnel.

Sources

1. Silappatikaram, 10.2.11-12. Bhaktivedant Vedabase. https://vedabase.io/en/library/sb/10/2/11-12/
2. Brajadulal Chattopadhyaya, ed. A Social History of Early India. Jointly published by CSC and Pearson Education for the Project of History of Indian Science, Philosophy and Culture. 2009; p. 238. https://en.wikipedia.org/wiki/Manimekalai
3. Tirukkural, 1030-1031. https://tamilnation.org/literature/kural/kurale2
4. Tiruvachakam by Manikkavachakar (7th century CE). https://www.ytamizh.com/thirukural/kural-1030/#google_vignette
5. Cutler, Norman (1987). Songs of experience: the poetics of Tamil devotion. USA: Library of Congress Cataloging-in-Publication-Data. ISBN 0-253-35334-3. https://en.wikipedia.org/wiki/Thiruvasagam

6. Vasudevan, Geetha. The royal temple of Rajaraja: an instrument of imperial Cola power, New Delhi: Abhinav Publications. 2003.
7. M. Athar Ali. Mughal India - Studies in Polity, Ideas, Society and Culture- (Oxford India Paperbacks) Oxford University Press (2008). https://www.scribd.com/document/799773559
8 Blochmann H. (tr.) (1927, reprint 1993). The Ain-I Akbari by Abu'l-Fazl Allami, Vol. I, Calcutta: The Asiatic Society, preface (first edition)
9. Shiwali Sharma, Usha Sharma, Shuchi Mitra, Khem Chand Sharma. A review of bhavaprakasha: an important ayurvedic treatise. Int. J. Res. Ayurveda Pharm. 2003;(4), 2023. https://ijrap.net/
10. Begley WE. The Taj Mahal: A Study of its Architecture and History. J Soc Architect Histor. 1979;38(2):144-57.
11. Koch E. The Construction of the Taj Mahal: A Study of the Labor Force. J Eco Soc Hist Orient. 2006;49(2):151-73.
12. AK Ganguly (Ed). Occupational Health in India. 2013.
13. Jindal SK, Wig J. Silicosis in developing countries. In: Banks DE, Parker JE (Eds). Occupational Health and Lung Diseases - An International perspective. London: Chapman and Hall; 1996.
14. Jindal SK. Occupational lung disease—Relevance in Indian scenario. In: Gupta SB. (Ed) Medicine Update. Mumbai: Association of Physician of India; 2002. pp. 641-45.
15. Tarlo S. Occupational Lung Disease. Goldman's Cecil Medicine. 2012:567-74.
16. Beckett WS. Occupational respiratory diseases. New Engl J Med. 2000;342(6):406-13.
17. Jindal SK. Silicosis in India: Past and present. Curr Opin Pulmon Med. 2013;19(2):163-8.
18. Ghosh PK. Industrial pulmonary disease in India. Ind Med Surg. 1964;33:732-7.
19. Jones WR. Silicotic lungs: the minerals they contain. J Hyg. 1933;33:307-29.
20. Jindal SK, Aggarwal AN, Gupta AN. Dust induced interstitial lung disease in the tropics. Curr Opin Pulm Med. 2001;7:272-7.
21. Supreme Court of India, Writ petition (Civil) No. 110 of 2006. No. 318926 dated 3.5.2009.
22. National Human Rights Commission. Special report to Parliament of India on silicosis. [online] Available from https://nhrc.nic.in/document/manuals/special-report-parliament-india-silicosis [Last accessed September; 2025].
23. Cullinan P, Muñoz X, Suojalehto H, Agius R, Jindal S, Sigsgaard T, et al. Occupational lung diseases: from old and novel exposures to effective preventive strategies. Lancet Respir Med. 2017;5(5):445-55.
24. Mason RJ, Slutsky A, Murray JF, Nadel JA, Gotway MB, Broaddus VC (Eds). Murray & Nadel's Textbook of Respiratory Medicine. Elsevier Saunders; 2016. pp. 1307-30.
25. Dhar R, Jindal SK. Occupational exposures and COPD: Significant issues in the Indian subcontinent. Respirology. 2022;27(6):62-4.

CHAPTER

12

Novel Respiratory Concepts and Diseases

The numerous discoveries made during the period of the European Renaissance resulted in the development of new ideas and concepts about diseases, their diagnoses, and treatments. Most medical philosophers of the past had emphasized on the practice of breaking down complex systems into smaller components to understand and treat diseases. The concept of "breaking down into components" or "reductionism" got firmly established during the 16th and 17th centuries, with seminal work on human anatomy by Andreas Vesalius and Rene Descartes' advocacy of questioning and rationalism. René Descartes, who conceptualized the body as a machine composed of separate parts, reinforced reductionist thinking.

Reduction and Rationalism

Descartes' skepticism had a lasting impact on modern science in general and medicine in particular, which encouraged researchers to break down complex systems into smaller and more manageable parts. Rationalism has a rich history since ancient times in both India and Europe, with various philosophers, scientists, and thinkers contributing to the new developments. But the change had never been as radical as during the post-Renaissance period. People started challenging the existing thoughts about everything, including medicine. There was a rapid change in the beliefs about the spectrum and etiology of diseases, as well as a more effective approach for their management.

There was a rapid broadening of the disease spectrum affecting humans. Apart from the ancient diseases such as tuberculosis and asthma, new and novel diseases were identified and explained. These diseases were differently classified based on different etiologies, clinical manifestations, natural history, and/or prognosis. It is not our intention to go into the details of these diseases but rather to focus on important historical developments.

Infectious Diseases

Developments related to tuberculosis, which continued to remain a significant cause of human suffering, have been separately discussed elsewhere in the book. Of nontubercular diseases, viral infections such as influenza top the list as the major cause of morbidity and mortality both globally and in India. Pneumonias due to various microorganisms continue to affect people of all ages, genders, ethnicities, and nationalities. There are several high-risk populations, including children, the elderly, malnourished, and the immunocompromised, who are more prone to these infections and likely to suffer from atypical organisms, fungi, and parasitic infections.

Infectious Outbreaks and Epidemics

Most cases of bacterial and fungal pneumonias occur sporadically. There are, however, few examples of bacterial outbreaks, while viral infections have tended to occur in outbreaks affecting a larger population in epidemic or pandemic proportions. Plague has been one of the worst examples of bacterial epidemics in the past, which has fortunately almost disappeared now. Another bacterial outbreak occurred in the form of a localized cluster of cases of pneumonia caused by *Legionella pneumophila* at an American Legion convention in Philadelphia in 1976.

Pneumonic Plague

Pneumonic plague, a highly infectious and deadly form of the plague, had spread like wildfire all over the world in several pandemics. The disease, believed to have originated in Central Asia over 2,000 years ago, was transmitted to humans through the bites of infected fleas that lived on rats and other rodents. One of the earliest recorded outbreaks of the plague occurred during the reign of Byzantine Emperor Justinian I. This pandemic, known as the Justinian Plague, is estimated to have killed between 25 and 100 million people, roughly 10–50% of the world's population of that time. The most devastating pandemic in human history was the Black Death, which spread across Europe, Asia, and North Africa, killing an estimated 75–200 million people. The plague spread rapidly due to urbanization, trade, and lack of sanitation. During the 16th to 19th centuries, pneumonic plague emerged as a distinct form of the disease. This form of the plague is highly infectious and can be transmitted person-to-person through respiratory droplets.

In India, the plague first appeared during the sixth century, with outbreaks reported from the western coastal regions. The disease spread rapidly along trade routes, affecting major cities like Bombay (now Mumbai) and Surat. One of the most significant plague outbreaks in Indian history occurred in Bombay (now Mumbai) in 1896–1897. The outbreak killed an estimated 200,000 people, leading to widespread panic and social unrest. In response to the Bombay (now Mumbai) outbreak, the British colonial government established the Indian Plague Commission to investigate the causes of the disease and develop public health measures. The commission's recommendations led to significant improvements in sanitation, hygiene, and disease surveillance.

In the 20th century, antibiotics and other treatments that became available have significantly reduced the incidence and mortality rate of pneumonic plague. However, small outbreaks continue to occur, particularly in Africa and Asia. Most recently, small pneumonic plague outbreaks occurred in Madagascar in 2013 and 2017. After India gained independence in 1947, the government continued to implement public health measures to control the plague. Despite these efforts, plague outbreaks occur, particularly in rural areas. In the 1990s, an outbreak occurred in the state of Gujarat, killing 56 people. More recently, in 2017, a plague outbreak was reported in the state of Maharashtra, affecting several districts.

Influenza Pandemics

Viruses constitute a major group of micro-organisms responsible for large outbreaks of respiratory infections from time to time. Viruses likely originated over 2 billion years ago, emerging from ancient cells or genetic material. They have evolved alongside their host organisms, developing strategies to infect, replicate, and transmit. Dmitri Ivanovsky identified the first virus, the *tobacco mosaic virus,* in 1892, while the term "virus" was coined in 1898 by Martinus Beijerinck, who also demonstrated that the virus was a contagious agent. Electron microscopy and the development of molecular biology techniques in the 20th century made it possible to visualize viruses as well as study their genetic basis, viral replication, and gene expression. Advances in genomics, proteomics, and bioinformatics have further facilitated the study of viral evolution, transmission, and pathogenesis. The emergence of acquired immunodeficiency syndrome (AIDS) and human immunodeficiency virus (HIV) in the last century and the recent COVID-19 pandemic highlight the impact of viral diseases on human health, the ongoing threat of viral diseases, and the importance of global health preparedness.

Viral infections like influenza are described in various forms throughout history, with evidence of outbreaks dating back to ancient civilizations in Egypt, Greece, and Rome. The disease was often referred to as "catarrh" or "grippe."

The disease has been responsible for some of the deadliest pandemics in human history. A worldwide pandemic that lasted for a decade toward the end of the 19th century killed an estimated 1 million people. The 1918 Spanish flu pandemic was one of the most devastating, killing an estimated 20–50 million people worldwide. In the 20th century, the Asian flu pandemic and the Hong Kong flu pandemic had killed over 1 million people each. The last Hemagglutinin (H) Type 1 and Neuraminidase (N) Type 1 (H1N1) pandemic at the beginning of the 21st century was equally devastating.

India has similarly suffered from several major outbreaks and pandemics. The 1918 Spanish flu pandemic had killed an estimated 17–18 million people, which was roughly 5% of the population. This pandemic was particularly deadly due to factors like malnutrition, poor healthcare infrastructure, and the virus's high virulence. The two mid-20th-century outbreaks of the Asian flu and the Hong Kong flu were equally devastating. These outbreaks were characterized by high rates of absenteeism and incapacitation, particularly in urban areas, which had greatly affected industrial productivity and the national economy.

In recent years, India has continued to experience seasonal outbreaks of influenza, including the H1N1 pandemic in 2009, although the overall mortality has declined compared to the earlier pandemics. The epidemiology of influenza in India is changing, with shifting patterns of seasonality, age distribution, and geographic spread. For example, the 2017 outbreak saw a higher number of cases and deaths among younger adults and in the nontraditional flu season months.

Overall, India's history with influenza highlights the need for continued vigilance, improved healthcare infrastructure, and enhanced surveillance to mitigate the impact of future outbreaks. Significant advances have been made in influenza prevention and treatment. Vaccination and self-hygienic measures have proved to be fairly effective in preventing influenza. The first inactivated flu vaccine was developed in the 1940s, and since then, various types of vaccines have been developed, including trivalent and quadrivalent vaccines. In addition, antiviral medications are also available to treat and prevent influenza.

Coronavirus Outbreaks and Coronavirus Disease 2019 Pandemic

Coronaviruses (CoV) are a large family of viruses that cause respiratory illnesses in humans and animals. Coronaviruses are responsible for 10–20% of common cold cases but can cause bronchitis and pneumonia, particularly in older adults and those with underlying health conditions. Small, localized outbreaks were reported at the beginning of this century from China (severe acute respiratory syndrome) and Saudi Arabia (Middle East respiratory syndrome) involving a few thousand individuals every time. But the most recent 2019 pandemic (COVID-19), caused by SARS-CoV-2, has been highly devastating, responsible for millions of cases and deaths.

Coronavirus disease 2019 was first detected in Wuhan, China, in December 2019. The virus is believed to have originated from an animal source, with many early patients linked to a seafood market in Wuhan that sold live animals, including bats and snakes. It was also suspected that the virus might have leaked from an advanced viral laboratory in the city. It rapidly spread worldwide in over 200 countries. The first cases from India were reported on January 30, 2020, from Kerala. The first peak towards the end of the year was followed by an even more severe second wave during early 2021. India accounted for over 45 million reported cases, the second-highest in the world, and over half a million reported deaths, the third-highest in the world. The pandemic had a significant impact on the national economy and healthcare systems with widespread lockdowns, travel restrictions, and increased unemployment.

India's response to the pandemic was marked by significant challenges, including inadequate healthcare infrastructure, vaccine shortages, and economic disruption. But the response was rapid with the adoption of preventive measures, wider use of rapid diagnostic tests, and antiviral treatments. The country also made notable progress in vaccination, testing, and relief measures. India launched its vaccination drive on January 16, 2021, with a focus on healthcare workers, frontline workers, and vulnerable populations. Multiple vaccines were made available, including COVAXIN, Covishield, ZyCoV-D, and Sputnik V. Over 1.7 billion vaccine doses were administered, resulting in full vaccination of more than 720 million people. Other relief measures included economic stimulus packages, welfare schemes, and tax relief.

Acquired Immune Deficiency Syndrome and Human Immunodeficiency Virus Infection

An unknown disease in the past, AIDS was first described among gay men in San Francisco in 1981. Michael Gottlieb, an immunologist at the University of California, Los Angeles, encountered a 31-year-old gay man who presented with symptoms of a rare and opportunistic parasitic infection, *Pneumocystis carinii*, PCP (now reclassified as a fungus, *Pneumocystis jirovecii*). The immunological tests revealed that the patient's immune system was severely impaired, with a low count of CD4+ T cells. Investigations at the Centers for Disease Control and Prevention (CDC) led to the issuance of an alert in the Morbidity and Mortality Weekly Report (MMWR) on June 5, 1981, describing the cluster of cases and requesting for reports of similar cases.

The CDC also established a case definition for the syndrome, which included symptoms such as pneumonia, Kaposi's sarcoma, and other opportunistic infections. The epidemiological investigation revealed that the cases were clustered among gay men in California and New York. It further led to the identification of the human immunodeficiency virus (HIV) as the causative agent in 1983–1984, independently by the French scientist Luc Montagnier and the American scientist Robert Gallo.

HIV is believed to have originated from a simian immunodeficiency virus in chimpanzees in Central Africa. It was thought that the virus probably jumped from animals to humans through hunting and handling of infected animals. AIDS cases were soon reported in other countries, including Canada, Europe, and Australia. It soon spread globally with the number of cases increasing exponentially. The disease is often associated with stigma, fear, and discrimination, particularly against marginalized communities. The discovery of HIV led to the development of diagnostic tests, treatment, and prevention measures. It enabled physicians to diagnose, monitor, and treat disease with antiretroviral therapy and pre-exposure prophylaxis. Antiretroviral therapy was introduced in the mid-1990s, significantly improving treatment options and survival rates. The treatment has now become more widely available, particularly in low- and middle-income countries. Prevention strategies, such as preexposure prophylaxis and voluntary medical male circumcision, have been implemented.

The first description of AIDS from India was reported in 1986 by Suniti Solomon and her student Sellappan Nirmala in six female sex workers in Chennai, Tamil Nadu. They had earlier collected 30 blood samples from sex workers in 1980, which later tested positive for

HIV. Throughout the 1990s and 2000s, India's HIV epidemic continued to grow, with high-risk groups such as female sex workers, homosexual men, and injection-drug users being disproportionately affected.

In recent years, India has made significant progress in controlling the epidemic. The Indian government established the National AIDS Committee within the Ministry of Health and Family Welfare in the late 1980s. This was followed by the creation of the National AIDS Control Organization (NACO) in 1992, which aimed to oversee policies and prevention and control programs related to HIV and AIDS. According to the National AIDS Control Organization, the estimated adult HIV prevalence in India has declined from 0.41% in 2000 to 0.22% in 2019. Additionally, the number of new HIV infections has decreased, and access to antiretroviral therapy has increased. Despite these advances, there is still much work to be done to address the stigma and discrimination faced by people living with HIV in India. The government has implemented various policies and programs to address these issues, including the HIV/AIDS (Prevention and Control) Bill 2014, which aims to prevent and control the spread of HIV and AIDS in the country.

Immunity, Autoimmunity, and Immunological Disorders

Immunology involves the study of immunity and immunological disorders. Immunity generally refers to a protective phenomenon in response to some infection or other extraneous agent. Ancient Greeks, such as Hippocrates, had recognized the importance of immunity and observed that people who recovered from certain diseases became immune to them. The ancient Chinese, Indians, and Africans practiced inoculation, exposing people to small amounts of a disease-causing agent to build immunity.

The earliest written description of immunity is available from the pre-Biblical Era (430 BCE) when Thucydides noted that people who had recovered from the plague did not get sick again after nursing the patients. The concept of immunity was further developed during the Middle Ages with contributions of Ibn Sina and Girolamo Fracastoro. It was the introduction of the smallpox vaccine by Edward Jenner in 1798 that marked the beginning of modern immunology.

Louis Pasteur's germ theory of disease, supplemented with Robert Koch's work, brought immunology to the forefront of disease prevention strategies. The major 20th-century additions to immunology, which revolutionized the field, include the discovery of the immune system's components, antibodies, and immunoglobulins. In the 1960s, immunochemistry assumed a dominant role in immunology. This led to the identification and discovery of the chemical structure of antibodies. The discovery of HIV and the understanding of AIDS further boosted the progress in the field of immunology.

The term immunity was coined by Russian biologist Ilya Ilyich Mechnikov, who advanced studies on immunology and received the Nobel Prize for his work in 1908 jointly with the German scientist, Paul Ehrlich, "in recognition of their work on immunity."

Autoimmunity

In certain situations, the immune system attacks the body's own cells and tissues—a concept defined as autoimmunity. The phenomenon was recognized in one way or the other way in ancient medical literature. Symptomatic suggestions of autoimmune diseases like rheumatoid arthritis and lupus are available in the Hippocratic corpus as well as the *Charaka Samhita* and *Sushruta Samhita*. Galen had also noted that some diseases seemed to be caused by an "internal poison" or "bad blood." In the Middle Ages, physicians like Thomas Sydenham and William Heberden described diseases with autoimmune features, such as lupus and rheumatoid arthritis. Persian physicians of the Unani system in India also described diseases with autoimmune features. The Swiss physician Paracelsus had proposed in the 15th century that some diseases were caused by internal factors, rather than external ones.

Paul Ehrlich, a German scientist, introduced the concept of "*horror autotoxicus*," at the turn of the 20th century, initially with the belief that the immune system would never attack the body's own cells. Later, he adjusted his theory to recognize the possibility of autoimmune tissue attacks. In the following decades, a number of conditions with autoimmune responses were recognized along with a greater understanding of autoantibodies. In recent times, the recognition of genetic factors contributing to autoimmunity and the development of new immunological techniques have further improved our understanding of autoimmune diseases.

There have been simultaneous developments related to management strategies. The introduction of immunosuppressive medications, such as corticosteroids and cyclophosphamide, has transformed the treatment of autoimmune diseases. The discovery of immunosuppressive drugs has also enabled organ transplantation, besides the treatment of autoimmune diseases. Advances in immunotherapy, including checkpoint inhibitors, have transformed cancer treatment. The development of precision medicine approaches has improved the treatment of immunological disorders. Gene editing technologies hold promise for treating genetic immunological disorders, while the integration of immunology, genomics, and computational biology has enabled a deeper understanding of the immune system.

Immunological and Inflammatory Disorders

Immunological and inflammatory disorders encompass a wide variety of disorders, from infections to autoimmune diseases to cancers. Although there are early references to immune-related conditions such as asthma and allergies in ancient medical texts, the long list of immune and autoimmune disorders that are now recognized to affect humans, is rather novel. In particular, there is a greater understanding of autoimmune connective tissue diseases (CTDs) such as rheumatoid arthritis and lupus, vasculitides, and several other idiopathic or inflammatory disorders.

Sarcoidosis

Sarcoidosis is an important condition characterized by granulomatous inflammation and scarring in the lungs and other organs, which was first described by Jonathan Hutchinson, an English surgeon, in a patient with skin lesions and lung involvement, while Schaumann, a Swedish physician, proposed the term "sarcoidosis" to describe the systemic disease. The discovery of immunoglobulins (antibodies) in the 1950s and 1960s helped us to understand the role of the immune system. Advances in imaging, such as high-resolution computed tomography and positron emission tomography, have improved diagnosis and monitoring. New treatments, including biologics and immunomodulators, have expanded therapeutic choices for patients with sarcoidosis.

The disease is of considerable importance in India because of the similarities of clinical, radiological, and histopathological features with those of tuberculosis, a common disease in India. Incidentally, the differentiation between the two diseases assumes greater importance because of different treatment approaches, which are somewhat antagonistic to each other. The first case of sarcoidosis from India was reported by MC Gupta in 1947. Thereafter, sporadic case reports had appeared in Indian medical literature during the 1950s and 1960s. The number of reports had markedly increased in the next decades, largely because of an increased awareness and improved diagnostic capabilities. Research on the epidemiology of sarcoidosis in India has provided insights into its prevalence, clinical characteristics, and outcomes.

Interstitial Lung Disease

Interstitial lung disease (ILD) is a collective term used for a group of over 200 conditions of different etiologies characterized by similar clinical and radiological features. Most conditions in the group show a progressively downhill course, although the speed of progression is widely variable. The initial condition, Hamman–Rich syndrome, first described in 1935, was characterized by a rapidly progressive form of ILD, now known as acute interstitial pneumonia. The term idiopathic pulmonary fibrosis (IPF) was first used in the 1940s to describe a chronic, progressive form of ILD. Classification and diagnostic criteria for different types have been repeatedly changed since the first classification system described in the American Thoracic Society Statement (1978).

The introduction of HRCT in the 1980s has revolutionized ILD diagnosis, allowing for more accurate categorization. Currently, the prototype ILD with pulmonary fibrosis is a group of conditions together listed as Idiopathic Interstitial Pneumonitis, of which both AIP and IPF are the relentlessly progressive forms. Several other types of ILDs, which have been recognized, include the CTD-related disorders, chronic hypersensitivity pneumonias, ILD induced by drugs and radiation, occupational exposure-related ILDs, and granulomatous inflammatory disorders. CTD-ILD with interstitial parenchymal involvement is frequently seen in conditions such as systemic sclerosis, rheumatoid arthritis, Sjögren's syndrome, systemic lupus erythematosus, mixed CTD, antisynthetase syndrome, and others. Autoimmune pulmonary alveolar proteinosis is another rare autoimmune disease that causes inflammation and scarring in the lungs.

The complex, multifactorial nature of the disease has led to the development of multidisciplinary approaches to diagnosis, treatment, and management. The development of antifibrotic medications has improved the treatment options for patients with IPF and other forms of ILD. Their role in IPF, however, is limited to slowing down the rate of decline in lung function. The search for a drug that can reverse or even stop the progression of fibrosis is still on. ILDs with a hypersensitivity or inflammatory background respond better with anti-inflammatory treatments. For example, the rheumatoid lung disease, which occurs as a complication of rheumatoid arthritis, scleroderma, lupus pneumonitis, and other CTDs, characterized by inflammation and subsequent scarring of the lungs, shows significant improvement with corticosteroids and/or other immunosuppressant drugs.

Some other rare conditions described in the mid-20th century include eosinophilic pneumonia, characterized by inflammation and eosinophilic infiltration in the lungs, eosinophilic granulomatosis with polyangiitis (previously known as Churg–Strauss syndrome), granulomatosis with polyangiitis (previously known as Wegener's granulomatosis), microscopic polyangiitis, and lymphomatoid granulomatosis.

Pulmonary Vasculitides

Vasculitides, vasculitis, or angiitis constitute a group of conditions characterized with inflammation of blood vessels of different organ systems. They were first characterized in the early 20th century, with Goodpasture's syndrome being the first recognized entity in 1919. This is a rare autoimmune disease that causes inflammation of vessels in the lungs and kidneys.

Most of the vasculitides involve multiple organs and present with clinical features related to that organ. Wegener's granulomatosis, a condition characterized by granulomatous inflammation of the blood vessels of the lungs, nose, and upper respiratory tract was renamed as granulomatosis with polyangiitis in 2010 when it was discovered that the German physician Friedrich Wegener had a strong Nazi connection as a member of "Sturmabteilung' the brownshirts—a paramilitary branch of the Nazi party that participated in violent conflicts. Churg–Strauss syndrome was revised to Eosinophilic Granulomatosis with Polyangiitis (EGPA) on evaluation of the eponyms due to the 2012 Revised International Chapel Hill Consensus Conference on nomenclature of vasculitides.

There are quite a few other important systemic vasculitides that do not generally involve the lungs but may rarely do so. Periarteritis nodosa, now known as polyarteritis nodosa, has been one of the earliest described conditions since 1866. Others include Takayasu arteritis, described by the Japanese physician, Mikito Takayasu, characterized by inflammation of the aorta and its branches, and Giant cell arteritis, with the characteristic giant cells in the blood vessel walls.

Miscellaneous Disorders

In addition to the groups of diseases described above, which were either unknown or inadequately described in the past, several rare and anecdotal disorders have been identified in the last two centuries. Advances in genetic research have improved our understanding of respiratory diseases, such as cystic fibrosis and asthma. Individually, these diseases may belong to the main groups: Infectious diseases, hypersensitivity and autoimmune disorders, diseases due to industrial, occupational, and environmental exposures, and congenital and genetic diseases. Respiratory neoplasms and respiratory sleep disorders constitute other important groups, which include a variety of different conditions. Severe respiratory illnesses requiring respiratory intensive/critical care and chronic disabling diseases requiring pulmonary rehabilitation are other important conditions that have emerged in the last century.

As medicine is expanding widely in its spectrum, it is also becoming more and more individualized. There is an obvious attempt to understand each disease as it manifests and responds to treatment in each individual patient, with the premise that 'one size does not fit all'. The development of personalized medicine has enabled targeted treatments for respiratory diseases based on individual morphological and/or genetic profiles, further enlarging the number and types of diseases.

Sources

1. Sakai T, Morimoto Y. The History of Infectious Diseases and Medicine. Pathogens. 2022;11(10):1147.
2. Cunha BA, Burillo A, Bouza E. Legionnaires' disease. Lancet. 2016;387(10016):376-85.
3. Whitfield J. Portrait of a serial killer. Nature. 2016. doi:10.1038/news021001-6.
4. Glatter KA, Finkelman P. History of the Plague: An Ancient Pandemic for the Age of COVID-19. Am J Med. 2021;134(2):176-81.
5. Roser M. (2020). The Spanish flu: The global impact of the largest influenza pandemic in history. [Online] Available from https://ourworldindata.org/spanish-flu-largest-influenza-pandemic-in-history [Last accessed September, 2025].
6. Spreeuwenberg P, Kroneman M, Paget J. Reassessing the global mortality burden of the 1918 influenza pandemic. Amer J Epidemiol. 2018;187(12):2561-7.
7. World Health Organization. (2021) Latest COVID-19 Information. [Online] Available from http://www.who.int/covid-19 [Last accessed September, 2025].
8. Lim WM. Editorial: History, lessons, and ways forward from the COVID-19 pandemic. Int J Quality Innov. 2021;5(2):101-8.
9. Hao YJ, Wang YL, Wang MY, Zhou L, Shi JY, Cao JM, et al. The origins of COVID-19 pandemic: A brief overview. Transbound Emerg Dis. 2022;69(6):3181-97.
10. Morens DM, Breman JG, Calisher CH, Doherty PC, Hahn BH, Keusch GT, et al. The Origin of COVID-19 and Why It Matters. Am J Trop Med Hyg. 2020;103(3):955-9.
11. Edouard Mathieu, Hannah Ritchie, Lucas Rodés-Guirao, Cameron Appel, Daniel Gavrilov, Charlie Giattino, et al. "COVID-19 Pandemic". 2020 Published online at OurWorldinData.org. Retrieved from: https://ourworldindata.org/coronavirus' [Online Resource]
12. Laxminarayan R, Jameel S, Sarkar S. India's Battle against COVID-19: Progress and Challenges. Am J Trop Med Hyg. 2020;103(4):1343-7.

13. Jindal SK, Jindal A, Moitra S. Problems of management of non corona respiratory diseases in the era of COVID 19. Int J Non Commun Dis. 2020;5:63-9.
14. Sharp PM, Hahn BH. Origins of HIV and the AIDS pandemic. Cold Spring Harb Perspect Med. 2011;1(1):a006841.
15. HIV and AIDS. Fact Sheet. World Health Organization. https://www.who.int/news-room/fact-sheets/detail/hiv-aids
16. Margo CE, Harman LE. Autoimmune disease: Conceptual history and contributions of ocular immunology. Surv Ophthalmol. 2016;61(5):680-8.
17. Agmon-Levin N, Lian Z, Shoenfeld Y. Explosion of autoimmune diseases and the mosaic of old and novel factors. Cell Mol Immunol. 2011;8(3):189-92.
18. Spagnolo P. Sarcoidosis: a Critical Review of History and Milestones. Clin Rev Allergy Immunol. 2015;49(1):1-5.
19. Jindal SK. Mycobacterial relationship of sarcoidosis: the debate continues. Expert Rev Resp Med. 2008;2:139-43.
20. Guler SA, Corte TJ. Interstitial Lung Disease in 2020: A History of Progress. Clin Chest Med. 2021;42(2):229-39.
21. Interstitial Lung Diseases: A Historical Note. In: Clinical Atlas of Interstitial Lung Disease. London: Springer; 2006.
22. Jindal SK, Gupta D. Incidence and recognition of interstitial pulmonary fibrosis in developing countries. Curr Opin Pulm Med.1997;3(5):378-83.
23. Dhooria S, Agarwal R, Dhar R, Jindal A, Madan K, Aggarwal AN, et al. Consensus Statement for the Diagnosis and Treatment of Idiopathic Pulmonary Fibrosis in Resource-Constrained Settings. Indian J Chest Dis Allied Sci. 2018;60(2):91-119.
24. Arkuszewski P, Cieślak-Arkuszewska A. Undisclosed facts in Friedrich Wegener's links with Nazism. Histopathology. 2025;86(3):317-26.
25. Sargin G. The Evaluation of Changing the Eponym Churg-Strauss Syndrome Due to the 2012 Revised International Chapel Hill Consensus Conference Nomenclature of Vasculitides. J Clin Med. 2024;13(12):3424.
26. Mora B, Bosch X. Medical eponyms: Time for a name change. Arch Intern Med. 2010; 170(16):1499-500.
27. Brown KK. Pulmonary vasculitis. Proc Am Thorac Soc. 2006;3(1):48-57.
28. Mehrotra AK, Swami S, Soothwal P, Feroz A, Dawar S, Bhangoo HD. Pulmonary Vasculitis: Indian Perspective. Indian J Chest Dis Allied Sci. 2016;58(2):107-19.
29. Bambery P, Bhushnurmath B, Jindal SK, Datta B. Pulmonary Vasculitis: An Indian Perspective. Seminars in Respiratory Medicine. 1991;12:115-23.
30. Robinson PN. Deep Phenotyping for Precision Medicine. Hum Mutat. 2012;33(5):777-80.
31. Goetz LH, Schork NJ. Personalized medicine: motivation, challenges, and progress. Fertil Steril. 2018;109(6):952-63.

CHAPTER

13

Respiratory Sleep Disorders

Sleep is the period of rest for both the mind and the body. On an average, one spends about one-third of daily life in sleep. Sleep, therefore, has tremendous importance both in health and disease. There are significant alterations in almost all normal physiological functions during sleep. It is natural therefore that the pathological states are also affected differently during sleep. In modern history, sleep has been extensively studied since mid-19th century starting with the experiments of Kohlschütter who applied systematically varying acoustic stimuli to study the depth of sleep. It is rather interesting to note that sleep is not only a restful period promoting recovery from troublesome conditions but sometimes associated with equally disturbing and distressful psychological and physical symptoms.

Respiratory Sleep Disorders

Respiratory conditions constitute an important group of respiratory sleep disorders that affect breathing during sleep, leading to disrupted sleep patterns, reduced oxygen levels, and other complications. Respiratory sleep disorders now include a large number of conditions with varied presentation. The prototype obstructive sleep apnea (OSA) is characterized by pauses in breathing due to airway obstruction, often caused by relaxed throat muscles or obesity. Loud snoring, nocturnal choking, morning headaches, fatigue, and daytime sleepiness are some other common symptoms.

Besides OSA, several other important conditions recognized in the broad group include the central sleep apnea (CSA), mixed sleep apnea, sleep-related hypoventilation, nocturnal limb movement disorder, rapid eye movement behavior sleep disorder, and insomnia. Childhood OSA is another worrying condition which is being more frequently recognized. OSA is frequently complicated by high blood pressure, diabetes, increased risk of cardiovascular diseases, stroke, and sudden death. OSA is frequently associated with overlap conditions and comorbidities further complicating the natural history.

Historical Perspectives

The concept of respiratory sleep disorders has evolved over time. Early mention of sleep-related breathing abnormalities can be found in texts belonging to the ancient civilizations including the *Ayurvedic Samhitas*. The Greek physician, Hippocrates had described a condition characterized by excessive daytime sleepiness and snoring while Aristotle had noted that some people would stop breathing during sleep, only to resume breathing later. Ancient Indian yogic and tantric practices had also emphasized the importance of breathing and sleep in maintaining overall health. Nothing much, however, was described beyond the occasional mention of sleep. The medieval physician, Avicenna, had described conditions resembling sleep apnea at the end of the first millennium CE.

It was only in the modern period that the problem was recognized in the true sense. The first medical publication on the subject by Alberti and Lust in 1745 described details of anatomical risk factors such as obesity and a short neck, which caused obstruction of the airway passages during sleep. There were no reports on respiratory *apnea* during sleep. Even Charles Des-Alleurs, a French medical doctor who had proposed a classification for respiratory disorders in his *Apnéologie méthodique* did not include sleep-related apneic events.

Interestingly, some of the early descriptions owe their origins to literary contributions. The American author, Nathaniel Hawthorne wrote about a person who would stop breathing during sleep in his novel "*The House of the Seven Gables*". Charles Dickens' famous 1836 novel, "*The Posthumous Papers of the Pickwick Club*" featured a character named Joe, a fat and somnolent boy, who was described as having a "confoundedly" large appetite and being prone to falling asleep. This character's depiction is often cited as the first literary reference to Pickwick syndrome, which can be possibly identified as obesity hypoventilation syndrome.

Modern Era Developments

In medical literature, the first reported case of obstructive sleep apnea was described in a child by William Osler in 1892. Osler, originally a Canadian citizen had spent much of his professional life at Johns Hopkins in Baltimore in the United States and is commonly known as "the father of modern medicine".

The child, a 7-year-old boy who presented with symptoms of excessive daytime sleepiness, loud snoring, and breathing difficulties during, would fall asleep during the day, even while sitting or standing. The boy underwent surgical removal of his tonsils and adenoids following which he showed significant improvement with reduced daytime sleepiness and snoring.

Osler's report marked the beginning of medical recognition of this condition, but it was not until the 20th century that childhood OSA began to receive more attention. Since then, our understanding of childhood OSA has grown significantly. We now know that it is a common condition affecting approximately 3% of children, with the peak prevalence occurring between 2 and 8 years old. Meanwhile, it was reported in adults in 1903 by French neurologist, Pierre Marie, who described a condition characterized by obesity, hypersomnia, and respiratory symptoms. Several reports in adults appeared in the subsequent decades. The American physician, Burwell, reported a series of cases featuring obesity, alveolar hypoventilation, and pulmonary hypertension in 1956. The syndrome was thereafter formally defined in the 1960s, with the establishment of criteria for diagnosis of obesity hypoventilation syndrome.

Wider acceptance of the disorders in the 1960s and 1970s led to the establishment of sleep laboratories to systematically study the sleep disorders, including OSA. Polysomnography (overnight sleep study) became the standard for diagnosis of various sleep disorders. The development of portable sleep monitors and home sleep apnea testing has further improved diagnosis and treatment of respiratory sleep disorders. Treatments such as lifestyle changes, continuous positive airway pressure therapy, and bilevel positive airway pressure have significantly improved outcomes for patients with sleep disorders. New treatments, such as oral appliances and hypoglossal nerve stimulation, have expanded treatment options. Surgical procedures to remove excess tissue or correct anatomical issues are employed as indicated. Recently, the US Food and Drug Administration (FDA) in December 2024 approved a weight reducing medicine, tirzepatide as the first drug to treat moderate-to-severe obstructive sleep apnea in adults with obesity.

Indian Developments

Mention of sleep and its impact on health and well-being can be found in ancient Indian texts such as the *Vedas*. Ayurvedic texts of Mauryan and post-Mauryan era also describe sleep disorders such as including insomnia (*Anidra*) and excessive sleep (*Atinidra*). *Ashtanga Hridayam*, the influential Ayurvedic text (400 CE) discusses sleep disorders and their treatments. The *Yoga Sutras* of Patanjali (2nd century CE) provided some insights into brain function, consciousness, and sleep, linking consciousness to a divine expression within individuals.

Ayurveda classified sleep into seven types based on their causes, and it also recognized the importance of prayer and invoking the goddess *Nidra Devi* for sleep. Sleep is considered one of the three pillars of health (*Trayopastambha*).

Ayurvedic texts emphasize the importance of a healthy lifestyle, including proper sleep habits, for maintaining overall well-being. Sleep disorders are attributed to imbalances in the *three doshas* (*Vata, Pitta, and Kapha*).

Descriptions of sleep disorders include difficulty falling asleep, waking up frequently, and excessive daytime sleepiness. Ayurvedic texts also recommend herbs such as *Brahmi, Jatamansi*, and *Tagara* for promoting relaxation and improving sleep. Lifestyle modifications with sleep hygiene practices, such as maintaining a consistent sleep schedule and creating a relaxing sleep environment are also considered essential. Ayurveda's approach to sleep disorders emphasizes the interconnectedness of physical, mental, and spiritual health.

Medieval Period scholars such as Chakrapani Datta (11th century CE) and Bhavamishra (16th century CE) further elaborated on sleep disorders and their treatments in commentaries on classical Ayurvedic texts. The Unani system of medicine, introduced to India during this period, also discussed sleep-related issues and their management. The prominent Unani physician, Hakim Ajmal Khan wrote about sleep disorders and their treatments in the context of Unani medicine. The introduction of Western medicine during the British period led to the establishment of modern sleep medicine in India leading to a more comprehensive understanding of sleep-related issues.

The post-Independence period was marked by a gradual increase in awareness, diagnosis, and treatment which almost paralleled the global history. In India, sleep practices and perceptions were influenced by traditional medicine and lifestyle besides the cultural and social factors. The rapid modernization and urbanization during the British period led to changes in sleep patterns and the emergence of new sleep-related issues. There was a significant increase in interest in sleep medicine. The first sleep laboratories were established in India in the 1960s and 1970s since when the Indian researchers began studying sleep disorders. In the mid-20th century, researchers such as Dr Baldev Singh at the All India Institute of Medical Sciences, New Delhi began studying sleep and wakefulness using more sophisticated tests and analyzing sleep patterns in patients referred from neurology and psychiatry departments.

Respiratory sleep disorders found little specific mention in most of the texts thus far. It was toward the end of the 20th century that respiratory sleep problems were recognized as an issue of major public health concern requiring increased awareness and education among healthcare professionals and the general public in view of the high prevalence of sleep disorders, particularly OSA. Efforts to raise awareness and promote recognition of the syndrome have led to earlier diagnosis and treatment.

Sources

1. Schulz H, Salzarulo P. The development of sleep medicine: a historical sketch. J Clin Sleep Med. 2016;12(7):1041-52.
2. Dickens C. The Posthumous Papers of the Pickwick Club; 1867 (reprint). p. 8.

3. Littleton SW, Mokhlesi B. The Pickwickian syndrome-obesity hypoventilation syndrome. Clin Chest Med. 2009;30(3):467-78.
4. Smith BJ. A sleep and a forgetting: William Osler's beliefs about aging and death. Can Fam Physician. 2015;61(2):167-8.
5. Burwell CS, Robin ED, Whaley RD, Bickelmann AG. Extreme obesity associated with alveolar hypoventilation: a Pickwickian syndrome. Am J Med. 1956;21:811-8.
6. Kryger MH. Sleep apnea. From the needles of Dionysius to continuous airway pressure. Arch Intern Med. 1983;143:2301-3.
7. Lavie P. Nothing new under the moon. Historical accounts of sleep apnea syndrome. Arch Intern Med. 1984;144:2025-8.
8. Lavie P. Who was the first to use the term Pickwickian in connection with sleepy patients? History of sleep apnoea syndrome. Sleep Med Rev. 2008;12:5-17.
9. Teschler H, Randerath W. Sleep-related breathing disorders - historical development, current status, future prospects. Pneumologie. 2010;64(9):583-9.
10. Vorona, Robert D et al. History and epidemiology of sleep-related breathing disorders. Oral Maxillofac Surg Clin North Am. 2002;14(3):273-83.
11. FDA.gov. (2024). [online] Available from https://www.fda.gov/news-events/press-announcements/fda-approves-first-medication-obstructive-sleep-apnea [Last accessed September 2025].

CHAPTER

14

Interventional Pulmonology

Interventions in medicine refer to procedures performed to prevent, diagnose, or treat a medical condition, disease, or injury. Factually, all kinds are treatments used in modern medicine involve one or the other kind of pharmacological or non-pharmacological intervention which can be either involving surgical, semi-surgical or non-invasive techniques. Broadly speaking, lifestyle and dietary modifications also involve therapeutic interventions. In common parlance, however, an interventional procedure employs an invasive, or at least a semi-invasive or minimally invasive methodology generally for purpose of diagnosis of an illness.

In pulmonary medicine, different invasive interventions focus on the use of bronchoscopic and pleural endoscopic procedures. Image-guided percutaneous procedures to obtain aspirates or biopsies from pleural or lung nodules and masses are also commonly used for histopathological diagnosis.

Pleural interventions commonly include procedures such as thoracentesis, pleural biopsy, chest tube placement, and pleurodesis. These are commonly done procedures for pleural effusions of all kinds as well as for empyema, pneumothorax, and other pleural diseases.

Pleural Drainage

There is little evidence of direct invasive pulmonary interventions in the ancient literature. Pleural drainage for empyema was described by Hippocrates in the ancient, pre-historic times. The Ebers Papyrus of Egypt as well as the *Sushruta Samhita* described the procedure for draining abscesses, which may have included pleural empyema. In India, the history of pleural drainage is a similar story of gradual development and growth. *Sushruta Samhita*, the ancient Ayurvedic text, described a procedure called "*Vrana shodhana*" or "wound cleansing", which involved draining abscesses and empyema. The Ayurveda had described various techniques for draining fluid from the pleural space, including the use of needles and tubes. Excavations at the ancient city of Taxila (now in Pakistan) uncovered surgical instruments, including Susruta's needle, dating back to the 6th century BCE which was used for draining empyema.

Subsequent contributions from ancient civilizations and medieval physicians point to the presence of the continued practice. Medieval Arabic physicians such as Al-Razi and Ibn Sina made significant contributions to the field of surgery, including the management of pleural empyema. During the Middle Ages, European physicians such as Guy de Chauliac and Ambroise Paré described various procedures for draining abscesses, including pleural empyema.

The 18th and 19th centuries saw significant advances in thoracic surgery including the development of procedures for draining pleural empyema. The use of chest tubes for draining pleural empyema became more widespread during this period. A closed drainage system was developed in the modern times in the 19th century to prevent the entry of air into the pleural space and reduce infection risk. Besides needle thoracentesis and chest-tube drainage, placement of intrapleural catheters is practised on more permanent basis for recurrent and persistent effusions such as in cases of malignancy. The development of imaging technologies such as X-rays, computed tomography (CT) scans, and ultrasound further improved the methods of diagnosis and management.

British physicians introduced modern medical techniques, including pleural drainage, to India. The first reported cases of pleural drainage in India were published in the Indian Medical Gazette in the late 19th century. Indian surgeons, PK Sen and RN Chakravarty, played a significant role in developing thoracic surgery including pleural drainage techniques. Chest tubes became widely available during this period, making pleural drainage a more common and effective procedure.

Advances in imaging technologies, such as ultrasound and CT scans, have improved the accuracy and safety of pleural drainage procedures. Small-bore catheters have become increasingly popular in India, offering a less invasive and more comfortable alternative to traditional chest tubes. Indian surgeons and physicians have gained significant expertise in pleural drainage, with many publishing research papers and presenting at international conferences.

Bronchoscopy

Bronchoscopy has a more recent history that spans over a century and a half beginning with Gustav Killian, a German physician who in 1897 removed a pork bone from a farmer's airway, using an esophagoscope. He had used a rigid tube with a built-in light source. Endoscopes into other body cavities were already being used by physicians earlier. Killian was however first to undertake medical inspection of the human airway. Alfred Kirstein, another German physician developed the first practical bronchoscope in 1898. The procedure was done in an awake patient using a local anesthetic agent, topical cocaine. Chevalier Jackson, an American otolaryngologist, used a refined rigid bronchoscope for inspection of the trachea and main bronchi and laid the foundation for the modern-day rigid bronchoscopy in the early 20th century.

Rigid bronchoscopes were used exclusively until the flexible bronchoscope was developed by the Japanese physician, Shigeto Ikeda in 1966. Soon, the first commercially available flexible bronchoscope was introduced in 1967 by André G de Vries, a Dutch physician. The initial flexible bronchoscope, with a diameter of 5–6 mm, employed fiberoptic bundles requiring an external light source for illumination. Being flexible, they had the ability to bend and could be used to visualize and enter the lobar and segmental bronchi for obtaining fluid and biopsy samples. Later, these were largely replaced with bronchoscopes using charge-coupled device (CCD) video chips at the inner end.

Introduction of video bronchoscopes enormously improved visualization and documentation capabilities. Various diagnostic and therapeutic procedures with the bronchoscopy were added in the late 20th and early 21st centuries. Today, bronchoscopy is used for both diagnostic as well as therapeutic indications.

Besides visual examination of the airways, the commonly used bronchoscopic diagnostic procedures include bronchial and transbronchial biopsies, needle aspirates, and broncho-alveolar lavage. Endobronchial ultrasound and electromagnetic navigation tools have further expanded the role of bronchoscopy for different conditions. Bronchoscopy in several ways has contributed to the success of lung transplantation programs. Therapeutic bronchoscopy is mostly used for patients of bronchial tumors for application of laser or electrical energy, cryotherapy, stent placements, and balloon dilatation for bronchial narrowing. Bronchoscopic lung volume reduction with use of endobronchial one-way valves is sometimes employed in patients with emphysema. Bronchial thermoplasty with use of heat energy to reduce airway smooth muscle and improve lung function in patients with severe asthma is now less commonly employed.

Indian Perspectives

In India, British physicians had introduced modern bronchoscopy and thoracoscopy techniques primarily with use of rigid instruments. While RN Cooper, a surgeon, performed early procedures in 1920s in Mumbai, rigid bronchoscopy in the post-Independence was first introduced by physicians, such as RN Chakravarty and S Roy in major cities such as Kolkata and Mumbai. It remained confined to large cities with limited availability of expertise. Physicians often depended upon cardiothoracic surgeons to perform rigid bronchoscopy. It was possible, another cardiac surgeon, PK Sen, who introduced flexible fiberoptic instruments in 1960s which completely revolutionized the clinical practice of respiratory medicine.

Flexible bronchoscopy, first introduced in 1970s in Mumbai and Chandigarh, soon became widely available with many hospitals and medical institutions acquiring the necessary facilities. Most Indian pulmonologist have adopted and contributed to the advances in bronchoscopy procedures and imaging technologies. Bronchoscopy has played a crucial role in the diagnosis and management of lung cancer and other lung diseases in India.

Thoracoscopy and Video-assisted Thoracic Surgery

Thoracoscopic diagnostic or surgical procedures with minimally invasive techniques, such as video-assisted thoracic surgery (VATS) are used to diagnose and treat various thoracic conditions. Thoracoscopic visualization of the thoracic cavity and biopsy procedures to collect tissue samples for histopathological examination helps to diagnose conditions such as pleural effusions, pneumothorax, or mediastinal masses as well as for examination of the lungs and pleura. Thoracoscopic surgery is also used for removal of lung tissue, including wedge resections, segmentectomies, and lobectomies; pleurectomy, thymectomy, esophagectomy, and several other kinds or surgeries involving thoracic structures.

Robotic thoracic surgery with use of robotic systems has enhanced precision and dexterity. Thoracoscopic procedures have revolutionized the field of thoracic surgery, providing patients with safer and more effective treatment options. Compared to open surgical techniques, VATS has the advantages of a shorter hospital stay and faster recovery time. Moreover, there is reduced postoperative pain and discomfort and less scarring.

Thoracoscopy perhaps was first done by Sir Francis Cruise in 1865 to examine the pleural space in a patient with empyema. But the credit goes to Hans Christian Jacobaeus, a Swedish physician who performed it to treat adhesions that limited the success of artificial pneumothorax which was earlier introduced by Forlanini in 1882 for the treatment of pulmonary tuberculosis. He had also inserted a galvanocautery instrument through a separate entry site to divide adhesions between the lung and chest wall. Soon the procedure was widely adopted with reports of series of 1,000 or more cases. In spite of the significant complications, it continued to be popular until after the introduction of streptomycin in 1945.

Thoracoscopy was initially used to diagnose and treat conditions such as pleurisy, empyema, and pneumothorax. The development of more sophisticated thoracoscopes, including rigid and flexible instruments, enabled better visualization and manipulation within the thoracic cavity. Eric Leyden introduced the first modern thoracoscope in the 1960s. Thoracoscopy became more widely used for diagnosing and treating conditions such as lung cancer, mesothelioma, and pleural effusions. Development of VATS by Robert in

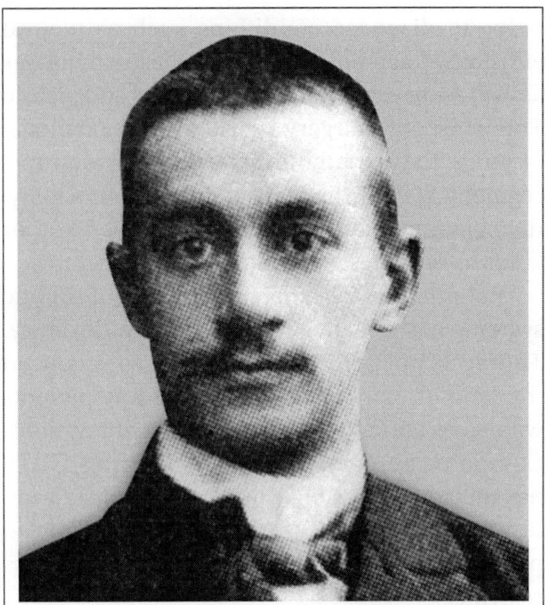

Hans Christian Jacobaeus, a Swedish internist performed first thoracoscopic exploration in 1910.

the 1990s enabled surgeons to perform complex thoracic procedures using smaller incisions and thoracoscopic guidance. VATS significantly advanced the field of minimally invasive thoracic surgery. The development of new surgical techniques, such as single-incision VATS and robotic-assisted thoracic surgery, has further expanded the applications of thoracoscopy.

Thoracoscopy, like bronchoscopy in India, was initially performed by cardiothoracic surgeons like PK Sen and RN Chakravarty in the 1950s and 1960s at a few major hospitals. VATS was introduced in the 1990s. Presently, thoracoscopy and VATS have become widely accepted and practiced for pleural, lung, and mediastinal diseases.

Other Percutaneous Interventions

Some other minimally invasive interventions include tests or procedures such as imaging studies or laboratory tests routinely employed to diagnose diseases. Percutaneous route is frequently used to approach pleural, mediastinal, and lung nodules. Either blind or image guided, transthoracic needle aspiration, and biopsy is commonly employed for evaluation. Similarly, some of the pulmonary therapeutic inventions may involve a minimally invasive technique such as pleural fluid aspiration, vaccination, desensitization therapy, and pulmonary rehabilitation. The minimally invasive techniques enable precise diagnosis and treatment with image guidance. They offer several other benefits such as the reduced risk of complications and faster recovery times. They also provide enhanced patient comfort and reduce the need for surgical interventions.

Indian Developments

The first image-guided needle aspiration and biopsy procedures were performed in the late 1980s and early 1990s. Interventions, such as percutaneous lung biopsy and percutaneous fiducial marker placement inside and around a tumor being treated for cancer have been commonly used. The concept of minimally invasive surgery had been around for decades, but its application in pulmonary medicine gained momentum in the 1990s and 2000s when Indian surgeons began adopting and adapting these techniques, paving the way for future advancements. VATS emerged as a significant development in minimally invasive thoracic surgery.

Indian surgeons started using VATS for various thoracic procedures including lung cancer surgery, empyema, and pleural diseases. In recent years, some Indian hospitals and research institutions have made significant strides in minimally invasive pulmonary techniques. For instance, some hospitals now offer advanced procedures such as balloon pulmonary angioplasty and pulmonary endarterectomy for chronic thromboembolic pulmonary hypertension.

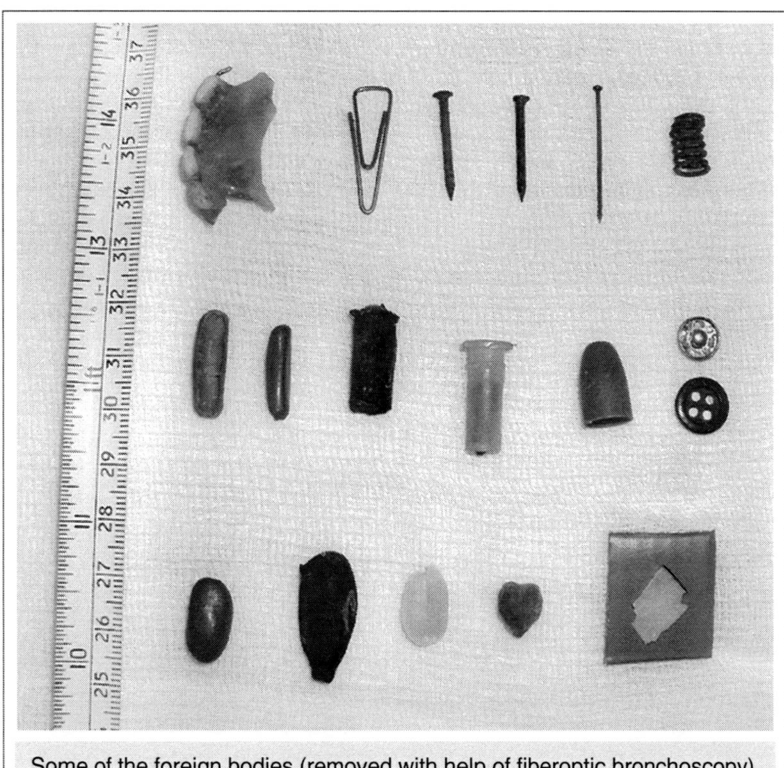

Some of the foreign bodies (removed with help of fiberoptic bronchoscopy).

Despite these advancements, there are still challenges to overcome, such as limited access to these techniques. But with the growing expertise and infrastructure in India, the future of minimally invasive pulmonary techniques looks promising. The future of minimally invasive interventions in pulmonology in India is promising, with a projected growth rate of 10–15% per annum. Artificial intelligence and machine will enhance diagnostic accuracy, predict patient outcomes, and optimize treatment plans. Growing awareness and private sector investment in healthcare infrastructure and technology will drive the growth of minimally invasive interventions.

Sources

1. Panchabhai TS, Mehta AC. Historical perspectives of bronchoscopy. Connecting the dots. Ann Am Thorac Soc. 2015;12(5):631-41.
2. Vaidya PJ, Leuppi JD, Chhajed PN. The evolution of flexible bronchoscopy. From historical luxury to utter necessity!! Lung India. 2015;32(3):208-10.
3. Ikeda S, Yanai N, Ishikawa S. Flexible bronchofiberscope. Keio J Med. 1968;17:1-16.
4. Braimbridge MV. The history of thoracoscopic surgery. Ann Thorac Surg. 1993;56(3):610-4.
5. Thomas PA Jr. A thoracoscopic peek: what did Jacobaeus see? Ann Thorac Surg. 1994;57(3):770-1.
6. Marchetti GP, Pinelli V, Tassi GF. 100 years of thoracoscopy: historical notes. Respiration. 2011;82(2):187-92.
7. Madan K, Tiwari P, Thankgakunam B, Mittal S, Hadda V, Mohan A, et al. A survey of medical thoracoscopy practices in India. Lung India. 2021;38(1):23-30.
8. Murthy V, Bessich JL. Medical thoracoscopy and its evolving role in the diagnosis and treatment of pleural disease. J Thorac Dis. 2017;9(Suppl 10):S1011-S1021.
9. Hoksch B, Birken-Bertsch H, Müller JM. Thoracoscopy before Jacobaeus. Ann Thorac Surg. 2002;74(4):1288-90.

10. Shah R, Sun L, Ridge CA. Image guided lung biopsy. Lung Cancer. 2024;192:107803.
11. Kim DY, Sun JS, Kim EY, Park KJ, You S. Diagnostic accuracy and safety of CT-guided percutaneous lung biopsy with a coaxial cutting needle for the diagnosis of lung cancer in patients with UIP pattern. Sci Rep. 2022;12:15682.
12. Sharma VK, Manjunath BG, Singh P, Chaudhry D. Interventional Pulmonology and Issues Related to the Lung Surgery. Lung India. 2022;39(Suppl 1):S21-3.
13. Sorino C, Feller-Kopman D, Mei F, Mondoni M, Agati S, Marchetti G, et al. Chest Tubes and Pleural Drainage: History and Current Status in Pleural Disease Management. J Clin Med. 2024;13(21):6331.
14. Walcott-Sapp S, Sukumar M. A History of Thoracic Drainage: From Ancient Greeks to Wound Sucking Drummers to Digital Monitoring. 2022. https://www.ctsnet.org/article/history-thoracic-drainage

CHAPTER 15

Resuscitation and Critical Care

In modern medicine, intensive or critical care has assumed a pivotal role in different medical and surgical specialties. Critical care essentially involves medical care for people who have life-threatening injuries and illnesses. Though it is a boon in saving innumerable lives, it sometimes serves as a bane by prolonging a vegetative life and delaying death. Starting with resuscitation of vital organ function, critical care includes several components of management of organ dysfunction and assisted life support systems. Resuscitation, more precisely cardiopulmonary resuscitation (CPR), is an emergency procedure involving the revival of cardiac and respiratory functions. Resuscitation, however, includes restoration of all other vital functions as well. Assisted respiratory support is one of the most important and critical steps in a critical care unit.

Historical Aspects

Resuscitation: Religions and Mythological Stories

The history of resuscitation is rather old, while intensive care globally is a recent phenomenon; a story of rapid evolution, driven by advances in medical science and technology. Resuscitation of the life of a person who has died has remained a fantasy in most ancient religious and mythological stories of different civilizations. The Hindu married women often recall the story of Savitri on the occasion of the *"karva-chowth"* fast. Savitri, a devoted wife, brought her husband Satyavan back to life by convincing the god of death, *Yama*, to return his soul. Bhishma, a legendary character of the *Mahabharata*, was revived by the god Krishna's divine intervention after he was mortally wounded in the war. All five *Pandava* brothers, who were the protagonists of the *Mahabharata*, were killed by their enemies but later revived by the god Krishna's divine intervention. In the Shiva *Purana*, there is a story of King Daksha, who was beheaded by the god Shiva but was later revived and given a goat's head. In the *Bhagavata Purana*, Sandipani Muni, the guru of Lord Krishna, was killed by a demon but later revived by Krishna's divine powers. The god Vishnu, in his incarnation as the tortoise *Kurma*, had helped to revive the gods and demons who died during the famous *Samudra Manthan*, i.e., churning of the ocean.

Greek and Egyptian mythologies also abound with stories of divine resuscitation. Orpheus, a musician and poet, journeyed to the underworld to reclaim his beloved wife Eurydice, who had died. He charmed the rulers of the underworld with his music, and they agreed to let him take Eurydice back to the world of the living. Asclepius, the god of medicine, was killed by Zeus but was later resurrected and became a god. Osiris, the god of the afterlife, was killed by his brother Set. His wife, Isis, gathered up his body parts and, with the help of the god Thoth, brought him back to life long enough to conceive their son Horus. In ancient Egyptian mythology, the pharaoh was believed to become a god in the afterlife. The myth of the resurrection of the pharaoh was central to the Egyptian concept of the afterlife. The Eight Immortals, a group of deities in Chinese mythology, were said to have achieved immortality through their good deeds and are often depicted as being resurrected or reincarnated. In Christianity, Jesus Christ had raised Lazarus from the dead in the Biblical Story of Lazarus (John 11:1-44).

These stories in different religions and mythologies illustrate the theme of resuscitation and revival, often involving divine intervention or supernatural power. But the concept persisted in historical accounts of later periods. In the 13th century, Robert of Artois, a French nobleman who was killed in battle, was revived by a surgeon. In medieval Indian folklore, Kabir, a poet and mystic, is said to have revived a Muslim saint who had died. Anne Green, a servant, was hanged for infanticide but was revived after being cut down from the gallows. In 1740, James Duport, a British clergyman who was killed in a carriage accident, was revived by a surgeon.

Dramatic stories of resuscitation and revival are known throughout the 19th and 20th centuries as well. Some of these examples defy existing knowledge and explanation, while others may imply misinformation and misquotation. Still others may indicate the presence of unusual circumstances. In 1857, an Indian soldier was hanged but was revived after being cut down from the gallows. In 1999, Anna Bågenholm, a Norwegian skier, was trapped under a layer of ice for 80 minutes and revived after being rescued.

Mouth-to-Mouth Resuscitation

All these stories of resuscitation with divine interventions from different parts of the world demonstrate the importance of preserving human life. In the present times, resuscitation consists of measures to restore spontaneous blood circulation and breathing in a person who has suffered from cardiorespiratory arrest. It involves repeated chest compressions often combined with mouth-to-mouth breathing in an effort to manually preserve intact brain function. Mouth-to-mouth respiration is sometimes known as Elisha breathing, derived from the act of Prophet Elisha of the Hebrew Bible and the Christian Old Testament. Elisha brought back to life the son of a *Shunammite* woman who had died. "Elisha laid on the boy, putting his mouth on the boy's mouth, his eyes on the boy's eyes, and his hands on the boy's hands; he prayed to God, asking Him to revive the boy" (2 Kings 4:18-37).

Roots of mouth-to-mouth resuscitation can also be traced to ancient scriptures and Ayurvedic texts, which described a technique called *"mukha-mārga,"*—blowing air into the mouth of a person who has stopped breathing. Sushruta Samhita also mentioned a similar technique called *"prāṇa-pratīkṣepa"* (restoring life force). References to both the methods can also be found in the later medieval Indian texts such as Vagbhata, Chakrapani, Rajavallabha, and Sharngadhara Samhita. The Mughal medical texts, Tibb-i-Akbari, written during the reign of Mughal Emperor Akbar, and Al-Hawi by the Indian physician Hakim Muhammad Sharif Khan, also mention both the techniques that involved blowing air into the mouth of a person who had stopped breathing.

The Moroccan traveler, Ibn Battuta, wrote about witnessing Indian villagers using mouth-to-mouth resuscitation to revive people who had stopped breathing during his travels to India (Travels of Ibn Battuta, 14th century). Historical accounts from the Mughal Empire (16th to 19th centuries) describe the use of mouth-to-mouth resuscitation to revive drowning victims. Other historical accounts are available in the travel stories of the French physician and traveler, Francois Bernier, who wrote about witnessing Indian physicians using mouth-to-mouth resuscitation to revive patients. Another French traveler and merchant, Jean-Baptiste Tavernier, also described Indian physicians using mouth-to-mouth resuscitation to revive drowning victims. British colonial officers and travelers wrote about witnessing Indian villagers using mouth-to-mouth resuscitation to revive people who had stopped breathing. It is also likely that European travelers and traders who visited India during the 16th to 18th centuries may have learned about these techniques and carried them back to Europe.

The modern mouth-to-mouth resuscitation techniques, which were influenced by ancient Indian practices, were developed in the 1950s by Peter Safar and James Elam, two American physicians. It soon became a standard technique in Western medicine, with the American Heart Association and other organizations promoting its use. Today, mouth-to-mouth resuscitation is an essential component of CPR, which is taught worldwide as a lifesaving technique. The Indian Red Cross Society has been promoting mouth-to-mouth resuscitation as a lifesaving technique since the 1950s.

Other Aspects of Critical Care

Ancient history is also replete with medical interventions related to critical care and resuscitation. For example, ancient Indian texts such as the *Charaka Samhita and the Sushruta Samhita* described critical care concepts, including respiratory support, fluid management, and wound care. The *Ebers Papyrus* described techniques for resuscitating drowning victims, including mouth-to-mouth respiration. Later physicians like Hippocrates and Galen described techniques for resuscitating patients, including the use of bellows for ventilation. Their works on anatomy, physiology, and pharmacology laid the foundation for later innovations and practices that are relevant to modern critical care medicine.

In the Middle Ages, scholars like Ibn Sina (Avicenna) and Ibn Rushd (Averroes) made significant contributions to medical knowledge in critical care concepts. The monasteries and convents provided care to the sick and injured, laying the groundwork for later hospital developments. As for all other fields in medicine, it was during the period of the Renaissance that Vesalius's work on human anatomy laid the foundation for later surgical and critical care advancements. Similarly, William Harvey's work on blood circulation revolutionized the understanding of cardiovascular physiology and critical care. The discovery of anesthesia in the 1840s by William Morton and Crawford Long enabled the development of modern surgery and critical care. In addition, other advancements in medical science, including the development of antibiotics and mechanical ventilators, allowed for the treatment of conditions previously deemed untreatable.

Mechanical Ventilation

Most of the milestone developments actually happened during the 19th century onwards. Physicians like John Dalziel and Friedrich Trendelenburg developed techniques for mechanical ventilation. The first mechanical ventilator, known as the "iron lung," was developed by John Dalziel, a Scottish physician, in 1832. He was inspired to create a mechanical respirator after observing patients struggling to breathe due to respiratory diseases. He experimented with various designs, eventually developing a tank-like device with a pump that created a partial vacuum to provide negative pressure ventilation and expand the lungs. The tank enclosed the patient's body while the patient's head protruded from the tank, allowing for breathing. Dalziel tested his iron lung on animals and later on human patients, refining his design based on the results. The iron lung was not widely adopted during his lifetime, but his innovative design laid the groundwork for future developments in mechanical ventilation. Philip Drinker's iron lung, developed in 1928, was heavily influenced by Dalziel's work.

The iron lung was used extensively during the polio epidemic in the first half of the 20th century in the United States. Paul Alexander, who contracted polio in 1952, developed paralysis below the neck when he was six. He remained in the iron lung since then and breathed his last in 2024. He had earned a law degree, practiced law, and also published a memoir, "Three Minutes for a Dog," typing each word with his mouth.

A mechanical ventilator called the "Pulmotor" was patented in 1907 by the German engineer Heinrich Drager. The first model was only a prototype, while further modifications of the breathing connector and the control mechanism led to the development of the positive pressure ventilator for patient use. It was powered by a hand crank, which created a partial vacuum to expand the lungs. The device used a bellows-like mechanism to deliver air to the patient through a mouthpiece or mask connected to the Pulmotor. The device was particularly useful in treating soldiers with cholera and pneumonia, which were prevalent during the war. The device was not widely available, and its use was limited to select military hospitals. Moreover, there were technological limitations. The Pulmotor influenced the development of future mechanical ventilators, paving the way for more advanced life-support technologies.

Essentially, the ventilator employs the principle of a "*bellows,*" a device used by blacksmiths to blow air into a fire. The 'bellow' ventilator is used to drive pressurized gas to a patient who cannot breathe. It employs a flexible gas reservoir that expands and contracts, i.e., *a bellows*, to deliver air to the patient to produce inspiratory flow. Bellows ventilators are often more reliable than other types of ventilators. The Engstrom ventilator, developed by Carl-Gunnar Engstrom in 1950, was another positive-pressure ventilator that used a piston-driven system.

The introduction of microprocessor-controlled ventilators in the 1980s in the modern era has revolutionized mechanical ventilation, allowing for precise control of ventilation parameters. Noninvasive ventilation (NIV) with the use of a facial mask or nasal interface instead of an endotracheal tube, initially introduced in the 1990s, became increasingly popular for managing respiratory failure. The new technology has improved patient-ventilator synchrony and outcomes. It has enabled the development of advanced ventilation modes, such as pressure-support ventilation and proportional assist ventilation. Another important step to optimize patient care includes the development of closed-loop ventilation systems, which use algorithms to adjust ventilation parameters in real-time. Multiple options of ventilation with portable and wearable ventilators for home care and emergency medicine have also become available.

Mechanical Ventilation in India

Mechanical ventilation in India became available in the first half of the 20th century with significant advancements in the latter half. The first mechanical ventilators imported from foreign countries were introduced primarily in major cities, such as Mumbai, Delhi, and Kolkata. The demand for ventilators increased significantly, driven by the growing need for critical care services in India. The development of indigenous ventilators helped in the expansion of services to a wider range of the population in various other cities and towns. The Indian government's "Make in India" initiative has also encouraged domestic manufacturing of ventilators, reducing dependence on imports.

Indian companies like Medtronic India, Philips Healthcare India, and Skanray Technologies are some of the companies engaged in developing ventilator solutions.

Noninvasive ventilation is becoming increasingly popular in India, particularly for managing respiratory failure in patients with chronic obstructive pulmonary disease. Overall, India has made significant progress in the development and adoption of mechanical ventilation technology, with a growing focus on indigenous innovation and manufacturing.

Intensive Care Units

The growing demand for specialized care and intense monitoring required for critically ill patients, supplemented with advances in medical technology, such as with reference to mechanical ventilation, led to the need for specialized wards, the intensive care units (ICUs). There were no dedicated ICUs in the hospitals in the early days. Instead, critically ill patients were scattered throughout the hospital, receiving care from various teams. However, the need for specialized care became apparent as the medical technology improved and the complexity of cases increased.

The concept of ICUs gained momentum in the 1950s and 1960s, particularly during the polio epidemics. Hospitals began setting up dedicated units to provide close monitoring and life-sustaining interventions for critically ill patients. Hospitals in Denmark and Sweden set up specialized units to care for patients with respiratory failure. The first ICU was established in 1953 at the Copenhagen Municipal Hospital in Denmark by Dr Bjørn Ibsen. The 1960s saw the development of cardiovascular ICUs, which focused on caring for patients with heart conditions. The introduction of mechanical ventilation in the 1960s revolutionized ICU care, enabling hospitals to support patients with respiratory failure. The 1970s witnessed significant advancements in monitoring and diagnostic tools, including the development of pulmonary artery catheters and echocardiography.

The next few decades saw further expansion and advancement with modernization and the introduction of specialized ICUs. These included cardiovascular ICUs, neurological ICUs, neonatal ICUs, pediatric ICUs, and others. Surgical ICUs and trauma units served the needs of accident and trauma victims as well as of patients with acute surgical emergencies. In recent years, the coronavirus disease 2019 (COVID-19) pandemic has highlighted the importance of ICUs worldwide. The surge in critically ill patients during the pandemic had exposed weaknesses in healthcare systems and the need for intensive care, particularly in resource-constrained areas.

Contemporary Intensive Care Units

Today, the ICUs employ advanced technologies related to the monitoring of different vital functions and assistive support for their dysfunction and failure. More importantly, the modern ICUs emphasize the importance of multidisciplinary teams, including intensivists, nurses, respiratory therapists, and other specialists who play a vital role in overall intensive care. Some of the more advanced facilities also incorporate innovative technologies like tele-ICU services for remote monitoring and consultation. This expansion of tele-ICU capabilities has improved access to specialized care, especially in the remotely situated, underserved regions. Such facilities have also proved to be helpful during natural disasters.

The history of intensive (or critical) care in India is closely tied to the global evolution of critical care medicine. India's journey with ICUs began taking shape with the first respiratory intensive care units (RICUs) in two hospitals in Mumbai by Farokh E Udwadia in the mid-1970s. Training in critical care medicine was provided in some of these RICUs as 1–3 months short-term courses. In the 1990s, the postdoctoral department (DM) (Pulmonary Medicine) course, started at Chandigarh, was expanded to DM (Pulmonary and Critical Care Medicine) with an additional year of course curriculum. In due course of time, DM (Critical Care) was also introduced as a separate super specialty.

Over the years, ICUs in India have become increasingly sophisticated, with various specialized units emerging to cater to specific medical requirements. These include coronary care units, pediatric ICUs, and neonatal ICUs, among others. ICU services expanded rapidly during the 1990s and 2000s, with the establishment of private hospitals and corporate healthcare chains. The Indian Society of Critical

Care Medicine (ISCCM) was founded in 1993 to promote the development of critical care medicine in India.

India continues to face several challenges in relation to ICU services. There is a significant shortage of critical care specialists and nurses. Moreover, ICUs are largely concentrated in urban areas, leaving rural areas with limited access to critical care. Many ICUs lack adequate infrastructure and resources, including ventilators, monitors, and trained staff. Continued efforts are being made to increase awareness and education about critical care medicine among healthcare professionals and the general public. There is a growing need to expand ICU services to rural areas and to increase the number of critical care specialists in India, as well as to improve infrastructure and resources.

Critical Care Nursing

The history of nursing dates back to thousands of years, with evidence of caregiving and healing practices found in ancient civilizations when nursing care was provided by priests, priestesses, family members, slaves, and other caregivers. The Hippocratic Oath emphasized the importance of compassion and confidentiality. Phoebe, a Christian nurse, is mentioned in the Bible (Romans 16:1-2) for her care of the sick and elderly during the first century CE. Another Roman nurse, Fabiola, is said to have established a hospital in Rome to provide care to the poor and sick during the fourth century CE. Monasteries and convents provided nursing care, with monks and nuns serving as caregivers. In Europe, nursing began to emerge as a distinct profession, with the establishment of nursing schools and training programs during the Middle Ages.

In the modern era, Florence Nightingale, a British social reformer, statistician, and nurse, is considered the founder of modern nursing. She had studied nursing in Germany at the Institute for the Care of Sick Gentlewomen in Kaiserswerth, returned to London, and became the superintendent of the Hospital for Gentlewomen. During the Crimean War (1853–1856), Nightingale traveled to Turkey to provide care to British soldiers. Nightingale established the first professional nursing school in London in 1860, which became a model for nursing education worldwide. She published "Notes on Nursing" in 1860, which remains a foundational text in the field of nursing. She used statistical analysis to demonstrate the importance of sanitation and hygiene in reducing mortality rates. Her experiences during the Crimean War led her to advocate for improvements in sanitation, hygiene, and patient care. Her birthday, May 12, is celebrated as International Nurses Day. Also, the Florence Nightingale Medal, established in 1912, is the highest international distinction for a nurse.

Caring for the sick in India has also been practiced since thousands of years and is deeply rooted in the country's rich cultural and spiritual heritage. *Dhanvantari*, the god of medicine, is often depicted with a nursing attendant. Buddhist monasteries provided care to the sick and injured, with monks and nuns playing a significant role in nursing. The school of Mahayana Buddhism, in particular, emphasized the importance of compassion and care for the sick. Both the original Ayurvedic texts describe surgical nursing care techniques, including wound dressing and patient hygiene.

Nursing during the medieval and Mughal periods was provided by the social workers and family members who played a significant role in caring for the sick. Spiritual practices, such as prayer and meditation, were integral to patient care. These traditional practices continue to influence modern nursing in India. Professional nursing was introduced during the late colonial period, while the Indian Nursing Council was established in 1947. The Indian Nursing Council regulates nursing education and practice in India.

The establishment of ICUs gave rise to the need for specialized nursing care tailored to critically ill patients. The 1960s and 1970s saw significant advancements in critical care nursing, with the establishment of the American Association of Critical-Care Nurses (AACN), which played a crucial role in defining the scope of practice, establishing standards of care, and promoting professional development for ICU nurses.

Undoubtedly, the development of ICUs has transformed the way critically ill patients receive care, significantly improving outcomes and saving countless lives. But intensive care in India faces significant challenges, including workforce conditions, education and training, and accessibility to usable clinical resources. The COVID-19 pandemic has further highlighted the importance of intensive care and the need for continued innovation and advancement in this field. High costs beyond the affordable limits of most Indians remain the major roadblock to intensive care. The serious issues related to moral and ethical dilemmas of critical care continue to bother the Indian medical, legal, and social fraternity of India, even more than elsewhere in the world.

Sources

1. Roos D. (2005). 6 Ancient Resurrection Stories. [Online] Available from https://www.history.com/news/resurrection-stories-ancient-cultures [Last accessed September, 2025].
2. Varma RR. Hindu mythology and medicine. BMJ. 2004;328(7443):819.
3. Trubuhovich RV. History of mouth-to-mouth rescue breathing. Part 2: the 18th century. Crit Care Resusc. 2006;8(2):157-71.
4. Baker AB. Artificial respiration: the history of an idea. Medical History. 1971;15(4):336-51.
5. In: Tossach W (Ed). Man dead in appearance recovered by distending lungs with air. Medical Essays and Observations. London and Edinburgh: T.W. and T. Ruddimans; 1744. pp. 605-8.
6. Hall M. Asphyxia, its rationale and its remedy. Am J Med Sci. 1856;32:224-7.
7. Hurt R. Modern cardiopulmonary resuscitation—not so new after all. J R Soc Med. 2005;98 (7):27-31.
8. Cooper JA, Cooper JD, Cooper JM. Cardio-pulmonary resuscitation: history, current practice, and future direction. Circulation. 2006;114 (25):2839-49.
9. www.bible.com. Acts - Chapter 2 (ESV). [Online] Available from https://www.bible.com/bible/compare/2KI.4.32-35 [Last accessed September, 2025].
10. Slutsky AS. History of Mechanical Ventilation. From Vesalius to Ventilator-induced Lung Injury. Am J Respir Crit Care Med. 2015;191(10):1106-15.
11. Kacmarek RM. The mechanical ventilator: past, present, and future. Respir Care. 2011;56(8):1170-80.
12. Tobin MJ. Mechanical ventilation. N Engl J Med. 199330 (15):1056-61.
13. Bauer PR. A Short History of Mechanical Ventilation. In: Bellani G (Ed). Mechanical Ventilation from Pathophysiology to Clinical Evidence. Cham: Springer; 2022.
14. Kelly FE, Fong K, Hirsch N, Nolan JP. Intensive care medicine is 60 years old: the history and future of the intensive care unit. Clin Med (Lond). 2014;14(4):376-9.
15. Ristagno G, Weil MH. History of Critical Care Medicine: The Past, the Present and the Future. In: Gullo A, Lumb PD, Besso J, Williams GF (Eds). Intensive Critic Care Med. Milano: Springer; 2009.
16. Prayag S. ICUs worldwide: critical care in India. Crit Care. 2002;6(6):479-80.
17. Devanandan S. N P Singh: History of the first intensive care unit in Delhi - reminiscences. Indian J Anaesth. 2010;54(6):574-5.
18. Kulkarni AP, Zirpe KG, Dixit SB, Chaudhry D, Mehta Y, Mishra RC, et al. Development of critical care medicine in India. J Critic Care. 2020;56:188-96.
19. Murkute U. Historical perspectives of critical care in India and worldwide. Indian J Hist Sci. 2024;59(4):297-305.
20. Jindal SK. Pulmonary and Critical Care Medicine -Objectives of training (Part I). Lung India. 1997;15:112-14.
21. Jindal SK. Pulmonary and Critical Care Medicine -curriculum & evaluation (Part II). Lung India. 1997;15:164-67.
22. Bambi S. Evolution of Intensive Care Unit Nursing. Nursing in Critical Care Setting. 2017;489-524.
23. Karimi H, Masoudi Alavi N. Florence Nightingale: The Mother of Nursing. Nurs Midwifery Stud. 2015;4(2):e29475.
24. Gnanadurai A. Critical Care Nursing in India. Crit Care Nurs Clin North Am. 2021;33(1):61-73.

CHAPTER 16

Oxygen: The Essence of Life

Oxygen constitutes around half of the earth's crust. It supports the survival of all living beings. Oxygen, as an essential component of air, reflects the story of evolution dating back millions of years. However, the use of oxygen for medical treatments with which we are concerned is rather recent, discovered only in the last two centuries.

History of Evolution of Oxygen

Evolution of oxygen has been a very slow process which can be identified with the appearance of life on the earth. Life on Earth is said to have begun in an oxygen-free environment some 3.5–4.5 billion years ago where organisms relied on anaerobic metabolism *(fermentation)*. The earliest evidence of energy production is attributed to emergence of *chemiosmosis* through the movement of ions across membranes. Almost a billion years later, the evolution of oxygen-producing cyanobacteria marked a significant turning point. These microorganisms harnessed sunlight to produce oxygen through *photosynthesis* resulting in a gradual increase of oxygen levels in the atmosphere. This dramatic event (which actually took place over millions of years) is commonly known as the *Great Oxygenation Event* which transformed the Earth's atmosphere and paved the way for more complex life forms.

Oxygen levels in the atmosphere slowly stabilized, fluctuating between 10 and 30% of modern levels. A rapid diversification of life occurred around 541 million years ago (*Cambrian Explosion*) resulting in the emergence of many animal phyla. Gradually, there was evolution of complex body plans including bilateral symmetry, segmentation, and appendages. Ecosystems became more complex, with the emergence of predators, prey, and symbiotic relationships. The evolution of more complex life forms, including plants and animals, helped to further stabilize oxygen levels. The first humans (Homo sapiens) appeared in Africa approximately 300,000 years ago. Today, oxygen makes up approximately 21% of the Earth's atmosphere.

Ancient Concepts of Breathing as Essential for Life

The subject has been briefly mentioned in the first chapter on breathing. Importance of air as essential for life was identified ever since the known history of ancient civilizations even though the concept of oxygen as we know it today was not understood. Ancient Chinese philosopher Zhuangzi discussed the importance of "*qi*" (life energy), which is associated with breath and air. Similarly, ancient Greece (5th century BCE) philosophers Empedocles and Aristotle (5th and 4th century BCE) recognized the importance of air for human life. Aristotle proposed that air is one of the four fundamental elements (along with earth, fire, and water) necessary for life. Erasistratus, in the 3rd century BCE, in Egypt had recognized the interplay between air and blood while Galen, in the 1st–2nd century CE had conceptualized a two-way movement of inspired air and effluent waste vapors.

Medieval Period

John Severinghaus in an elegant article describes eight "sages" between the 13th and 18th centuries who discovered that the air we breathe contains something that we need and use. The Arab physician Ibn al-Nafis described the process of respiration and the role of lungs in exchanging air. But the concept of oxygen as we understand it today did not appear. Michael Servetus (16th century) in France described the pulmonary circulation and its effect on blood color. The others included Michael Sendivogius, John Mayow, Carl Wilhelm Scheele, Lavoisier, Joseph Priestley, and Henry Cavendish.

Early scientific discoveries in Europe between 1500 and 1800 CE helped to clarify some of the issues. Leonardo da Vinci made detailed observations about human respiration and recognized the importance of air for life. William Harvey's discovery of blood circulation (1628) laid the foundation for understanding the role of oxygen in human physiology while Robert Boyle's experiments with air pressure and volume helped establish the concept of air as a physical substance. Finally, Carl Wilhelm Scheele, Joseph Priestley, and Antoine-Laurent Lavoisier discovered oxygen in the late 18th century.

Indian Perspectives

The idea of "*prana*" or life force was mentioned in the Vedas, which dates back to around 1500 BCE. *Prana* was believed to be the vital energy that sustains life. The Vedic age scripture, *Rigveda,* mentions the concept of "*prana*" which was associated with breathing and air. The ancient Indian physician Charaka mentioned the importance of breathing and respiration in his medical text, the Charaka Samhita, the foundational text of Ayurveda. It described the concept of "*prana*" or "*pranavayu,*" which refers to the vital force or energy essential for life. While "*prana*" is not directly equivalent to oxygen, it is related to the idea of breathing and the essential energy required for life. Charaka's work emphasized the importance of proper breathing along with diet and exercise to maintain overall health and well-being.

It is important to note that "*prana*" and "*pranavayu*" respectively mean "life" and "life-air" even in modern Sanskrit and Hindi languages. Here are a few Sanskrit verses from Charak Samhita that relate to *prana or pranavayu*:

1. Charak Samhita, Sutrasthana 11.34:
   प्राणः प्राणवायुर्जीवनं सर्व प्राणिनाम्
   "Pranah pranavayur jivanam sarva prani nam."
   (*Prana* is the same as *pranavayu* (life-giving air), and it sustains all living beings.)

2. Charak Samhita, Sutrasthana 12.8:
   वायुस्तेन जीवति सर्वम्तेन जीवति
   "Vayus tena jivati sarvam tena jivati."
   [All living beings live due to the presence of *vayu* (air), and they sustain their life through it.]

Indian alchemists and physicians also continued to explore the properties of air and respiration. But the understanding of oxygen as a distinct element was still lacking. Incidentally, the role of Sarangadhara, a 13th century Indian physician is often missed from the list of seven sages partly because of the linguistic barriers and poetic expressions in Sanskrit which did not allow widespread communication. Sarangadhara had explicitly described the concept of respiration:

> नाभिस्थ : प्राणपवन : स्पृष्ट्वा हृत्कभलान्तरम् ।।
> कण्ठाद्बहिर्विनिर्याति पातुं विष्णुपदामृतम् ।
> पीत्वा चाम्बरपीयूषं पुनरायाति वेगतः ।।
> प्रीणयन्देहमखिलं जीवयश्चुठरानलम् ।

[The "*vayu*" (i.e., air) located in the "*hrdaya*" (Chest) goes out, and after drinking the "*Ambarapiyush*" (nectar), it goes back very quickly. It touches the interior of "*hrdaya*", promotes the "*Jatharanatha*" (life), and nourishes the entire body.] It describes the sequences leading to the inhalation of ambrosia, the nectar-like substance vital to life, from the outside air, its circulation through the heart to the brain and all other parts of the body. This "nectar like substance" is likely to be what we now know as oxygen.

Discovery of Oxygen

Antoine Lavoisier, a French chemist, is credited with the discovery of oxygen in 1778. Oxygen in fact was discovered earlier in 1774 by an English chemist named Joseph Priestley by heating mercuric oxide. He found that this gas supported combustion and respiration, which he called "*dephlogisticated air*." He also discovered other gases, including carbon dioxide, nitrogen, and ammonia. But Priestley faced persecution in England and, therefore, emigrated to the United States. He is often considered as one of the founders of modern chemistry. Almost at the same time, Carl Wilhelm Scheele, a Swedish pharmacist and chemist, noticed that a gas was released while heating manganese oxide with sulfuric acid. He called it the "fire air" (later known as oxygen). Priestley published his findings in a series of 6 volumes "Experiments and Observations on Different Kinds of Air" from 1774 onwards. Scheele's manuscript, however, was not published until 1777, 3 years after Priestley's publication. As a result, Priestley is often credited with the discovery of oxygen, although Scheele had actually discovered earlier. He was called as "hard-luck Scheele" by Isaac Asimov since a number of his chemical discoveries were later credited to others.

Priestley had also demonstrated that the gas supported life of a mouse better than the air. He commented: *"It might be salutary to the lungs in certain cases when the common air would not be sufficient to carry off the phlogistic putrid effluvium fast enough"*. In the 18th century, chemists believed in the phlogiston theory, which stated that a fire-like element called phlogiston was released during combustion. Lavoisier, however, was sceptical of this theory. Lavoisier repeated Priestley's experiment and discovered that the gas produced was not only essential for combustion but also necessary for respiration. He named this gas "oxygen," derived from the Greek words "*oxys*" (acid) and "*genes*" (generator), as he believed it was a fundamental component of acids. He compared respiration with the process of combustion and demonstrated that animal respiration involved the absorption of oxygen by the lungs from the inhaled air and elimination of carbon dioxide and water. Lavoisier also showed the essential nature of oxygen for human life that oxygen consumption increased with increased body activity. Lavoisier, who was an aristocrat by birth, was executed during the French Revolution in 1789.

Lavoisier's discovery of oxygen also marked a significant turning point in the history of chemistry. He disproved the phlogiston theory and established oxygen as a fundamental element. His work laid the foundation for modern chemistry and paved the way for future discoveries. He is often referred to as the "Father of Modern Chemistry" for his contributions to the field. The discovery of oxygen revolutionized the field of chemistry and paved the way for major breakthroughs in understanding the natural world. It also revolutionized the understanding of respiration and the role of oxygen in human life. It soon started to be used for therapeutic indications.

Other Related Developments

The 19th century witnessed several other clinical and physiological discoveries which clarified the need and use of oxygen for therapeutic purposes. In particular, the assessment of oxygen and carbon dioxide in the blood made it possible to precisely discover the clinical indications for oxygen use. Some of the initial methods included the vacuum extraction technique by Magnus and some other manometric or volumetric methods employed by Van Slyke, Scholander, and others. These methods were rather slow and elaborate for routine performance. Further refinements led to the development of highly accurate and fast response analyzers. Role of hemoglobin in the transport of oxygen by the blood described by Hoppe-Seyler and the identification of tissue respiration in the cells described by Pfluger helped in further understanding. Dalton gave the atomic theory of respiratory gases, while Paul Bert described the oxygen-dissociation curve in the early 1870s. The curve initially depicted as "hyperbolic" was changed to the sigmoid shape later by Bohr. The "Bohr effect" and the "Haldane effect" were reported later in the early 20th century.

Therapeutic Use of Oxygen

Oxygen for medical management was first used by Thomas Beddoes in the early 1800s. He collaborated with James Watt, the inventor of the steam-engine to build a pneumatic piston to store and deliver oxygen. Oxygen was commercially produced first time in 1895 by Carl Von Luide using fractional distillation of liquid air. Soon after, oxygen became a "cure-all" medicine for a large number of illnesses without any specific oxygen deficiency. There was no consistent or demonstrable benefit for most patients. Soon, oxygen became unpopular and achieved a kind of notoriety. Even eminent physicians such as William Osler were fearful of its toxicity than benefits. However, later developments, supported by firm clinical and experimental evidence, established that oxygen deficiency in a disease state was responsible for severe physiological disturbances which could be corrected with supplemental oxygen.

It was mostly during the 20th century when it was realized that therapeutic administration of oxygen had a significant role in the treatments of cardiac and respiratory diseases. John Haldane, who had used oxygen to treat chlorine poisoning during World War I, had made his tell-tale statement that *"hypoxia not only stops the machine but wrecks the machinery"*. Meakins reported that apart from the cure of infection, oxygen therapy was perhaps the most important factor in the treatment of pneumonia. There was a great resurgence of interest in improving the methods and devices used for oxygen administration. Different types of masks, oxygen tents, and cannulae were developed during the world wars. Medical and technological developments from the latter part of 20th century onwards have made oxygen as a highly valuable part of therapy for patients with cardiorespiratory illnesses and many other critical conditions in the emergency, intensive care units as well as for domiciliary care on long-term basis.

Oxygen toxicity had been long suspected almost since the first use by Von Liebig, Pasteur, Bent, and others. But increase in indications for oxygen raised greater concerns about its toxic effects on the lungs. Different investigators started recognizing respiratory failure as "oxygen toxicity lung" and "respirator lung" due to excessive oxygen use and release of "oxygen-free radicals". Devison factually compared the oxygen molecule to a grenade which could cause tremendous damage once the safety pin was pulled out.

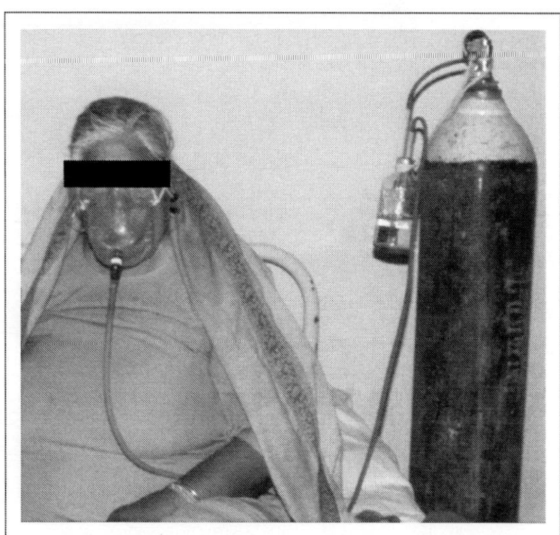

Oxygen administration to a patient in mid-20th century.

Portable oxygen concentrators were developed, allowing patients to receive oxygen therapy outside of hospitals. There were also advancements in oxygen delivery systems, including nasal cannulae, masks, and ventilators. Oxygen therapy has revolutionized the treatment of various medical disorders both in emergency and chronic conditions. It is not only used for respiratory but also for cardiovascular and other conditions characterized with hypoxia and oxygen deficiency. It is also used as a life-saving treatment for emergency medicine (e.g., cardiac arrest, trauma) and carbon monoxide poisoning. Development of long-term, domiciliary use for several chronic diseases has significantly improved patient outcomes, reduced mortality rates, and enhanced quality of life for millions worldwide. Oxygen therapy is now considered as a "medicine" for both acute and chronic maintenance therapy.

Long-term, Domiciliary Oxygen

Importance of continuous use of oxygen for the reversal of hypoxemia in patients with chronic obstructive lung disease was first described by Alvan Barach in the 1920s. Later in the 1950s, ambulatory oxygen was shown to improve exercise tolerance by Cotes in UK. It was also shown to reverse or at least reduce polycythemia and pulmonary hypertension in two studies on domiciliary use of oxygen in patients of chronic obstructive lung. A significant improvement in overall survival was also shown. Studies by the Medical Research Council (MRC) and the National Institute of Health (NIH) in 1980–1981 are considered landmark studies in the use of domiciliary oxygen thus firmly establishing the beneficial role of long-term oxygen therapy. Indications for domiciliary oxygen soon expanded to include several other chronic lung diseases associated with hypoxemia or breathlessness. Presently, the modality of treatment is widely used, sometimes without any proven evidence. Oxygen use at home has now assumed the role of a maintenance drug for many debilitating diseases in patients with chronic congestive heart failure, malignancies, and other non-respiratory illnesses.

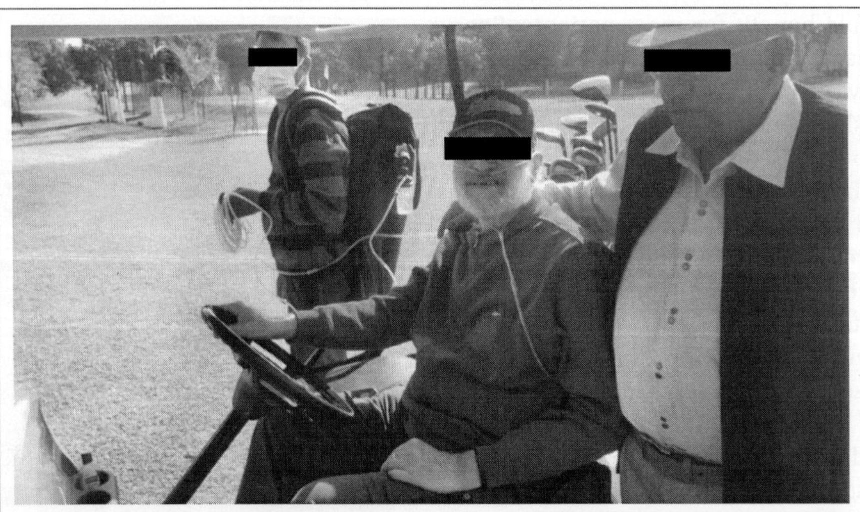

21st Century: One of our patients on ambulatory oxygen playing golf.

Hyperbaric Oxygen

Hyperbaric oxygen therapy (HBOT), which involves breathing oxygen in a pressurized chamber, is also gaining popularity for several serious and sometimes life-threatening conditions. Hyperbaric air chambers to treat different ailments have been used since 1662 in one or the other form with varying degrees of enthusiasm and antagonism. It was in the early 20th century when hyperbaric oxygen was first used to treat decompression sickness in deep sea-divers. Later, the scope of therapy was extended to cover several other clinical indications. This treatment is used to enhance the body's natural healing process by increasing oxygen flow to damaged tissues. HBOT promotes wound healing especially to treat diabetic foot ulcers, radiation injuries, and other nonhealing wounds by increasing oxygen flow to the damaged tissues. HBOT also stimulates the immune system, helping the body fight off infections. There are many other proven or presumptive indications for which HBOT is being used at present.

Indian Perspectives

In Ayurveda, oxygen is associated with the concept of "*prana*" (life force). Some Ayurvedic practitioners emphasize the importance of proper breathing techniques to balance *prana*. Hindus in India believe in the concept of *Pancha Bhuta,* or the five elements—earth, water, fire, air, and ether. Oxygen is associated with the air element, which is considered vital for life. *Prana* refers to the life force or vital energy. Oxygen is essential for sustaining life and is often associated with *Prana*. Fire is considered sacred, and oxygen is essential for combustion. Most Hindu religious ceremonies are performed with "*havana*", the sacred fire. In some Hindu traditions, the dying person is placed near an open window or outside to facilitate the flow of fresh air and oxygen, believed to aid in the transition of the soul. As the final death rites (*Antyeshti),* the body is cremated (*Agni Sanskar*), and the fire is believed to purify the soul.

Oxygen, therefore, is valued as more than a simple treatment for hypoxia. It is sometimes administered as a terminal act to a dying person. There are also mistaken beliefs that oxygen deficiency is a common health issue, leading to unnecessary use of oxygen supplementation. Some Indians believe that oxygen bars can cure various ailments, including respiratory issues and stress. Certain companies in India market "oxygen-rich" water, claiming it has various health benefits. Nevertheless, experts argue that the human body cannot absorb oxygen from water. Some people believe that inhaling oxygen directly from cylinders can help alleviate respiratory issues. Apparently, most such beliefs are exaggerated claims largely for commercial reasons.

Even the medical use of oxygen in the hospital had been practiced erroneously and commonly identified with placement of a nasal catheter (or a face mask) attached with a tube to an oxygen cylinder for a patient with a serious illness. There are a number of errors associated with assessment of uses and misuses of oxygen. It is commonly believed by the nursing staff even in large hospitals that oxygen is a gas that improves patient's dyspnea. There are no protocols for oxygen therapy in most hospitals.

As per modern medical practices, oxygen therapy is employed as per standard indications in various medical conditions. In post-colonial India, the country's healthcare infrastructure expanded and oxygen therapy became more widely available. Oxygen therapy began to be used in Indian hospitals, particularly in urban areas especially for the treatment of respiratory diseases. In recent years, India has made significant strides in increasing access to oxygen including in rural areas. It is important to consider oxygen as a drug and have oxygen treatment protocols and educational programs. Like that for a drug, a proper oxygen prescription should specify the oxygen concentration to be administered, flow to be used, source and the method of oxygen delivery. Need for aerosolization should also be defined. Finally, monitoring for continuation should be regularly reviewed at fixed intervals.

COVID-19 Crisis in India

The COVID-19 pandemic during 2020–2022 highlighted the importance of oxygen therapy in India. Indian hospitals faced a crisis situation due to oxygen shortages. In May 2021, India's hospitals were at break point leading to global newspaper headlines. One of the biggest challenges was to provide enough medical oxygen for the sickest patients, unable to breathe unaided, as the demand rose tenfold. Some hospitals posted "oxygen out of stock" signs, while others asked patients to search for treatment elsewhere. Oxygen support became one of the rate-limiting steps for medical care during the pandemic.

The government, however, took rapid corrective steps and upgraded the oxygen-infrastructure to provide better care for patients. The Indian government allocated funds to support the expansion activities, procurement of oxygen equipment, and training of healthcare workers. The government introduced policy reforms to streamline the production, storage, and distribution of oxygen, ensuring a more efficient and responsive system. The Indian government and private sector collaborated to increase oxygen production, setting up new oxygen plants and augmenting existing ones. Many hospitals, including in rural areas, installed oxygen generation plants to reduce reliance on oxygen cylinders and ensure a steady supply. Some of the large navy and corporate hospitals in cities such as Mumbai, Chennai, and Delhi have also established HBOT treatment centers.

The pandemic also accelerated the adoption of innovative technologies, such as oxygen generators and cryogenic oxygen tanks. Indian innovators and start-ups designed affordable oxygen concentrators, making oxygen therapy more accessible to those in need. In addition, the government and medical organizations conducted training programs for healthcare workers on oxygen therapy, including the use of oxygen concentrators and ventilators. Public awareness campaigns were also launched to educate people about the importance of oxygen therapy, its proper use, and the prevention of oxygen-related complication.

The COVID-19 pandemic has indeed served as a watershed moment for oxygen therapy in India, highlighting the need for a robust and responsive oxygen infrastructure. In the pre-COVID-19 era, only 1,000 MT was available for medical usage. This was increased up to 19,940 MT through the strengthening of in-house oxygen manufacturing, low-cost innovations, and enhanced storage facilities. National Oxygen Stewardship Program' was initiated to build the capacity of health care workers. It is essential to maintain the momentum gained during the pandemic and continue to strengthen it further. Integrating oxygen therapy into primary healthcare services can help ensure timely and effective treatment for patients with respiratory illnesses.

Oxygen therapy today is widely available in India, with both public and private healthcare providers offering oxygen services. The COVID-19 crisis has significantly facilitated the improvement of the facilities and overall awareness. However, challenges persist, particularly in rural and resource-poor areas. Efforts are ongoing to improve access to oxygen therapy, increase awareness about its benefits, and develop more innovative and cost-effective solutions.

Sources

1. Holland HD. The oxygenation of the atmosphere and oceans. Philos Trans R Soc Lond B Biol Sci. 2006;361(1470):903-15.
2. Dole M. The Natural History of Oxygen. J Gen Physiol. 1965;49(1):5-27.
3. Crowe SA, Døssing LN, Beukes NJ, Bau M, Kruger SJ, Frei R, et al. Atmospheric oxygenation three billion years ago. Nature. 2013;501(7468):535-8.
4. Rutten MG. The history of atmospheric oxygen. Space Life Sci. 1970;2:5-17.
5. Dickerson RE. Chemical evolution and the origin of life. Sci Am. 1978;239:70-86.

6. Dwarkanath C. The development of Indian Medicine - Sarangadhara's contribution. New Delhi: Central council for Research in Ayurveda and Sidha Ministry of Health and Family Welfare, Govt. of India; 1991.
7. Sarangadharacharya P. The Sarangadhara Smihta. Bombay: Nirnaya-Sagar Press; 1920.
8. Fitting JW. From Breathing to Respiration. Respiration. 2015;89:82-7.
9. Franklin KJ. A Short History of Physiology, 2nd edition. London: Staples; 1949.
10. West JB. Carl Wilhelm Scheele, the discoverer of oxygen, and a very productive chemist. Am J Physiol Lung Cell Mol Physiol. 2014;307(11):L811-6.
11. Severinghaus JW. Eight sages over five centuries share oxygen's discovery. Adv Physiol Educ. 2016;40(3):370-6.
12. Heffner JE. The Story of Oxygen. Respiratory Care. 2013;58(1):18-31.
13. Barach AL. The therapeutic use of oxygen. JAMA. 1922;79:693-8.
14. Grainge C. Breath of life: the evolution of oxygen therapy. J Royal Soc Med. 2004;97:489-93.
15. Priestley J. Experiments and observations on different kinds of air (1775). Alembic Club Reprints, Part 1, No. 7. Chicago: University of Chicago Press; 1906.
16. Perkins JF Jr. Historical development of respiratory physiology. in: Fenn WO, Rahn H (eds). Handbook of Physiology. Section 3: Respiration, vol. 1. Bethesda, MD: American Physiological Society; 1964. pp. 1-62.
17. McKie D. Antoine Lavoissier: Scientist, Economist, Social Reformer. New York: Schuman; 1952.
18. Warren CP. The introduction of oxygen for pneumonia as seen through the writings of two McGill University professors, William Osler and Gonatham Meakins. Can Respir J. 2005;12:81-5.
19. Sternbach GL, Varon J. The discovery and rediscovery of oxygen. J Emerg Med. 2005;28:221-4.
20. Simons E, Oelz O. Mont Blanc with oxygen: the first rotters. High Alt Med Biol. 2001;2:545-9.
21. Cotes JE, Gilson JC. Effect of oxygen on exercise ability in chronic respiratory insufficiency. Lancet. 1956;1:872.
22. Meakins J. Observations on the gases in human arterial blood in certain pathological pulmonary conditions and their treatment with oxygen. J Pathol Microbiol. 1921;24:79-90.
23. Flenley DC. Long term home oxygen therapy. Chest. 1985;87:99-103.
24. Levine BF, Bigelow DB, Hamstra RD, Beckwitt HJ, Mitchell RS, Nett LM, et al. The role of long term continuous oxygen administration in patients with chronic airway obstruction with hypoxaemia. Ann Intern Med. 1967;66:639.
25. Medical Research Council Working Party. Long term domiciliary Oxygen therapy in chronic hypoxic cor pulmonale complicating chronic bronchitis and emphysema. Lancet. 1981;1:681.
26. Neff TA, Petty TL. Long term continuous oxygen therapy in chronic airway obstruction. Mortality in relationship to cor pulmonale, hypoxia and hypercapnia. Ann Intern Med. 1970;28:784.
27. Nocturnal oxygen Therapy Trial Group. Continuous or nocturnal oxygen therapy in hypoxaemic chronic obstructive lung disease: a clinical trial. Ann Intern Med. 1980;93:391.
28. Petty TL. Historical highlights of long-term oxygen therapy. Respir Care. 2000;45:29-36.
29. Mirza M, Verma M, Sahoo SS, Roy S, Kakkar R, Singh DK. India's Multi-Sectoral Response to Oxygen Surge Demand during COVID-19 Pandemic: A Scoping Review. Indian J Community Med. 2023;48(1):31-40.
30. Gowda NR, Siddharth V, Kumar P, Vikas H, Swaminathan P, Kumar A. "Constrained Medical Oxygen Supply Chain in India During COVID-19: Red-tapism, the Elephant in the Room?". Disaster Med Public Health Prep. 2022;17:e296.
31. Jindal SK. Historical aspects. In: Jindal SK, Agarwal R (Eds). Oxygen Therapy, 3rd edition. New Delhi: Jaypee Brothers Medical Publishers; 2022.

CHAPTER 17

Thoracic Surgery and Lung Transplantation

Thoracic surgery is a specialized field of respiratory medicine that focuses on surgical procedures for management of conditions affecting the thoracic organs, including the lungs, trachea, chest wall, and the mediastinal organs. The heart and the great vessels which also lie in the thoracic cavity constitute a separate superspecialty. In recent years, thoracic surgery has undergone significant advancements, driven by improvements in surgical techniques, diagnostic imaging, and perioperative care. One of the most notable developments is the increased use of minimally invasive surgical (MIS) approaches, such as video-assisted thoracic surgery (VATS) and robotic-assisted surgery. Despite these advancements, thoracic surgery remains a challenging field.

Historical Aspects

Thoracic surgery has a long and undulating history in the practice of respiratory medicine. While surgery for thoracic trauma has been practiced for several millennia in one or the other form, its role in the management of infections such as empyema and tuberculosis (TB) has shown a wavy course in the past. Some of the major advances in anesthetic and surgical techniques in modern medicine, especially in the last few decades, have advanced the role of thoracic surgery for previously unknown indications. On the other hand, there is a significant shift toward medical management for many of the common previously described conditions.

The earliest recorded information on surgical procedures, including thoracic surgery, is available from ancient Egypt in the Edwin Smith *Ebers Papyrus,* which describes surgical procedures for thoracic injuries, including rib fractures and lung injuries. The ayurvedic texts of *Charaka and Sushruta Samhita* from India described surgical procedures for treating chest injuries and diseases such as pleural effusions. Sushruta who lived around 600 BCE is believed to have practiced surgery in the ancient Indian city of Varanasi. He described surgical procedures for treating chest wounds, including the use of surgical instruments. Sushruta used various herbal preparations and other natural substances to induce anesthesia and manage pain during surgery. Today, he is considered as one of the earliest surgeons in recorded history. Thoracic injuries were common due to battles and accidents. Sushruta developed a procedure to treat these injuries, which involved surgically opening the chest cavity. The *Sushruta Samhita* describes eight types of surgical procedures including excision, drainage, suturing, and others.

Detailed recommendation of stepwise methodology adopted by Sushruta is available in some of the verses. Some examples of the verses for surgical indications are given as under:

- *For puncture wounds of the chest, Sushruta Samhita, Chikitsa Sthana, Chapter 13 (Verse 6):*
    - "पृथङ्गुणं यदि यत्नात्क्षेप्तव्यमणुः शिरोऽंशकं।।"

"In case of puncture wounds that cause a hole in the thoracic cavity, air should be prevented from entering by sealing the wound and applying appropriate treatments to prevent infection or further complications."

- *Surgical procedures for pleural effusion:*
    - *Sushruta Samhita, Chikitsa Sthana, Chapter 10 (Verse 38):*
        - "शोषवहं कृतं छेदनं सम्यग् उपचारं चालयेत्॥"

"When the chest is filled with excess fluid or pus, the surgeon should use a sharp instrument to evacuate the accumulated fluid, ensuring the wound is properly treated and kept sterile."

- *Managing fractured ribs and chest deformities:*
    - *Sushruta Samhita, Sutra Sthana, Chapter 15 (Verse 16):*
        - "विबन्धनं च यथान्यं गात्रेषु समन्यकं॥"

"A fractured rib should be repositioned and fixed using a bandage or splint, so that the rib heals in the correct alignment."

- *Management of thoracic tumors or growths:*
    - *Sushruta Samhita, Chikitsa Sthana, Chapter 4 (Verse 11):*
        - "विकारवष्टवः पुष्टमाणवर्द्धयाः॥"

"In cases of growths or tumors in the chest, the surgeon should carefully remove the growth, ensuring that the surrounding tissues are preserved and the thoracic cavity is not further damaged."

Sushruta's contributions to thoracic surgery were groundbreaking for his time, and his techniques were adopted by other ancient civilizations, including the Greeks and Romans. His work laid the foundation for modern thoracic surgery.

In Europe, the Greek, and Roman physicians like Hippocrates and his followers had described various thoracic surgical procedures. Besides managing chest wall injuries, they are also known to have performed rib resections and thoracocentesis.

Thoracic surgery remained largely stagnant in the early and late Middle Ages in Europe perhaps due to the influence and restrictions of the Catholic Church. However, middle eastern physicians such as Al-Zahrawi wrote about chest drainage and lung resections. The Unani physicians, such as Ibn Sina (Avicenna), wrote on surgical procedures, including those related to the chest. The Indian craftsmen are said to have developed sophisticated surgical instruments, including those used in thoracic surgery.

Modern Era European Developments

There was lack of scientific advancements until the period of the Renaissance, when Andreas Vesalius' work on human anatomy laid the foundation for modern thoracic surgery. In modern period, thoracic surgery can be traced to 1499 to Rolandus, a surgeon from Parma, who resected a piece of lung infected with worms between two ribs. Ambroise Paré, a renowned French *barber-surgeon,* is said to have described the use of thoracotomy to treat empyema. Most

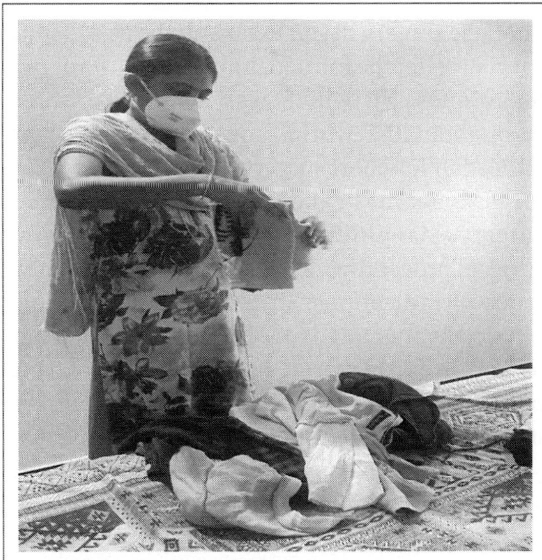

A patient of lung transplantation done for allergic bronchopulmonary aspergillosis, 1 year after surgery fully involved in household activities. *Courtesy*: Dr Srinivas Rajagopala, Apollo Hospital, Chennai.

of the surgical procedures during this period were related to treatment of war wounds and abscesses.

Meanwhile, there were landmark developments in medicine during the 19th century, which included the discovery of bacteria by Louis Pasteur and of *Mycobacterium* by Robert Koch. These developments coupled with introduction of anesthesia by William Morton and Crawford Long enabled more complex thoracic surgeries including major chest wall debridements, thoracoplasty, and others. Introduction of antiseptics by Joseph Lister significantly reduced postoperative infections. Advances in diagnostic imaging with help of X-rays, CT scans, and MRI machines improved diagnosis and surgical planning. The introduction of cardiopulmonary bypass by John Gibbon enabled more complex cardiac and thoracic surgeries.

Tuberculosis—The Mother of Thoracic Surgery

Thoracic surgery began to take shape as a distinct specialty after the introduction of modern surgical techniques. TB which was a major problem throughout the world, constituted the prime indication for chest surgery. For this very reason, TB is sometimes called the mother of thoracic surgery. Many different kinds of conservative surgical procedures were employed for different types of indications. In the late 19th century, physicians attempted to collapse the infected lung to "rest" it and allow it to heal. It was believed that only a resting lung could heal itself, and therefore it should be deflated to give it a chance to heal.

Although the benefit of lung collapse was first suggested in 1771 by Edmond Claude Bourru, in Paris, it was in 1888 when Carlo Forlanini, an Italian physician of Pavia, first practiced the procedure by causing artificial pneumothorax by introducing nitrogen gas into the pleural space. In 1890, Max Schede, a German surgeon, performed thoracoplasty, unilateral partial rib resection to reduce thoracic cavity volume and collapse tuberculous cavities. Thereafter, the procedure was widely adopted in Europe and the United States. This was done by injecting air or gas into the pleural space. Sometimes phrenic nerve crushing was also used to collapse the lung. Thoracoplasty that involved the removal of a few ribs to collapse the lung was another common procedure. Lobectomy or pneumonectomy was sometimes done in case of a destroyed part or the whole lung.

It was advocated by French surgeon, Theodore Tuffier that the collapsed lung should be maintained to allow the resting lung to recover. The pleural space thus created due to surgical pneumothorax was filled with other material such as the oil ("oleothorax"). Occasionally, this was achieved by "plombage" with the use of Lucite (polymethylmethacrylate) balls devised by David Wilson of Duke University, USA.

The introduction of streptomycin and isoniazid in the 1940s and 1950s revolutionized TB treatment. Surgical interventions gradually declined as drug therapy became the primary treatment. In the 1950s and later, almost all forms of surgical treatment were abandoned in favor of medical treatment. In India, it even led to a shortage of thoracic surgeons. For several decades in the latter half of the 20th century, it became difficult to avail thoracic surgical treatments for genuine indications. Rise of drug-resistant TB and the HIV epidemic led to a renewed interest in surgical interventions. Surgical interventions were more frequently required for cases of multidrug-resistant TB or complicated TB, such as localized disease, aspergillomas, tubercular empyema, or bronchopleural fistulas. Moreover, there was expansion of nontubercular indications including lung nodules and lung cancer.

Video-assisted Thoracic Surgery

Thoracic surgery got a further boost with the development of MIS techniques such as VATS, anesthesia, and intensive care, which improved outcomes and reduced morbidity. A minimally

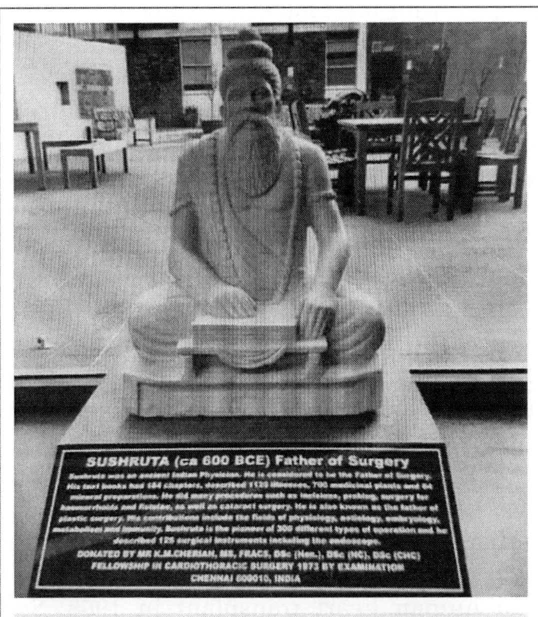

Statue of sage *Sushruta*, Father of Surgery at the head office of Royal Australasian College of Surgeons in Melbourne, Australia.

invasive procedure uses small incisions and a camera to visualize the lesions. MIS techniques in particular have revolutionized the field of thoracic surgery, offering patients reduced trauma, less postoperative pain, and faster recovery times. These approaches also enable surgeons to perform complex procedures with greater precision and accuracy. Advances in diagnostic imaging and staging have improved patient selection and outcomes. Robotic-assisted surgery is another specialized type of minimally invasive surgery using a robotic system to assist the surgeon.

Minimally invasive surgical techniques are used to diagnose and treat various conditions affecting the thoracic cavity. Some common indications include the diagnosis of undiagnosed pleural effusion, thoracic tumors, and pulmonary nodules: VATS is highly useful in the overall management of pleural conditions including empyema, hemothorax, and pneumothorax. MIS techniques are helpful to diagnose and stage lung cancer, thymoma, or other thoracic tumors. Therapeutic indications extend to removal of lung and mediastinal tumors, such as cysts, thymoma, teratomas, and others. VATS is also used to treat esophageal cancer, achalasia, esophageal diverticula, and repair chest wall defects or deformities.

Lung Cancer Surgery

Another area of significant progress was related to the treatment of lung cancer. Lung cancer surgery led to a significant increase in the scope of thoracic surgery beyond the conventional borders, which were limited to TB and other infective conditions. Surgical resection remains the primary treatment for early-stage lung cancer. This includes wedge resection, segmentectomy, lobectomy, or pneumonectomy, depending upon the location and spread of tumor. Sometimes, sleeve resection involving removal of a section of airway and surrounding tissue, followed by reattachment of the remaining airway, is also done. The type of surgery performed depends on the stage and location of the tumor, as well as the patient's overall health. Surgery may be combined with other treatments, such as chemotherapy or radiation therapy. Additionally, the development of stereotactic body radiation therapy (SBRT) and other ablative therapies has expanded treatment options for patients with inoperable or advanced-stage disease.

Other Surgical Options

Surgical options for diagnosis and/or management of obstructive and parenchymal lung diseases have opened up entirely new frontiers for thoracic surgeons. Surgery involving resection of large bullae, as well as for lung-volume reduction, has met with at least partial success in patients with disabling emphysema. A bullectomy involves removing large air-filled cysts (bullae) that compress normal lung tissue. Lung volume reduction surgery (LVRS) is a surgical procedure to remove damaged lung tissue, typically performed to help improve lung function and breathing in people with severe emphysema involving the upper lung lobes. LVRS can significantly improve overall quality of life, but the results may vary. Some patients do not experience significant improvements. Bronchoscopic lung volume reduction is also used as an alternative procedure.

Pleurectomy, which involves removing part or all of the pleura, is typically performed for patients with pleural fibrosis or pleural plaques. Surgical procedures are not the primary treatment option for diffuse interstitial lung diseases or pulmonary fibrosis, but may be necessary in certain cases. Lung biopsy is required in doubtful cases to decide the line of therapy or to monitor disease progression. It is essential to carefully evaluate the risks and benefits of surgery for each individual patient.

Lung transplantation for advanced lung destruction is an entirely new area of thoracic surgery, which is rapidly developing all over the world including in India.

Contemporary Thoracic Surgery in India

Presently, India is home to numerous thoracic surgery departments, with surgeons performing minimally invasive surgery and complex procedures, including lung transplantation. Initial thoracic surgery was generally restricted to cardiac problems. The first department of Cardiothoracic Surgery was started in 1948 at Christian Medical College, Vellore by the American missionary Thoracic Surgeon, Rev H Betts who performed the first patent ductus arteriosus (PDA) ligation in 1950. In the mid-20th century, dedicated thoracic surgery departments were established in Indian hospitals, marking a significant milestone in the specialty's development. Over the years, India has made significant advancements in thoracic surgery, with the establishment of specialized departments and institutions.

Indian surgeons, such as Ram Nath Chatterjee, made significant contributions to the development of thoracic surgery in India. The Association of Surgeons of India (ASI) also played a vital role in the country. The ASI's Thoracic Surgery Section was established in 1954, and it provided a platform for thoracic surgeons to share their knowledge and expertise. The Indian Association of Cardiovascular-Thoracic Surgeons (IACTS) was formed in 1990, and it has been instrumental in promoting the development of cardiothoracic surgery in the country.

One of the earliest and most influential thoracic surgeons in India was Prafulla Kumar Sen, who performed India's first closed mitral valvotomy. He also performed the country's first human heart transplant in 1968. Sen was a trailblazer in the field of cardiothoracic surgery, and his work laid the foundation for future generations of surgeons. Today, India is recognized as a major hub for thoracic surgery, with many world-class hospitals and medical institutions offering advanced treatment options for patients with thoracic diseases. Advanced thoracoscopic and robotic surgeries, which have reduced recovery times and improved outcomes, are now done at several centers in the country.

Thoracic surgery in India is a specialized field that deals with surgery of the thoracic organs including the lungs, heart, and other organs in the chest cavity. The Master of Chirurgiae (MCh) in Cardiovascular Thoracic Surgery is a 3-year postgraduate course that requires candidates to have an MS degree in Surgery. Similar to courses in other superspecialties of surgery, Post-MS, DNB in CTV Surgery is also offered by the National Board of Examinations. Unlike cardiac surgery which constitutes the primary area of interest, lung surgery has received step-motherly treatment. Lately, there is an increased interest in lung surgery and a trend toward development of separate superspecialty courses in Thoracic Surgery.

Lung Transplantation

Lung transplantation is a major surgical procedure that involves replacing one or both lungs with healthy donor lungs. A number of pulmonary diseases such as pulmonary fibrosis and emphysema are relentlessly progressive leading to a stage of damaged end-stage lung. Some of the infective conditions such as extensive bronchiectasis and cystic fibrosis may also lead to an end-stage condition when nothing more than palliative therapies can be offered. Innovative treatments such as the use of tissue engineering and regenerative medicine to repair or replace damaged thoracic tissues are yet in an exploratory stage.

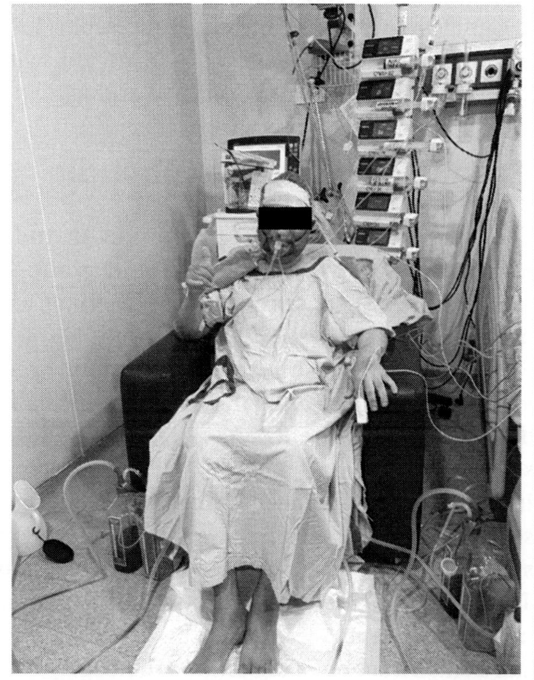

Postoperative period following lung-transplantation surgery.
Courtesy: Dr Srinivas Rajagopala, Apollo Hospital, Chennai.

Historical Perspectives

One can trace the instances of solid organ transplantation and xenotransplantation described in different mythological stories. In Hindu mythology, Lord Ganesha is said to have received an elephant's head after he was decapitated by Lord Shiva in a mistaken belief. He is often depicted to showing signs of side effects from steroid-like medication. In another story, Lord Shiva gave a goat's head to Daksha, the "*Prajapati*" *(a divine king-rishi),* as punishment for his evil deeds.

Mythology apart, the present-day transplantation story began with animal experimentation as early as the beginning of the 20th century when Alexis Carrel transplanted a kitten's lung into the neck of an adult cat, which died 2 days later due to sepsis. About 40 years later, Vladimir Demikhov first transplanted heart and lungs in a dog. It was James Hardy who was ultimately successful in surgically removing lungs and reimplanting them in the same animal at the University of Mississippi. He successfully performed the first lung transplant in 1963 using a nonheart beating donor. The recipient died 18 days later from renal failure and infection. George Magovern and Adolph Yates carried out the second human lung transplant, but the patient died within a few days.

The first "successful" lung transplant where the recipient survived for about a year was reported by Fritz Derom in 1971. There was rapid expansion thereafter with newer developments such as *en bloc* transplantation of the heart and one lung with a single distal tracheal anastomosis, double lung transplant, and sequential double lung transplantation. Bruce Reitz performed the first successful double lung transplant in 1986, which marked a significant milestone in the development. Introduction of lung preservation techniques, such as flush perfusion and cold storage, improved the viability of donor lungs. There have other related developments such as the improved immunosuppression regimens and the introduction of extracorporeal membrane oxygenation as a bridge to transplant, which helped to significantly improve the outcome. Today, lung transplantation is performed worldwide, with thousands of transplants performed annually.

Lung Transplantation in India

The first heart–lung transplantation in India was performed by KM Cherian and group in 1999, while first successful lung transplant was performed by Jnanesh Thacker on July 11, 2012 in Hyderabad. Subsequent to this, there were few reports of heart and lung or lung transplants discretely from different parts of the country. Now, several hospitals and medical institutions across India have begun offering lung transplantation services. The development has been gradual, with significant milestones achieved in the last decade. The country has seen an increase in the number of lung transplants performed annually, albeit still a small fraction of the estimated need.

The Indian government has implemented policies and laws to promote organ donation, such as the Transplantation of Human Organs Act (THOA) in 1994, which allowed for cadaveric organ donation. The availability of donor lungs is limited, leading to a significant gap between the demand for transplants and the available organs. Moreover, the high cost of lung transplantation and postoperative care is a significant barrier for many patients in India. Today, lung transplantation is available in several major cities across India, including Hyderabad, Delhi, Mumbai, Chennai, and Bengaluru.

The current success rates of lung transplantation are quite promising. According to the International Society for Heart and Lung Transplantation Registry, the 1-year and 5-year survival rates for adult lung transplant recipients are around 85% and 59%, respectively, for those transplanted since 2010. In India, the success rates are also improving, with an estimated average of 475 lung transplants performed every year from 2021 to 2023. The country has seen a significant increase in lung transplants, partly due to the COVID-19 pandemic, which has led to an increase in cases of post-COVID acute respiratory distress syndrome (ARDS) and end-stage lung disease requiring lung transplants. It is worth noting that the success rates of lung transplantation can vary depending on several factors, including the underlying disease, the recipient's overall health, and the expertise of the transplant team.

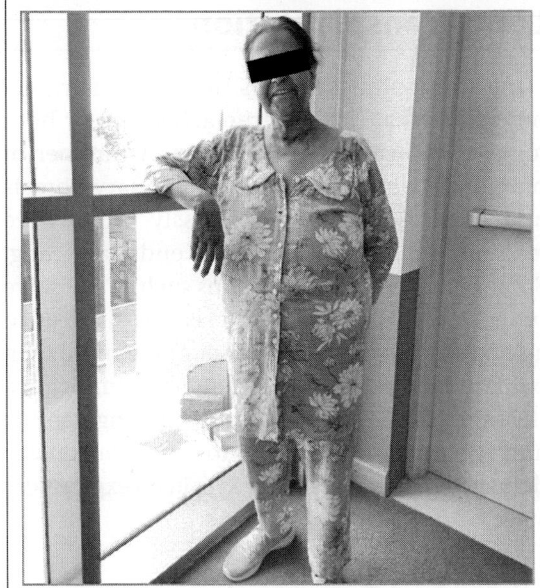

Patient post lung transplantation.
Courtesy: Dr Apar Jindal, Gleneagles Health City, Chennai.

Lung transplantation is presently the only life-saving medical procedure that has revolutionized the treatment of end-stage lung diseases. The surgery involves replacing a diseased or damaged lung with a healthy one from a donor, offering a new lease on life for such individuals. Lung transplantation significantly improves survival rates for individuals with advanced lung diseases, improves the quality of life, enables recipients to breathe more easily, engage in physical activities and enjoy a better overall quality of life. Continuous improvements in surgical techniques, immunosuppressive regimens, and postoperative care have contributed to better outcomes and increased survival rates.

There are significant challenges to transplantation all over the world. Limited availability and high cost of the facility are particularly important in India. Shortage of suitable donor lungs remains a significant challenge, leading to prolonged waiting times for transplantation. Lung transplant recipients require lifelong immune suppression to prevent rejection, which increases the risk of infections. Successful lung transplantation requires comprehensive postoperative care, including rehabilitation programs to optimize lung function and overall health. Personalized immunotherapy strategies aim to minimize the risks associated with immunosuppression and improve long-term outcomes. Ex vivo lung perfusion technology allows for the evaluation and rehabilitation of donor lungs outside the body, potentially increasing the availability of suitable donor organs.

It can be concluded that thoracic surgery in India has made significant strides in the recent years. From the days of sage Sushruta some 600 BCE, aptly called the Father of Surgery, India has now marched to the current era of advanced surgical procedures such as the lung transplantation. Keeping its pace with rest of the world, it seems to have regained its position, albeit for different indications than those which were common in the first half of the 20th century prior to the advent of tubercular chemotherapy. Factually, the field continues to evolve fast. The role and success of thoracic surgery, driven by advances in surgical techniques, diagnostic imaging, and perioperative care, is likely to expand further.

Sources

1. Sushruta Samhita, Chikitsa Sthana, Chapter 14, Verse 15*.
2. Sushruta Samhita, Sharira Sthana, Chapter 5, Verse 4*.
3. Sushruta Samhita, Chikitsa Sthana, Chapter 14, Verse 17*.
4. Khaitan PG, D'Amico TA. Milestones in thoracic surgery. J Thorac Cardiovasc Surg. 2018;155:2779-89.
5. Idhrees M, Narayan P, George M, Radhakrishna P, Abraham SJ, Velayudhan B. The motivators and barriers to a career in cardiothoracic surgery: a cross-sectional study among surgical residents in India. Indian J Thorac Cardiovasc Surg. 2022;38(6):613-23.
6. Molnar TF. Tuberculosis: mother of thoracic surgery then and now, past and prospectives: a review. J Thorac Dis. 2018;10(Suppl 22):S2628-42.
7. Bryder L. The Medical Research Council and treatments for tuberculosis before streptomycin. J R Soc Med. 2014;107(10):409-15.
8. Daniel TM. The history of tuberculosis. Respir Med. 2006;100:1862-70.
9. Odell JA. The history of surgery for pulmonary tuberculosis. Thorac Surg Clin. 2012;22(3):257-69.
10. Herzog H. History of tuberculosis. Respiration. 1998;65:5-15.
11. Yendamuri S. Thoracic surgery in India: challenges and opportunities. J Thorac Dis. 2016;8(Suppl 8):S596-600.
12. Indian Association of Cardiovascular-Thoracic Surgeons. [online] Available from https://www.iacts.org/content/history [Last accessed September, 2025].
13. Luh SP, Liu HP. Video-assisted thoracic surgery--the past, present status and the future. J Zhejiang Univ Sci B. 2006;7(2):118-28.
14. Migliore M. Initial History of Uniportal Video-Assisted Thoracoscopic Surgery. The Ann Thorac Surg. 2016;101:412-3.
15. Abbas AE. Surgical Management of Lung Cancer: History, Evolution, and Modern Advances. Curr Oncol Rep. 2018;20(12):98.
16. Montagne F, Guisier F, Venissac N, Baste JM. The Role of Surgery in Lung Cancer Treatment: Present Indications and Future Perspectives-State of the Art. Cancers (Basel). 2021;13(15):3711.
17. Singh N, Agrawal S, Jiwnani S, Khosla D, Malik PS, Mohan A, et al. Lung Cancer in India. J Thorac Oncol. 2021;16(8):1250-66.
18. Shields T (Ed). General Thoracic Surgery. Lippincott Williams & Wilkins; 2004. p. 524.
19. Dabak G, ŞeSnbaklavacı Ö. History of Lung Transplantation. Turk Thorac J. 2016;17(2):71-5.

20. Panchabhai TS, Chaddha U, McCurry KR, Bremner RM, Mehta AC. Historical perspectives of lung transplantation: connecting the dots. J Thorac Dis. 2018;10(7).
21. Sunder T. The evolution of lung transplantation in India and the current scenario. Indian J Thorac Cardiovasc Surg. 2022;38(Suppl 2):211-28.
22. Khaitan PG, Thomas A, D'Amico TA. Milestones in thoracic surgery. J Thorac Cardiovasc Surg. 2018;155:2779-89.
23. Attawar S, Manoly I, Shah U. Lung Transplantation in India: a Brief Review, Landmarks, Indian Scenario, and our Experience. Indian J Surg. 2023:1-12.

CHAPTER 18

Environment, Climate, and Respiratory Medicine

The environment, through the air we breathe, affects the respiratory system function out of all the body systems. Environmental factors can exacerbate existing respiratory diseases as well as contribute to the development of new conditions. The environment also affects respiratory health through changes in climatic conditions such as the heat waves and cold snaps which can exacerbate respiratory conditions. Climate change can worsen air quality by increasing particulate matter (PM) and ozone levels as well as alter pollen patterns resulting in an increase of exposure to allergens.

Environmental Risk Factors

Some key environmental factors that impact respiratory health include air pollutants such as the PM and gases, occupational dusts (silica, asbestos, and coal), chemical (pesticides, solvents, and heavy metals), and bioaerosols. PM, especially PM2.5 and PM10, can penetrate deep into the lungs, causing inflammation and damage. Environmental gaseous pollutants such as nitrogen dioxide (NO_2), ozone (O_3), and volatile organic compounds (VOCs) can exacerbate respiratory conditions such as asthma and chronic obstructive pulmonary disease (COPD). Exposure to bioaerosols (such as molds, bacteria, and viruses) can cause respiratory infections. Excessive moisture and mold growth can also contribute to indoor allergens such as dust mites, pet dander, and cockroaches which can trigger persistent respiratory symptoms.

Indoor air pollution from sources such as cooking, heating, and tobacco smoke is another important risk factor for exacerbation of respiratory diseases.

Environmental risk factors are particularly significant in low-income communities who are disproportionately exposed to environmental pollutants because of poor housing conditions, habitat in slums and crowded areas, and proximity to industrial sites. Children, the elderly, and people with preexisting respiratory conditions account for more vulnerable populations with greater susceptibility to environmental pollutants. It is important for respiratory physicians to consider these environmental factors when diagnosing and managing respiratory illnesses.

Historical Aspects

Environmental as an important consideration for respiratory disease has been largely recognized in the modern era. But the significance has been known for several millennia in the ancient Indian, Greek, Roman, and other civilizations. Noted physicians such as Hippocrates had variously described the adverse effects of air pollution from industrial activities and urbanization. Ancient Indian texts mention air pollution from industrial activities such as metalworking and mining. Both Charaka and Sushruta of that era wrote extensively on respiratory diseases and their environmental causes:

- *Rigveda (1500 BCE)*: Book 5, Hymn 73 mentions the ill effects of polluted air on human health.
- *Mahabharata (400 BCE)*: Book 3, Chapter 68 describes the symptoms of respiratory diseases caused by air pollution.
- Charaka Samhita (400 CE) describes respiratory problems in miners and metalworkers, highlighting the occupational hazards of these professions.
- Sushruta Samhita (600 CE) mentions the effects of air pollution on respiratory health.

Medieval India was also marked by various environmental factors that contributed to respiratory issues. Besides the information available from medieval Indian medical texts, travelers such as Ibn Battuta and Marco Polo wrote about the poor air quality and respiratory issues they encountered during their travels in India. Marco Polo's travelogue, "Il Milione" (The Travels of Marco Polo), written in the 13th century, provides valuable insights into the environmental conditions. While Marco Polo's accounts are often anecdotal and based on his personal experiences, they offer a unique perspective on the environmental challenges faced by medieval Indian societies. Here is a relevant passage from Marco Polo's travelogue:

"In the province of Cormos [Kerala], the air is so bad that it causes a kind of asthma, which is very common among the inhabitants. The reason is that the country is very hot and humid, and the people are obliged to burn a great quantity of wood and other fuels, which makes the air thick and unwholesome."

— Marco Polo, "Il Milione" (The Travels of Marco Polo), Book 3, Chapter 34

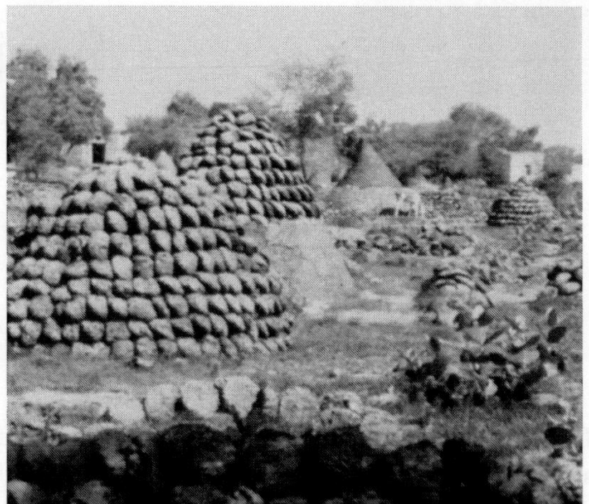

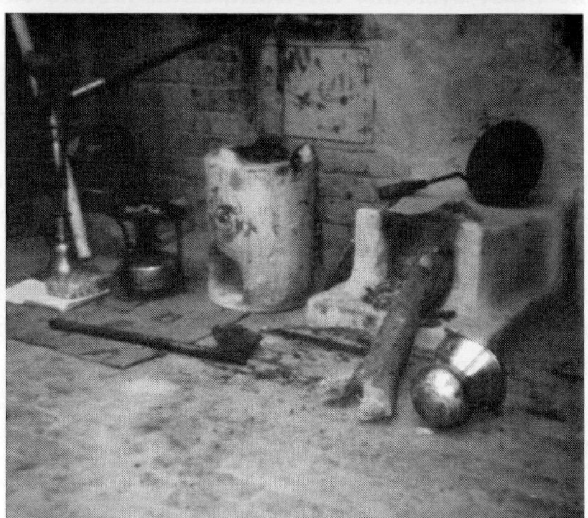

Dried dung and other solid fuels are commonly used as domestic fuels. Environmental smoke is responsible for respiratory and several other health effects.

Widespread use of biomass fuels such as wood, dung, and crop residues for domestic cooking and heating release pollutants such as PM, carbon monoxide, and VOCs. Indian homes often had poor ventilation, leading to the accumulation of indoor air pollutants. There were frequent dust storms, particularly in the arid and semi-arid regions, which contributed to respiratory problems. The subcontinent's climate was characterized by high humidity and frequent floods, which created ideal conditions for mold growth and exacerbated respiratory symptoms. Moreover, medieval India saw the growth of industries such as textiles, metalworking, and pottery, which emitted pollutants such as PM, sulfur dioxide, and nitrogen oxides. Miners were exposed to hazards like silica dust, leading to conditions like silicosis.

Modern Era

The Industrial Revolution in the beginning of the 19th century brought air pollution from coal burning and other industrial exhausts. A significant increase was noticed in the incidence of coal miners' pneumoconiosis (black lung disease) and other occupational lung diseases. Epidemiological air pollution studies in the 1950s and 1960s demonstrated the link between air pollution and respiratory diseases, such as bronchitis and lung cancer. The period also witnessed the introduction of tobacco smoking adding to indoor environmental pollution. The 1970s and 1980s saw increased concern about indoor air pollutants, such as radon, asbestos, and VOCs. Different research studies highlighted the role of environmental allergens and pollutants in asthma and allergic diseases. All these concerns and observations slowly led to the need for clean environment and workplace safety. The landmark 1964 US Surgeon General's report established the connection between cigarette smoking and lung cancer.

The Industrial Revolution in India during the British colonial era in India as well led to increased air pollution from coal burning, textile mills, and other industries. Industrial exhausts and accidental leakages were other important causes of environmental degradation. The Bhopal methyl isocyanate (MIC) gas tragedy of 2000 has been one such major example.

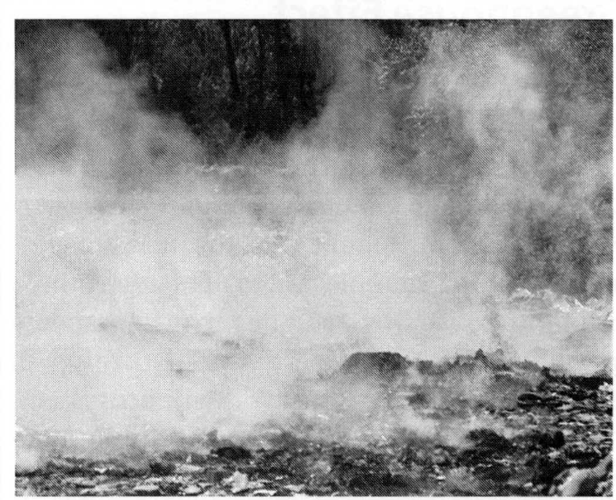

Outdoor burning of dried crop residues producing large amounts of environmental smoke is common in Indian villages during postharvesting seasons.

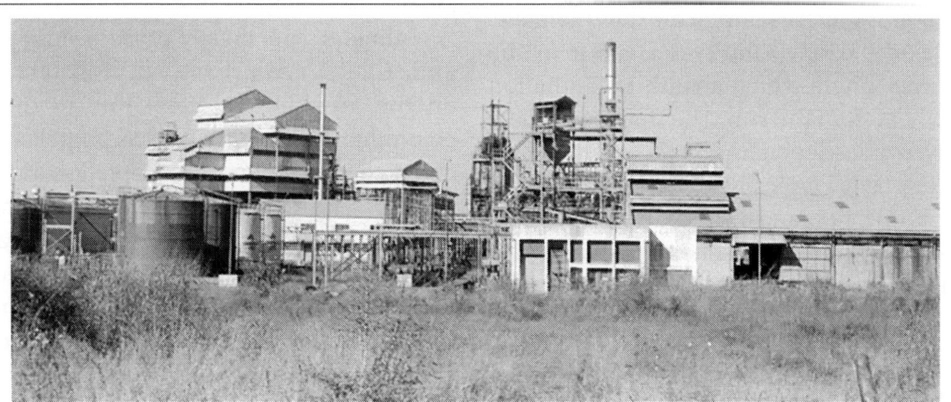

Bhopal disaster, 2 December 1984. One of the worst disaster in India occurred due to accidental leakage at Union Carbide Chemical Factory which caused massive environment leak of methyl isocyanate (MIC) gas causing death of >2,000. The immediate deaths happened due to asphyxiation and pulmonary edema while residual lung damage caused pulmonary fibrosis and other complications.

The Air (Prevention and Control of Pollution) Act, 1981, was enacted to regulate air pollution from industrial sources in post-Independence era. The Factories Act, 1948, and the Mines Act, 1952, mandated occupational health services for workers in factories and mines.

Climate Change and Greenhouse Effect

Climatic change and global warming emerged as another important issue concerning environment and overall health toward the end of the 20th century. Climate change refers to the long-term warming of the planet due to an increase in average global temperatures. This warming is primarily caused by activities that release large amounts of greenhouse gases disturbing the delicate balance in the earth's fragile ecosystem.

The greenhouse effect is a double-edged sword. It is a natural process that is essential for maintaining a habitable temperature on earth and protecting against the harmful effects of ultraviolet (UV) radiation. This is attributed to the ozone layer in the stratosphere, the second-lowest layer of the earth's atmosphere, approximately 15–30 kilometers above the earth's surface. This is formed by gases such as carbon dioxide, methane, nitrous oxide, ozone, and water vapor in the earth's atmosphere which absorb UV radiation and trap heat from the sun. The thickness of the ozone layer varies depending on the location, with the thickest layers typically found over the polar regions. Its thickness and distribution change with the seasons, with the largest depletion occurring over Antarctica during the Southern Hemisphere spring.

Ozone Holes

The ozone layer plays a vital role in protecting life on earth. Ozone layer depletion creates "ozone holes" allowing UV radiation to reach the earth's surface. This depletion is attributed to several human activities, particularly the burning of fossil fuels and deforestation which have significantly increased the concentration of these greenhouse gases, leading to an enhancement of the greenhouse effect. Propellant gases can have a significant impact on the ozone layer, particularly those that contain chlorine and bromine. As an example, satellite propellants can have a significant impact on the ozone layer. While regulations and mitigation efforts are in place, continued research and development of alternative propellants are necessary to minimize the effects of satellite propellants on the ozone layer.

Impact on Respiratory Health

Climate change has many other far-reaching and devastating effects including extreme weather events, severe heat waves, droughts, and storms; rising sea levels threatening coastal communities and loss of biodiversity. Epidemics of infectious diseases, heat stress, allergies, and other health problems are also important. The impact of climate change including due to heat stress, air pollution, and allergen exposure on respiratory health and diseases such as asthma, COPD, and hypersensitivity pneumonias has become a growing concern.

Inhalers, specifically those used for asthma and COPD, can have an indirect impact on the greenhouse effect due to the use of chlorofluorocarbons (CFCs) as propellants which could contribute to ozone depletion and climate change. The production of inhalers, including the manufacturing, transportation, storage, and disposal of inhalers also contribute to greenhouse gas emissions. While inhalers do contribute to greenhouse gas emissions, it is essential to consider the overall health benefits they provide. By adopting mitigation strategies and developing more sustainable inhaler technologies, it is possible to reduce their environmental impact while maintaining their therapeutic benefits.

International agreements, such as the Montreal Protocol, have led to a gradual recovery of the ozone layer. After 1990, the Montreal Protocol phased out CFCs in inhalers, replacing them with alternative propellants such as hydrofluoroalkanes. Alternate strategies which are being investigated include the use of compressed air as propellant and powder-based inhalers. Optimizing inhaler design to reduce wastage and minimize emissions during production and transportation; encouraging better disposal practices, such as recycling or proper waste management, can also help reduce emissions. Some pharmaceutical companies are exploring carbon offsetting initiatives to compensate for the emissions associated with their products.

Mitigation and Adaptation Strategies

Strategies involving slow transition to clean or renewable energy sources, increasing energy efficiency, and electrifying transportation are advocated to mitigate the global warming impacts. Clean energy is generated from natural resources that are replenished over time and do not harm the environment. The primary goal of clean energy is to reduce our reliance on fossil fuels, decrease greenhouse gas emissions, and mitigate climate change. It is also important to develop climate-resilient infrastructure, implement climate-smart agriculture, and enhance disaster preparedness. Continued efforts to protect the ozone layer, such as enforcing the Montreal Protocol and developing alternative technologies, are also crucial. It requires a collective effort, involving governments, industries, and individuals.

A low-carbon economy is becoming an increasingly important part of the global clean energy mix. Carbon points, also known as carbon credits or carbon offsets, are tradable certificates or permits that represent the right to emit a certain amount of greenhouse gases, typically measured in tons of carbon dioxide equivalent (tCO_2e). Organizations and governments implement different projects that reduce greenhouse gas emissions, such as renewable energy installations, energy efficiency improvements, or reforestation efforts. The verified emissions and reductions are converted into carbon credits, which are traded on carbon markets or sold to companies or individuals looking to offset their emissions. Companies or individuals purchase carbon credits to offset their own emissions, effectively reducing their carbon footprint. Overall, carbon points can be an effective tool for reducing greenhouse gas emissions, but their implementation requires careful consideration of the challenges and criticisms associated with carbon markets.

There are innumerable challenges to the clean energy efforts. Widespread adoption of clean energy requires significant investment in new infrastructure, including transmission lines, storage facilities, and charging stations. While the cost of clean energy technologies has decreased, they are still more expensive than traditional fossil fuel-based power plants. Some of the clean energy sources such as solar and wind are intermittent, requiring energy storage solutions to ensure a stable power supply. Supportive policies and regulations are crucial for promoting the adoption of clean energy technologies.

International Agreements for Clean Environment

A number of multilateral environmental agreements (MEAs), movements, and awareness programs have been launched at different levels in the last few decades. India has both launched and participated in several initiatives to promote a clean environment and tackle climate change. Some of the key initiatives are discussed here.

Montreal Protocol (1987) to phase out substances that deplete the ozone layer and the Paris Climate Accord [or Paris Climate Deal to limit global warming to well below 2°C (and pursue efforts to limit it to 1.5°C)] are two important agreements between the international communities. While the details of all such agreements are beyond the scope of this book, a summary list is included for purpose of brevity. These agreements demonstrate global cooperation and commitment to protecting the environment and mitigating the impacts of pollution.

- *Stockholm Convention (1972)*: Aimed at controlling and eliminating persistent organic pollutants (POPs).
- *United Nations Framework Convention on Climate Change (UNFCCC) (1992)*: Addresses climate change through country-specific commitments.
- *Kyoto Protocol (1997)*: Sets binding emissions targets for developed countries.
- *Convention on Long-range Transboundary Air Pollution (CLRTAP) (1979)*: Addresses air pollution in Europe and North America.
- *Protocol to the 1979 Convention on Long-range Transboundary Air Pollution Concerning the Control of Emissions of Nitrogen Oxides or Their Transboundary Fluxes (1988)*: Targets nitrogen oxide emissions.
- *Basel Convention (1989)*: Regulates the transboundary movement of hazardous waste.
- *Rotterdam Convention (1998)*: Promotes shared responsibilities in international trade of certain hazardous chemicals.
- *Minamata Convention (2013)*: Aims to reduce mercury emissions and releases.

Regional Agreements

- *European Union's Air Quality Directive (2008)*: Sets limits for air pollutants in EU member states.
- *North American Agreement on Environmental Cooperation (1993)*: Addresses environmental concerns, including air pollution, in North America.

Activist Movement for a Clean Environment and Climate

- *Rachel Carson's Silent Spring (1962)*: A seminal work, exposed the dangers of pesticides, sparking widespread concern about environmental pollution.
- *First Earth Day (1970)*: Organized by Gaylord Nelson, it raised awareness about environmental issues and mobilized public action.
- *James Hansen's Congressional Testimony (1988)*: Warned about the dangers of climate change, bringing the issue to the forefront of public discourse.
- *Rio Earth Summit (1992)*: Produced the United Nations Framework Convention on Climate Change (UNFCCC), an international treaty addressing climate change.
- *An Inconvenient Truth (2006)*: Al Gore's documentary raised public awareness about climate change and its consequences.
- *Copenhagen Climate Summit (2009)*: Failed to produce a binding international agreement, but sparked widespread protests and activism.
- *Fridays for Future (2018)*: Greta Thunberg's solo protest in front of the Swedish parliament inspired a global movement of student-led climate strikes.
- *Extinction Rebellion (2018)*: A nonviolent direct action movement demanding government action on climate change.
- *Climate Strikes (2019)*: Global protests, led by youth activists, demanded immediate action on climate change.

Some of the key players and organizations of these movements include Greenpeace (founded in 1971, has been at the forefront of climate activism) and The Climate Justice Alliance (a coalition of organizations advocating for climate justice and human rights).

Indian Scenario

India's rapid industrialization and urbanization have led to severe air pollution crises, particularly in metropolitan cities such as Delhi and Mumbai. According to the World Health Organization, India has one of the highest burdens of respiratory diseases, including asthma, COPD, and lung cancer. According to a 2020 study, air pollution causes approximately 1.2 million deaths annually in India. Approximately 18% of India's population suffers from respiratory disease. Different reports clearly highlighted the need for sustained efforts to address air pollution, occupational health, and respiratory disease prevention.

India is a signatory to most of the international agreements listed earlier and collaborations which aim to address the global burden of diseases, with a focus on environmental factors, climate change, and health equity. The Indian government has launched initiatives like the National Clean Air Programme (NCAP) to reduce air pollution and improve respiratory health. Stricter air pollution regulations have been implemented to reduce emissions and protect public health. It has launched several programs and plans to promote a clean environment and tackle climate change. The Air (Prevention and Control of Pollution) Act, 1981, was enacted to regulate air pollution from industrial sources.

National Air Quality Monitoring Programme was launched in 1984 to monitor air quality in Indian cities. National Ambient Air Quality Standards were established in 1994 to regulate air quality. The NCAP was launched in 2019 to reduce PM levels in Indian cities.

Some of the other key initiatives include the following:

- *National Solar Mission (NSM)*: Aims to promote the development and use of solar energy in India
- *National Mission for Enhanced Energy Efficiency (NMEEE)*: Focuses on improving energy efficiency in various sectors, including industry, transportation, and buildings
- *National Mission on Sustainable Habitat (NMSH)*: Aims to promote sustainable urban planning and development, with a focus on reducing greenhouse gas emissions.
- *Faster Adoption and Manufacturing of Hybrid & Electric vehicles in India (FAME India)*: Encourages the adoption of electric and hybrid vehicles to reduce dependence on fossil fuels.
- *Bharatiya Prakritik Krishi Paddhati Programme*: Promotes natural farming practices to reduce the use of chemical fertilizers and pesticides.
- *Panchamrit Strategy*: A five-point plan to reduce India's carbon footprint, including increasing nonfossil energy capacity to 500 GW by 2030, meeting 50% of energy requirements from renewable energy by 2030, and achieving net-zero emissions by 2070.
- *Pradhan Mantri Ujjwala Yojana (PMUY)*: Aims to provide clean cooking fuel to women from Below Poverty Line (BPL) families, reducing their reliance on polluting fuels.
- *National Clean Air Programme (NCAP)*: Seeks to reduce PM levels in the air by 20–30% by 2024
- *Green India Mission*: Aims to increase forest cover, reduce greenhouse gas emissions, and promote sustainable forest management.

Pradhan Mantri Ujjwala Yojana

The PMUY is a game-changing initiative launched by Prime Minister Narendra Modi in 2016 to provide clean cooking fuel to women from BPL families. The scheme aims to safeguard the health of women and children by providing them with liquefied petroleum gas (LPG) connections, thereby reducing their reliance on polluting fuels such as coal and wood.

Key Features of PMUY

The scheme provides free LPG connections to women from BPL families, with a support of ₹1,600 per connection. The scheme was initially launched to cover 5 crore BPL families, but its scope was later expanded to include 8 crore poor households. It also includes special provisions for migrant families, who can avail of the benefits without submitting ration cards or address proof. The scheme has led to a significant increase in LPG coverage. By providing clean cooking fuel and reducing their exposure to polluting fuels, the scheme is beneficial in providing benefits especially related to lung health, in particular for women and children.

The scheme has also contributed to the economic empowerment of women, enabling them to spend more time on productive activities rather than collecting firewood.

One of the key challenges facing the scheme is sustainability as many beneficiaries struggle to afford refills. The scheme needs to be expanded to cover more households, particularly in rural areas where access to clean cooking fuel is limited. Raising awareness about the benefits of clean cooking fuel and the importance of safe handling and usage of LPG connections is also important for the scheme's success. Overall, the *PMUY* is a critical initiative that has transformed the lives of millions of women and children in India. While challenges remain, the scheme's impact and potential for future growth make it a vital component of India's development agenda.

Generally speaking, environmental pollution and climate change play a highly significant role in overall health issues and burden of respiratory diseases in India. Clean air and clean energy are needed for good health. Reducing greenhouse gas emissions and transitioning to cleaner energy sources are critical for mitigating the impact of climate change on respiratory health. Continued research and awareness campaigns are necessary to address the complex issues.

Sources

1. Michael W. "Vedas and Upaniṣads". In: Flood G (Ed). The Blackwell companion to Hinduism (1st paperback ed.). Oxford: Blackwell Publishing;2005. pp. 68-71.
2. Kisari Mohan Ganguli (Translator). The Mahabharata of Krishna-Dwaipayana Vyasa, Volume1, Books 1, 2, and 3. 2005 [EBook #15474] https://www.gutenberg.org/files/15474/15474-h/15474-h.htm
3. Mukhopadhyaya GN. History of Indian Medicine (3 volumes). https://www.exoticindiaart.com/book/
4. Sharma PV. Caraka Samhita, 4 Volumes. Chaukhamba Orientalia, Varanasi. [online] Available from https://www.exoticindiaart.com/
5. Bhishagratna KKL. [online] Available from www.worldhistory.org.
6. Pati B, Harrison M. The Social History of Health and Medicine in Colonial India. Routledge Studies in South Asian History. [online] Available from http://ndl.ethernet.edu.et/bitstream/
7. Gibb HAR. Ibn Battuta Travels In Asia And Africa. 1325-54. [online] Available from https://www.amazon.in/Battuta-Travels
8. The Travels of Marco Polo. Translated by Ronald Latham. London: Penguin Classics. (1958). [online] Available from https://en.wikipedia.org/wiki/The_Travels_of_Marco_Polo
9. Rangarajan M. Environmental History of India. Ranikhet, India: Permanent Black; 2018
10. Singh U. A History of Ancient and Early Medieval India From the Stone Age to the 12th Century. Pearson, Delhi. https://tehattagovtcollege.ac.in/Pdf/Resources/
11. Haidar M. Medical Works of the Medieval Period from India and Central Asia. Diogenes,2008;55. https://journals.sagepub.com/
12. Vishwanath V. M Environmental Practices in Medieval India: Unearthing Sustainability and Ecological Wisdom. Golden Research Thoughts. 2014;4:3.
13. Prakasha KP. The History of Ancient and Medieval Periods - An Environmental Study. International Jour Multidisciplinary Educational Research. [online] Available from https://s3-ap-southeast-1.amazonaws.com/ijmer.
14. Shetty SS, Deepthi D, Harshitha S, Sonkusare S, Naik PB, Kumari NS, et al. Environmental pollutants and their effects on human health. Heliyon. 2023;9(9):e19496.
15. Laumbach RJ, Kipen HM. Respiratory health effects of air pollution: update on biomass smoke and traffic pollution. J Allergy Clin Immunol. 2012;129(1):3-11.
16. World Health Organization. (2024). Ambient (Outdoor) Air Pollution. [online] Available from

https://www.who.int/news-room/fact-sheets/detail/ambient-(outdoor)-air-quality-and-health [Last accessed September, 2025].

17. Mortimer K, Gordon SB, Jindal SK, Accinelli RA, Balmes J, Martin WJ 2nd. Household Air Pollution Is a Major Avoidable Risk Factor for Cardiorespiratory Disease. Chest. 2012;142(5):1308-15.
18. Gordon SB, Bruce NG, Grigg J, Hibberd PL, Kurmi OP, Lam KB, et al. Respiratory risks from household air pollution in low and middle income countries. Lancet Resp Med. 2014;2(10):823-60.
19. Jindal SK, Jindal A. COPD in Biomass exposed nonsmokers: a different phenotype. Expert Rev Respir Med. 2021;15(1):51-5.
20. Khilnani GC, Tiwari P. Air pollution in India and related adverse respiratory health effects: past, present, and future directions. Curr Opin Pulm Med. 2018;24:108-16.
21. Hystad P, Duong M, Brauer M, Larkin A, Arku R, Kurmi OP, et al. Health effects of household solid fuel use: findings from 11 countries within the prospective urban and rural epidemiology study. Environ Health Perspect. 2019;127:57003.
22. Jindal SK, Aggarwal AN, Jindal A. Household Air Pollution in India and Respiratory Diseases: Current Status and Future Directions. Curr Opinion Pulm Med. 2020;26(2):128-34.
23. Gerardi DA, Kellerman RA. Climate Change and Respiratory Health. J Occup Environ Med. 2014;56 Suppl 10:S49-54.
24. Bayram H, Rice MB, Abdalati W, Akpinar Elci M, Mirsaeidi M, Annesi-Maesano I, et al. Impact of Global Climate Change on Pulmonary Health: Susceptible and Vulnerable Populations. Ann Am Thorac Soc. 2023;20(8):1088-95.
25. Smith KR, Sagar A. Fossil fuel subsidies and health. Lancet Glob Health. 2015;3:e674.
26. Ministry of Petroleum and Natural Gas. Pradhan Mantri Ujjwala Yojana (PMUY). Janpath, New Delhi: Ministry of Petroleum and Natural Gas; 2024.

CHAPTER

19

Ethics and End-of-Life Care

Ethics in respiratory medicine involve complex moral and philosophical issues that arise in the care of patients with respiratory diseases. Most of the ethical issues in respiratory medical practice are similar to those applied in other specialties of medicine. Informed consent is important to ensure that the patient understands the risks and benefits of a particular treatment especially when it is invasive, semi-invasive or a new mode of therapy and/or of doubtful benefits. Maintaining patient confidentiality and privacy as well as respecting patients' cultural and personal values are also important ethical issues.

Similarly, there are several important end-of-life (EOL) care issues which need critical decisions in consultation with patients and their families. These include the decisions regarding withholding or withdrawing life-sustaining treatments such as mechanical ventilation. It is a major ethical dilemma to decide whether to initiate or continue mechanical ventilation in patients with advanced disease or resort to palliative care with symptom management and emotional support. The issue of lung transplantation and decisions regarding treatment choice, organ allocation, allocation of limited resources, such as ICU beds and post-transplant care also involve complex ethical issues.

History of Respiratory Ethics

The history of ethics in respiratory medicine reflects the evolution of respiratory care, and changing societal values. Ancient medical texts from various cultures demonstrate that medical ethics have been an integral part of healthcare for thousands of years, with principles that remain relevant today. The ancient Egyptian\Ebers Papyrus contains the oldest known reference to a physician's ethical obligations, including respect for human life, and confidentiality.

In European medicine, medical ethics were well described in ancient Greek texts and incorporated in the iconic Hippocratic Oath which emphasized as below:

"Whatever I see or hear in the course of the treatment... I will keep to myself." (Confidentiality)

"I will do no harm or injustice to my patients." (Nonmaleficence)

"I will give no deadly medicine to anyone, even if asked." (Beneficence)

The Oath clearly emphasized the importance of four fundamental principles as applied to the practice of medicine: (1) Autonomy (respecting patients' rights to make informed decisions about their care); (2) beneficence (providing care that promotes patients' well-being and best interests); (3) nonmaleficence (avoiding harm or injury to patients); and (4) justice (ensuring fair and equitable distribution of resources and care).

Ancient and Medieval Indian Perspectives

The concurrent Vedic civilization of the Indian sub-continent clearly emphasized the importance of confidentiality, informed consent, non-maleficence and others as evident from the following statements contained in Charaka and Sushruta Samhita, the ancient Ayurvedic texts. These examples demonstrate that the Charaka Samhita, written over 2,000 years ago, contained many principles of medical ethics that remain relevant today.

- *"The physician should not disclose any information about the patient, whether it be good or bad, to anyone else." (Charaka Samhita, Sutrasthana, 8.64)*
- *"The physician should explain the treatment and its effects to the patient, and obtain their consent before proceeding." (Charaka Samhita, Sutrasthana, 8.66)*
- *"The physician should not cause harm to the patient, even if it is unintentional." (Charaka Samhita, Sutrasthana, 8.65)*
- *"The physician should avoid using treatments that are likely to cause harm to the patient." (Charaka Samhita, Chikitsasthana, 1.4)*
- *"The physician should act in the best interest of the patient, and strive to provide the best possible care." (Charaka Samhita, Sutrasthana, 8.63)*
- *"The physician should be compassionate and sympathetic towards patients, and provide care with kindness and empathy." (Charaka Samhita, Sutrasthana, 8.67)*
- *"The physician should respect the patient's autonomy and decision-making capacity, and involve them in the treatment process." (Charaka Samhita, Sutrasthana, 8.68)*
- *"The physician should provide care to all patients, regardless of their social status, caste, or creed." (Charaka Samhita, Sutrasthana, 8.69)*

Mahavagga, the Buddhist text (500 BCE) advocated the ethical conduct of physicians. Buddhism laid great stress on the moral principles of compassion (*"A physician should be compassionate and sympathetic towards patients"*) and honesty (*"A physician should be honest and transparent in their dealings with patients"*).

Medieval India's medical ethics were shaped by a rich cultural heritage, influential texts, and key principles. Most religious cultures in India during the medieval period including Hinduism, Buddhism, and Jainism, emphasized on *ahimsa* (nonviolence, emphasizing the importance of avoiding harm to living beings); *dharma* (righteousness, the concept of dharma guided medical practitioners to act with integrity, compassion, and fairness), and *seva* (service). These principles guided medical practitioners to act with compassion, integrity, and fairness. *Madhava Nidanam*, a treatise on pathology and diagnosis, discussed the ethical aspects of medical practice. The principles were also discussed in Ibn Sina's Canon of Medicine and advocated in Unani medicine introduced in India from the Middle East and Central Asia.

Modern Era Medical Ethics

In the modern era, the development of medical ethics can be attributed to Thomas Percival, an English physician and philosopher whose work, "Medical Ethics; or, a Code of Institutes and Precepts, Adapted to the Professional Conduct of Physicians and Surgeons" (1803), is considered a foundational text in the development of modern medical ethics. Percival's interest in medical ethics was sparked by his experiences as a physician and his observations of the medical profession. He was concerned about the lack of formal guidelines for medical professionals and the potential for conflicts of interest, particularly in the areas of patient care and medical research. His book on medical ethics consisted of four chapters, each elaborating on the duties of physicians to their patients; to each other; to the public and in relation to the Law.

Percival emphasized the importance of confidentiality, respect for patients' autonomy, and the duty to provide compassionate care. He stressed upon the need for professional courtesy, respect for colleagues' opinions, and

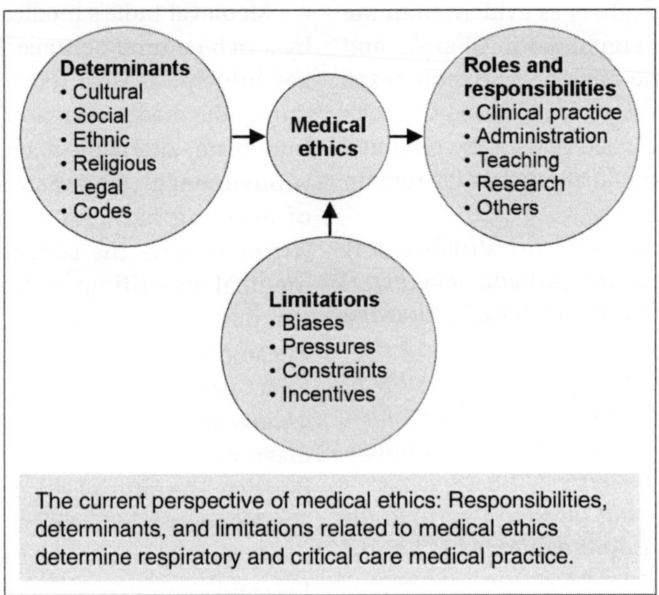

The current perspective of medical ethics: Responsibilities, determinants, and limitations related to medical ethics determine respiratory and critical care medical practice.

the importance of maintaining a united front in the face of adversity. Percival also highlighted the responsibility of physicians to promote public health, prevent disease, and provide education on health-related matters. He also elaborated on the intersection of medicine and law, including issues related to medical testimony, malpractice, and the regulation of medical practice.

Percival's book provided a formal code of conduct for medical professionals, outlining their duties and responsibilities to patients, colleagues, and society. Subsequently, "Medical Ethics" became a standard textbook in medical schools, shaping the education and training of future physicians. It further influenced the development of professional medical organizations, such as the American Medical Association (AMA), which adopted its first "Code of Medical Ethics" (1847) and established guidelines for medical professionals.

Post World Wars

The two great wars, particularly the 2nd World War witnessed major violations of human rights and medical malpractice. Post World War II, the international community adopted the Nuremberg Code in 1947 in response to Nazi atrocities. The Nuremberg Code established principles for human experimentation, emphasizing informed consent and respect for human subjects. Built upon the Nuremberg Code, the Helsinki Declaration (1964) was adopted which provided guidelines for medical research involving human subjects. In the United States, the National Institutes of Health (NIH) developed guidelines for human experimentation, which later influenced the development of institutional review boards (IRBs). The Belmont Report (1979), commissioned by the US Department of Health, Education, and Welfare, outlined principles for human subjects research, including respect for persons, beneficence, and justice. Similarly, the President's Commission for the Study of Ethical Problems in Medicine and Biomedical and Behavioural Research (1978–1983) commission addressed various bioethical issues, including informed consent, human subjects research, and access to healthcare.

Meanwhile, the medical community was confronted with a large number of complex issues posing critical ethical dilemmas. The dilemmas, attributed to rapid technological advances and increasing commercialization, kept on rapidly multiplying. International health initiatives have emphasized the need for ethical standards in healthcare, particularly in resource-poor settings. The human rights and feminist movements highlighting the importance of respecting patients' dignity, autonomy, and rights became more active and forceful. The rise of consumerism in healthcare has created new ethical challenges, such as balancing patient demands with medical professionalism. On the other hand, rising malpractice litigation has led to increased scrutiny of medical professionals and a greater emphasis on ethical standards.

Government regulations and accreditation standards have increased accountability and driven the development of formal medical ethics guidelines.

Introduction of Life-sustaining Treatments

The development of organ transplantation and other life-sustaining treatments have created ethical dilemmas around end-of-life care. In respiratory medicine, the dependence on mechanical ventilation and lung transplantation has frequently raised serious ethical questions around withholding/withdrawing treatment. End-of-life care and palliative medicine with discussions about life-sustaining treatments, advance care planning, and compassionate care is an important issue in advanced lung diseases such as chronic obstructive pulmonary disease (COPDs), interstitial fibrosis, and lung cancer. Resource allocation because of the restricted access to limited resources, and to resort to distributive justice have become important ethical issues with respect to these high-end treatments involving ICU beds and lung transplantation. Treatment of lung cancer is an equally significant issue.

Palliative and End-of-Life Care

End-of-life care in respiratory medicine focuses on alleviating symptoms, such as pain and breathlessness in patients with advanced respiratory diseases. It also includes discussions and decisions around withholding/withdrawing life-sustaining treatments, advance care planning, and compassionate care. The Hospice movement, led by Dame Cicely Saunders, emphasized compassionate care for terminally ill patients including those with respiratory diseases. The Hospice movement and the emergence of palliative care (1960s–1980s) have led to the development of multidisciplinary teams, including doctors, nurses, and social workers, who provide comprehensive care for patients with advanced illnesses.

Continuation of curative treatments and hospitalizations for advanced, end-stage diseases was not only futile but also painful and costly. It led to the emergence of palliative and hospice care in Europe. In UK, it was already in existence in the 20th century with St Christopher's Hospice in 1967. Hospice care emerged in the USA, with the establishment of the first hospice in 1974. Towards the end of the century, palliative care teams were established focusing on symptom management and quality of life for patients with advanced diseases.

The World Health Organization defined palliative care emphasizing the importance of symptom management and quality of life. The European Respiratory Society (ERS) published guidelines for palliative care in respiratory disease, highlighting the need for integrated care. Respiratory palliative care became more prominent, with the development of guidelines and services for patients with advanced respiratory diseases. In 2013, the American Thoracic Society (ATS) issued a statement on palliative care in respiratory disease, emphasizing the importance of early integration of palliative care. Currently, the European countries as well

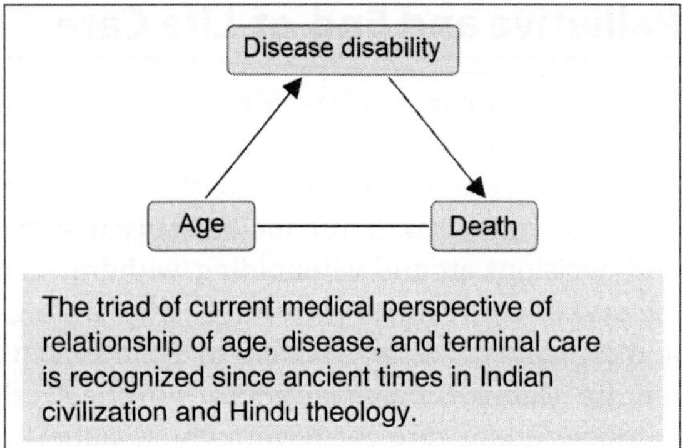

The triad of current medical perspective of relationship of age, disease, and terminal care is recognized since ancient times in Indian civilization and Hindu theology.

as the USA have implemented various models of palliative care, including integrated care pathways and multidisciplinary teams. The last decade has seen an increase in palliative care programs, with a focus on integrated care and multidisciplinary teams.

Modern India

Evolution of medical ethics in modern India has followed the trend parallel to what happened elsewhere in the world. Post Independence, India adopted the Indian Medical Council Act (1956) to regulate medical education and practice. The Indian Medical Association (IMA) introduced a code of ethics for medical practitioners, emphasizing confidentiality, informed consent, and nonmaleficence.

Distributive Care

Indian physicians face enormous ethical challenges in their day-to-day clinical practice. Addressing concerns around patient safety, medical errors, and quality of care has assumed paramount importance. Respiratory physicians daily face the issue of rationing of resources in view of the limited availability of ventilators and ICU beds. Decisions about allocation can be complex, particularly in cases where demand exceeds supply. Ensuring fairness and transparency in allocation processes is crucial. Decisions about who receives life-sustaining treatment can be challenging. Disparities in healthcare access and affordability can lead to unequal treatment opportunities. Rural-urban disparities and lack of specialized care in rural areas exacerbate this issue.

Informed Consent

The issue of informed consent is also difficult since patients may not fully understand their diagnosis, treatment options, or prognosis. Moreover, language barriers and low literacy rates also complicate this issue. Decisions about withdrawing life-sustaining treatment when it is no longer beneficial can be difficult, especially in cases where patients lack advance directives. Families may insist on continued treatment despite medical advice. Cultural and familial expectations significantly influence the decision-making process. Truth-telling and disclosing bad news to patients and families requires balancing the need for honesty with the potential harms. Cultural norms around truth-telling vary in different social and religious groups.

Conflict of Interest

Conflicts of interest pose major challenges in today's medical practice. Healthcare providers may face conflicts between patient interests and financial incentives especially since the pharmaceutical and equipment companies influence treatment decisions through aggressive marketing. Research ethics are crucial to balance the need for medical advancements with the potential risks and benefits to participants. It is important to ensure informed consent and protect the vulnerable populations in research studies.

Addressing these ethical dilemmas requires a multidisciplinary approach, including education, policy development, and open communication among healthcare providers, patients, and families. The Indian Council of Medical Research (ICMR) introduced guidelines for biomedical research, emphasizing informed consent, confidentiality, and respect for human subjects. Many Indian institutions have now established bioethics committees to address emerging ethical issues especially with reference to medical research, clinical trials, and animal-experimentation. All research protocols including post-graduation are required to be approved by the Institutional Ethics Committee or Review Board. The Committee is also required to provide support and guidance for healthcare professionals facing ethical dilemmas.

Palliative and End-of-Life Care in India

End-of-life issues in respiratory medicine in India involve addressing the unique needs of patients with advanced respiratory diseases. Symptomatic and end-of-life care is essential in improving the quality of life for these patients, focusing on symptom management, emotional support, and spiritual care. Management of symptoms involves a multidisciplinary approach including use of restricted drugs such opioids for pain and breathlessness management, anxiolytics and antidepressants for emotional support or noninvasive ventilation for respiratory support. Developing palliative care services and infrastructure is important for managing these patients with terminal illnesses.

Respiratory end-of-life care remains a challenging issue. Burnout among healthcare providers is an important issue which requires management for the emotional and psychological toll of caring for critically ill patients. It is important to ensure that healthcare providers receive adequate support and resources to maintain their well-being. Violence against doctors especially those working with critically ill patients is an entirely new element which has interjected the traditional doctor–patient relationship. Inclusion of medical practice in the Consumer Protection Act has made doctors more vulnerable resulting in a significant increase in the cost of medical care.

The concept of Hospice care emerged in India, with the establishment of the Shanti Avedna Sadan in Mumbai (1965) and the Cancer Institute in Chennai (1952). Palliative care was introduced in India, primarily focusing on cancer patients. These were established in a few hospitals, including the Tata Memorial Hospital in Mumbai (1986) and the All India Institute of Medical Sciences (AIIMS) in New Delhi (1990s). Palliative respiratory care in India has made significant progress, but there is still a long way to go. In the 1990s, palliative care initiatives started gaining momentum, with the formation of organizations such as the Pain and Palliative Care Society (PPCS) in Kerala and the Indian Association of Palliative Care (IAPC). Today, palliative care services are available in many parts of India, with some states such as Kerala and Maharashtra having made significant progress in integrating palliative care into their healthcare systems.

There is still a significant gap in access to palliative care. One of the significant challenges faced by palliative care providers in India relates to the restrictive Narcotic Drugs and Psychotropic Substances (NDPS) Act, which limits access to essential medications such as morphine and other narcotics, or sometimes even strong sedatives. However, after years of advocacy, the Act was amended in 2014, making it easier to access these medications. To address the gaps in palliative care, there is a need for increased awareness, education, and training of healthcare professionals. The government also needs to prioritize palliative care and allocate adequate resources to support its development. Organizations like the IAPC and Pallium India are working tirelessly to promote palliative care and advocate for policy changes.

Respiratory Palliative Care

Respiratory palliative care began to take shape, with the establishment of respiratory medicine departments in various hospitals. It has developed more rapidly since 2010s with the growing recognition of the importance of early integration for patients with advanced respiratory diseases. Care is becoming more personalized, with a focus on patient-centered goals, values, and preferences. Several advances in respiratory care on domiciliary basis have made it possible to continue the treatments for longer periods. For example, long-term oxygen therapy (LTOT) is shown to significantly improve the quality of life for patients with chronic respiratory diseases. Similarly, noninvasive ventilation (NIV) is being increasingly used to manage respiratory failure in such patients.

Withdrawal of Life-supports

Withdrawal of life-supports such as mechanical ventilation is another important issue in respiratory end-of-life care. There are two notable judgements which have dealt with some of the issues. The Gujarat High Court in Ranjanben Ramesh Bhatt v. State of Gujarat (2004) case ruled that patients have the right to informed consent and refusal of treatment. In another case, Common Cause versus Union of India (2018), The Supreme Court of India recognized the right to die with dignity allowing individuals to choose how they want to die. Both these judgements had raised more questions than answer the difficult issues related to withholding or withdrawing life-supports.

The court modified these guidelines in 2023, removing the condition that mandated a magistrate's approval for withdrawal or withholding of life support to a terminally ill person. This decision aimed to make the guidelines more workable and less cumbersome. The Court recognized "to die with dignity" as a fundamental right and that individuals can make informed decisions about their end-of-life treatment through living wills. Passive euthanasia was permitted in certain circumstances, allowing for the withdrawal or withholding of life support. Guidelines for end-of-life care were established to ensure that patients receive dignified and compassionate care. The Supreme Court made strong efforts to balance individual autonomy with the need to protect vulnerable patients, and to provide clarity on end-of-life care issues in India.

In summary, the life support treatments can be withdrawn in India under specific circumstances as below:
- If a patient has a terminal illness with no reasonable medical probability of recovery.
- If a patient is in a permanent vegetative state.
- If further medical intervention or treatment would only artificially prolong the process of dying.
- If a patient with decision-making capacity refuses treatment.
- If a patient has an advance medical directive or "living will" that specifies their wishes regarding life support.
- If a patient lacks decision-making capacity, a surrogate decision-maker can make decisions regarding life support withdrawal.

It is important to note that the withdrawal of life support treatments in India must be done in accordance with the guidelines established by the Ministry of Health and Family Welfare, which emphasize the importance of medical boards, patient consent, and palliative care.

In summary, medical ethics raise questions around data privacy and informed consent besides addressing health disparities and access to care. It is essential to make efforts to reduce inequities in access to respiratory care and promote health justice. It is important to focus on patient-centered care and respect for patients' autonomy, values, and preferences. The history of development of medical ethics guides us to the need of incorporating these principles into medical education and training programs. It is also required to strengthen palliative-care services for terminally ill patients with incurable diseases. Establishing robust ethics committees and ensuring that they are functional, effective, and independent is an important step to guide the physicians as well as the researchers to follow the ethical practices.

Sources

1. Berdine G. (2015). The Hippocratic Oath and Principles of Medical Ethics. [online] Available from https://pulmonarychronicles.com/index.php/pulmonarychronicles/article/view/185/438 [Last accessed September, 2025]
2. Civilsdaily. Medical Ethics of Charka. [online] Available from https://www.civilsdaily.com/news/medical-ethics-of-charaka [Last accessed September, 2025]
3. Tawalare KA, Nanote KD, Gawai VU, Gotmare AY. Contribution of Ayurveda in foundation of basic tenets of bioethics. Ayu. 2014;35(4):366-70.
4. Indian Journal of Medical Ethics. Handbook on Medical Ethics. Medical ethics - as prescribed by Caraka, Susruta and other ancient Indian physicians. [online] Available from https://ijme.in/articles/medical-ethics-as-prescribed-by-caraka-susruta-and-other-ancient-indian-physicians [Last accessed September, 2025]
5. Parmar P, Rathod G. A Comparative Analysis of the Hippocratic Oath and Charak Oath in Medical Ethics. Int Arch Integr Med. 2024;11(7):10- 3
6. Percival T. Medical ethics. In: John HP (Ed). Medical Ethics. France: World Medical Association; 1849. pp. 49–57, esp section 8 p. 52.
7. Markose A, Krishnan R, Ramesh M. Medical ethics. J Pharm Bioallied Sci. 2016;8(Suppl 1):S1-S4.
8. Will JF. A Brief Historical and Theoretical Perspective on Patient Autonomy and Medical Decision Making. Chest. 2011;139(6):1491-7.
9. Indian Medical Council (Professional Conduct, Etiquette and Ethics) Regulations, 2002. Amended up to 8th October 2016. https://www.nmc.org.in/wp-content/uploads/2017.
10. Singh MM, Garg US, Arora P. Laws applicable to medical practice and hospitals in India. Int J Res Found Hosp Healthc Adm. 2013;1:19-24.
11. Jindal SK. Old age, disease and terminal care: A Hindu perspective. In: Discourses on Aging and Dying. In: Chatterjee SC, Patnaik P, Chariar VM (Eds). New Delhi: Sage Publications India Pvt. Ltd.; 2008. pp.217-25.
12. Jindal SK. Caring for respiratory disease in India in the COVID era (Ed). Expert Review Respir Med. 2021;13:1-3.
13. Jindal SK. Privatization of health care: non ethical dilemmas. Issues Med Ethics. 1998;6:85-6.
14. Shweta K, Kumar S, Gupta AK, Jindal SK, Kumar A. Economic analysis of costs associated with a Respiratory Intensive Care Unit in a tertiary care teaching hospital in Northern India. Indian J Crit Care Med. 2013;17(2):76-81.
15. Jindal SK. Ethical issues related to Investigations and Therapeutic Interventions in the ICU: High Cost of Care. Ethics in Clinical Practice. Ann Nat Acad Med Sci. 2004;VI:41-5.
16. Sallnow L, Smith R, Ahmedzai SH, Bhadelia A, Chamberlain C, Cong Y, et al. Report of the Lancet Commission on the Value of Death: Bringing death back into life. Lancet. 2022;399:837-84.
17. Jindal SK. Ethical issues in the care of the terminally ill patients (ed). Chest India. 2005;6:1-2.
18. Jindal SK. Issues in the care of the dying. Ind J Med Ethics. 2005;2:79-80.
19. Law Commission of India. 196th report (2006). Medical treatment of terminally ill patients (for the protection of patients and Medical practitioners). [online] Available from http://lawcommissionofindia.nic.in/reports/rep196.pdf [Last accessed September, 2025]
20. Mani RK, Simha S, Gursahani R. Simplified Legal Procedure for End-of-life Decisions in India: A New Dawn in the Care of the Dying? Indian J Crit Care Med. 2023;27(5):374-6.
21. Jenifer Jeba S, Kuriakose J. End-of-Life Care. In: Jindal SK (Ed). Text Book of Pulmonary & Critical Care, 3rd edition. New Delhi: Jaypee Brothers Medical Publisher; 2025.

CHAPTER

20

Saga of Developments in Armed Forces Medical Services

Lt Gen (Retd) Dr BNBM Prasad

The Army Medical Corps

The Army Medical Corps (AMC) is a specialist corps in the Indian Army and includes the medical services of the Navy and the Air Force; primarily meant for providing medical services to all army personnel, serving and veterans along with their families. AMC has a colonial past dating back to 1613, when a small medical unit/establishment called the "Indian Medical Service (IMS)" was founded with a handful of staff to cater for the East India Company. With the company's increased military activities, "The Bengal Presidency Medical Service", which was the first of the military service of the three Presidencies in India, was established on January 1, 1764. Since then the Corps has come a long way from its modest beginning, expanding to meet the contingencies of conflicts and wars leading to the creation of a homogenous medical corps, the Indian Army Medical Corps (IAMC) for offering dedicated medical services to the Army on April 3, 1943. In the postindependent India, it came to be known as The Army Medical Corps with effect from January 26, 1950. Final feather in the AMC beret came when the then President of India, Dr Sarvepalli Radhakrishnan presented "The President's Colour Award", the highest award to the corps on its raising day on April 3, 1966.

Combat doctors are comrades in arms who fight both the enemy and disease with the same ferocity and do anything and everything which can make the soldier fit and fine again. AMC had many legends who served the sick including Mahatma Gandhi and Major Ronald Ross. The father of the nation founded a voluntary body, Natal Ambulance Corps in South Africa with around 1,100 volunteers primarily to assist British Army in the Anglo-Boer War of 1899–1902 as stretcher bearers for casualty evacuation. Major Ronald Ross, the Almora-born British doctor, served the AMC for 25 years and while serving at Secunderabad, he made the groundbreaking discovery of mosquito-borne transmission of malaria in 1897 for which he was awarded the Nobel Prize in 1902 for Medicine and Physiology. Field Marshal Sam Manekshaw wanted to become a doctor and serve AMC like his father but destiny took him to Indian Military Academy (IMA) while his brother late Air Vice Marshal JHF Manekshaw became an Aviation Medical specialist in the Indian Air Force, playing a pivotal role in the advancement of Aviation Medicine in India.

Lt Gen (Retd) Dr BNBM Prasad MD DNB DM FNCCP FCCP FRCP
Former DGHS, Armed Forces and President's Honorary Surgeon
Former Professor and Head, Pulmonary Medicine
Amrita Institute of Medical Sciences
Kochi, Kerala, India

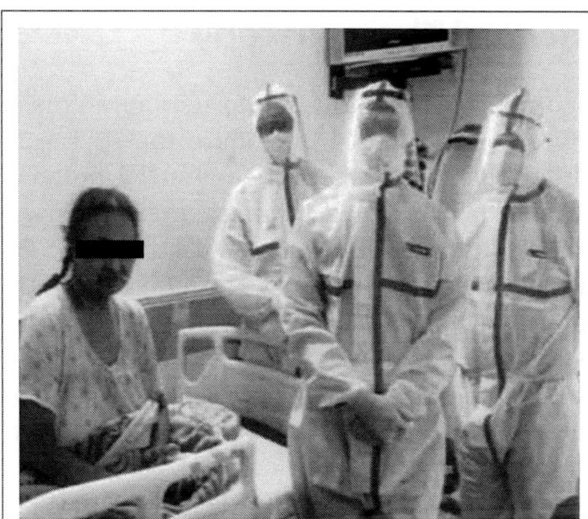

COVID intensive care unit (ICU) established in one of the army hospitals.

We shall focus here on the specific contributions to *respiratory medicine* and related areas.

Tuberculosis Care

Army Medical Corps has been the leading light in tuberculosis (TB) care in India for many decades extending back to the pre-chemotherapy era when TB sanatorium in idyllic conditions were established at Deolali (Nasik), Aundh (Pune), Ranchi, Dehradun, Abbottabad (Pakistan), and Kasauli to treat TB patients with fresh air, diet, rest, and respiratory rehabilitation. An "Indo Burmese General Hospital" was raised in 1942 which was later transformed in 1946 as Military Hospital Aundh (Pune) for the TB care of both the Indian and the British troops. In due course of time, it was converted to the present-day Army Institute of Cardiothoracic Sciences (AICTS), formerly known as Military Hospital Cardiothoracic Center (MH CTC). Asia's first lung resection was done at this historic TB sanatorium by a renowned army surgeon, Major Leigh Collis, on December 10, 1945, laying the foundation stone for the growth of thoracic surgery in India. Since then, this institution has grown to become a center of excellence in tubercular surgery. Armed forces TB hospitals are some of the best in the world and this was echoed by then Defense Minister George Fernandes during his visit to Military Hospital Namkum (Ranch).

Aviation Medicine

"The Institute of Aerospace Medicine" (IAM) at Bangalore was established in 1957, in the present Hindustan Aeronautical Limited (HAL) premises, for imparting training in aviation medicine, indoctrination of air crews in aviation medicine and carrying out in the aeromedical aspects of design and development of aircraft. In the early eighties, the institute was involved with Indo-Soviet manned space program in the evaluation and selection of space crew, i.e., Sqn Ldr Rakesh Sharma and Wg Cdr Ravish Malhotra. Recently in 2025, Group Captain Shubanshu Shukla, the first Indian to visit the international space station (ISS) and successfully complete 20 days of space odyssey as the mission pilot for Axiom Mission 4, underwent rigorous training for ISRO's Gaganyaan Space Mission. Today this institution has state-of-the-art facilities and is the nodal center for aeromedical research, training, consultancy and evaluation in India.

High Altitude Medical Research Centre, Leh

Many low-land young soldiers, otherwise fit, on sudden induction to high-altitude regions of Himalayas during Indo-China Conflict 1962 developed severe breathlessness, with some even succumbing within few days of high-altitude stay due to unexplained pulmonary edema. Army researchers, notably Lt Gen Inder Singh and Brig ND Menon, attributed this condition to lack of adaptation to high-altitude environment and due to severe hypoxia-induced pulmonary vasoconstriction resulting in noncardiogenic pulmonary edema. Similarly in areas like the

Siachen glacier, where there is severe hypobaric hypoxia, extreme cold and with constant threat to one's life due to avalanches, cold injuries and high altitude-related medical complications are common. Following the Indo-China Conflict 1962, the High Altitude Medical Research Centre (HAMRC) at Leh was established to address high-altitude health issues among people working and living there. This institute has state-of-the-art facilities including hypobaric chambers to manage life-threatening conditions and is the leading High Altitude Medical Research Institute of international standing.

Institute of Naval Medicine—INHS Asvini, Mumbai

Deep-sea divers as well as those deployed in submarines get exposed to hyperbaric conditions risking them to acute barotrauma like pneumothorax and decompression sickness, the bends or Caisson disease, following decompression of body gases on coming to the sea surface. The Institute of Naval Medicine focuses on underwater medicine and is the leading institute that provides state-of-the-art medical care including hyperbaric oxygen therapy to diving-related illnesses.

Pulmonary Interventions

The scope of respiratory medicine expanded significantly in the 1990s to include a wide range of respiratory and other systemic diseases, interventional procedures, and critical care. As result, the first postdoctoral course (DM) Pulmonary and Critical Care was introduced at the Postgraduate Institute of Medical Education and Research, Chandigarh and the author was privileged to enroll in the program as the "first" from the armed forces. Subsequently, he was able to introduce and promote the development of new areas in the specialty.

Medical Thoracoscopy

I got much needed booster to start a minimally invasive endoscopic procedure that is a safe alternative to complex video-assisted thoracic surgery (VATS) for the management of many pleural diseases. The first medical thoracoscopy was performed at Military Hospital Dehradun in 1994 by making use of an unused cystoscope held by the surgery department of the hospital. The initial procedure was exciting and fruitful for mycobacterial as well as histopathological confirmation of TB pleural effusion. At MH (CTC) Pune, I took up a pilot project titled "The role of medical thoracoscopy in the diagnosis of exudative pleural effusions of undetermined etiology" in the year 1996 under aegis of Armed Forces Research Committee (AFMRC). It finally paved the way for establishing medical thoracoscopy as a standard procedure in *armed forces chest centers.*

Pleural Drainage

I began using commonly available infant feeding tubes (5 to 8F) in 1992 at Military Hospital Dehradun where I was posted then. Subsequently when I moved to MH (CTC) Pune, where cardiac catheterization facilities existed, I started using reusable right-heart pigtail catheters since they were easily available without any additional cost. The problems with repurposed catheters were many—length, lack of side holes, puncture needle, guidewire, connectors, and underwater drainage issues. Meanwhile in the year 1996 while working at MH (CTC), Pune, I started getting a steady supply of specialized pleural catheters as per my patient's requirements.

COVID Warriors

The contribution of Indian Armed forces during COVID-19 pandemic was immense and the most invaluable. The department of respiratory medicine, AICTS has managed thousands of severe COVID-19 cases and had contributed in the validation of rapid detection kits, the formulation of national consensus statement for respiratory procedures, and the national COVID vaccine program—COVAXIN. The department had formulated and standardized technique of instillation of live COVID-19 virus in airways of rhesus macaques. Post-virus instillation, sequential bronchoscopy and bronchoalveolar lavage and assessment of sequential radiological investigations of the enrolled rhesus macaques was carried out in this trial.

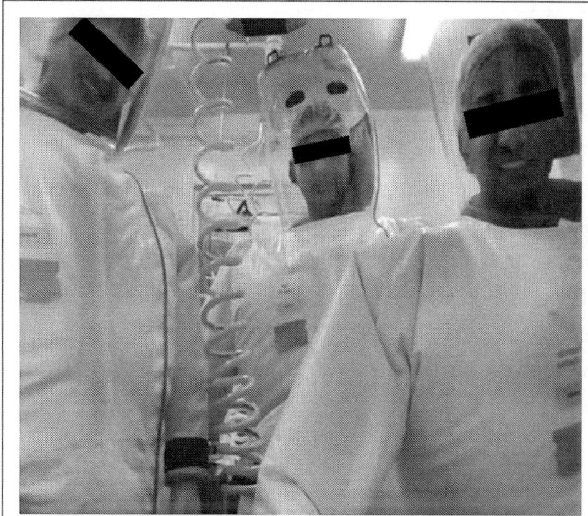

Army medical officers' team in the rhesus macaques bronchoscopy suite.
Courtesy: Col Vikas Marwah.

Army Medical Corps during its glorious existence has relentlessly contributed to the growth of health care, medical education, and research in India including in the specialty of *respiratory medicine*. Historically, military hospitals across the subcontinent under British rule were the centers of standardized

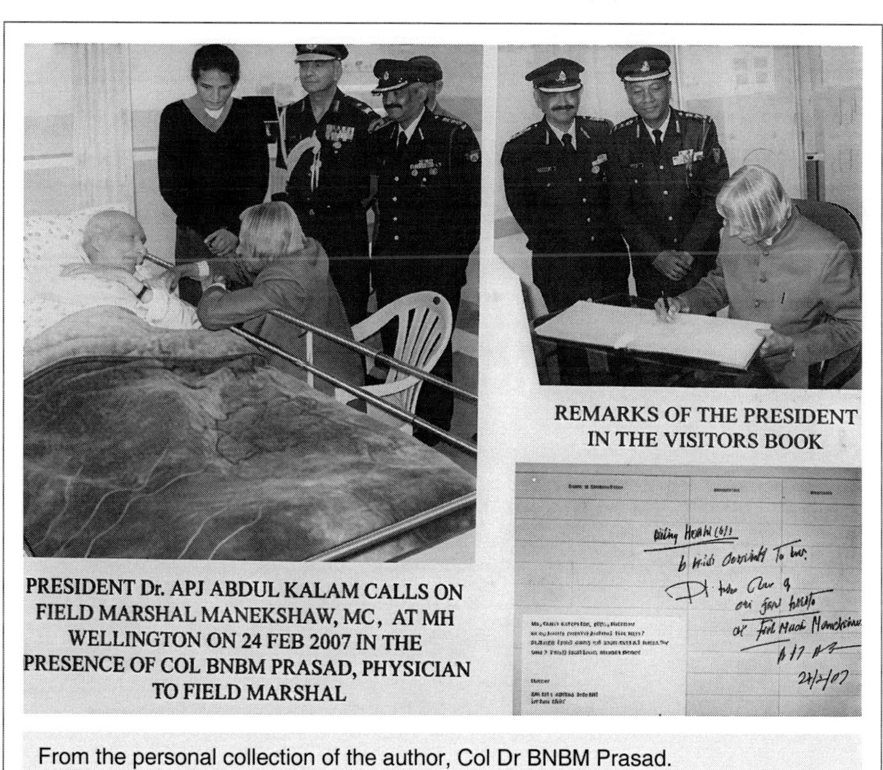

From the personal collection of the author, Col Dr BNBM Prasad.

care exclusive to soldiers, which was then not available to civilians. Army hospitals excelled in combat medicine, TB care, disaster management, and tackling with pandemics. They laid the foundation for the National Health Mission in the postindependent India. The journey of AMC from Bengal Presidency Medical Services to the present-day AFMS has been glorious—setting standards and keep moving while serving the sick and the needy to live up to the motto *"Sarve Santu Niramaya"* meaning "*Let all be free from disease and disability*".

Sources

1. Ghosh A, History of the Armed Forces Medical Services. New Delhi: Orient Longman; 1988. p. 349.
2. Medical Thoracoscopy. NACCON 99: 38th Annual Conference of National College of Chest Physicians (India), Udaipur; 1999.
3. Drainage of Intra-Thoracic Collections: Role of Small Catheter Chest Tubes. NACCON 99: 38th Annual Conference of National College of Chest Physicians (India), Udaipur; 1999.
4. Treatment of Empyema Thoracis by Percutaneous Catheter Drainage versus Surgical Tube Thoracostomy. CHEST 1999—65th Annual International Scientific Assembly of American College of Chest Physicians, Chicago; 1999.
5. Menon ND. High-Altitude Pulmonary Edema: A Clinical Study. N Engl J Med. 1965;273:66-73.
6. Singh I, Kapila CC, Khanna PK, Nanda RB, Rao BD. High-Altitude Pulmonary Oedema. Lancet. 1965;1(7379):229-34.
7. Singh I. High-altitude Pulmonary Edema: Am Heart J. 1965;70(4):435-9.

CHAPTER

21

Respiratory Research Innovations

Medical research plays a vital role in advancing our understanding of human health and disease, leading to improved treatments and outcomes. It helps to unravel the underlying causes of diseases and provides new insights into human physiology, anatomy, and genetics which lead to the development of more accurate and efficient diagnostic tools. It finally enables the development of effective treatments such as the discovery of new medications and interventions as well as tailored treatments and therapies based on individual characteristics. Medical research also helps in the development of preventive measures such as vaccines, screenings, and lifestyle interventions. In summary, it is essential to improve patient outcomes, enabling individuals to lead healthier and more fulfilling lives. Research in respiratory medicine is as vital as in all other medical fields.

Respiratory Research in India

The tradition of medical research in India is quite old as evidenced by the documented knowledge on a number of health problems in ancient medical texts, some of which have been mentioned in the earlier chapters. Most of this information was documented in *Sanskrit* which was restricted to scholars. Moreover, the centuries of internal strife and external aggressions led to stagnation of progress and a gradual decline. William Dalrymple, a contemporary historian, has elegantly pointed to some such issues in his book, "The Golden Road" with respect to the fall of culture, economy, trade, and political rule in India. The same reasons are likely to be relevant for nonprogression and dissipation of medical sciences.

There has been a resurgence of interest in medical sciences in modern postcolonial India. Publication of "research" papers in professional journals was given significant importance as criteria for selection and promotion in faculty jobs. According to latest available data, more than 312,250 papers are annually published in medical and health sciences. It is difficult to estimate the number of publications in respiratory medicine. Moreover, it is not possible to talk about the quality of these publications and their contribution to the overall development of health sciences. Similarly, India also introduced the necessary requirement for completion of a "Thesis/Dissertation" for all its postgraduate courses. It will be difficult to point out any meaningful or significant research work achieved through this program. At best, the thesis completion can be considered an introduction to research methodology. The whole programs require revamping for better outcomes.

The era has also seen a rapid progression in new developments related to respiratory medicine. Clinical research in modern respiratory medicine in India has been a significant step forward, but there is much work to be done to address the country's respiratory health challenges. A large number of research reports on subjects in respiratory medicine regularly appear in different professional journals from India and abroad.

But most Indian respiratory research is limited to observational, epidemiological, or descriptive studies on clinical spectrum of diseases.

In this chapter, we have tried to introduce the readers to some such studies which are either innovative or have made significant impact on clinical respiratory medicine. We also tried to include studies published in credible professional journals which have tended to describe diseases on a relatively wider scale in the country or which recognized an issue for the first time. Some of the consensus statements or guidelines have been separately listed. There are also reports on asthma, tobacco smoking, passive-smoking and lung diseases, nonsmoking risk factors, air-pollution, chronic obstructive pulmonary disease (COPD), interstitial lung disease (ILD), and lung cancer which have contributed to our knowledge and understanding of disease spectra in India.

There are other publications reporting results of individual observations or ad hoc research (projects on different issues related to disease mechanisms, diagnostic tests, pharmacological, and interventional treatments). Many of the published papers include interesting case reports, reviews and other kinds of teaching material. It cannot be denied that most such papers and many of the studies which are not listed here have also contributed to the overall progress of respiratory medicine in the country.

Basic Sciences

1. Paintal AS. Mechanism of stimulation of type J pulmonary receptors. J Physiol. 1969;203(3):511-32.
2. Paintal AS, Damodaran VN, Guz A. Mechanism of excitation of type J receptors. Acta Neurobiol Exp (Wars). 1973;33(1):15-9.

Discovery of juxtacapillary or J-receptors in the lungs by AS Paintal from V.P. Chest Institute, Delhi has been a groundbreaking finding. His work has had a lasting impact on our understanding of respiratory and cardiovascular physiology, and his contributions continue to influence research in these fields.

He discovered these sensory nerve endings, also known as juxtacapillary receptors or pulmonary C-fiber receptors, which are located within the alveolar walls of the lung, close to the pulmonary capillaries. Paintal's research showed that J-receptors respond to various stimuli, including pulmonary edema, pulmonary emboli, pneumonia, congestive heart failure, and barotrauma, which lead to decreased oxygenation and increased respiration. The stimulation of J-receptors triggers a reflex response, characterized by apnea, rapid breathing, bradycardia, and hypotension. Paintal's work suggested that J-receptors play a role in the sensation of dyspnea or difficulty breathing. Beyond J-receptors, he also worked on various aspects of respiratory and cardiovascular physiology, making significant contributions to our understanding of the neural control of breathing and circulation.

Tuberculosis

Several landmark studies on tuberculosis (TB) treatment strategies were undertaken at the Tuberculosis Chemotherapy Center, Madras which was established with the mandate to study the feasibility of domiciliary treatment. The work done at the Center had helped to define and implement the TB treatment strategies for TB Control Program in India. Some of the key findings included the treatment success with shorter duration of courses administered on domiciliary basis without any additional risk to the contacts. It is beyond the scope of this chapter to go into the details of these publications. Interested readers should go through these studies in the scientific journals.

1. Lotte A, Hatton F, Perdrizet S, Rouillon A. A concurrent comparison of intermittent (twice weekly) isoniazid and streptomycin and daily isoniazid plus PAS in the domiciliary treatment of pulmonary tuberculosis.

Tuberculosis Chemotherapy Centre, Madras. Bull World Health Organ. 1964;31(2):247-71.

The results of this study demonstrated that the intermittent regimen was at least as effective as the standard oral regimen. These findings suggest a possible change in drug administration for TB in developing countries.

2. Dawson JJY, Devadatta S, Fox W, Radhakrishna S, Ramakrishnan CV, Somasundaram PR, et al. A 5-year study of patients with pulmonary tuberculosis in a concurrent comparison of home and sanatorium treatment for one year with isoniazid plus PAS. Bull World Health Organ. 1966;34(4):533-51.

This report on progress of some newly diagnosed, sputum-positive pulmonary TB over a 5-year period showed the success of home treatment. The relapse rates over the follow-up period were 7% for the home patients and 10% for the sanatorium patients. These findings were very encouraging.

3. Tuberculosis Chemotherapy Centre. Isoniazid plus thioacetazone compared with two regimens of isoniazid plus PAS in the domiciliary treatment of pulmonary tuberculosis in South Indian patients. Bull World Health Organ. 1966;34(4):483-515.
4. Evans C, Devadatta S, Fox W, Gangadharam PR, Menon NK, Ramakrishnan CV, et al. A 5-year study of patients with pulmonary tuberculosis treated at home in a controlled comparison of isoniazid plus PAS with 3 regimens of isoniazid alone. Bull World Health Organ. 1969;41(1):1-16.
5. Tuberculosis Chemotherapy Centre. A concurrent comparison of isoniazid plus PAS with three regimens of isoniazid alone in the domiciliary treatment of pulmonary tuberculosis in South India. Bull World Health Organ. 1960;23(4-5):535-85.
6. Ramakrishnan CV, Rajendran K, Mohan K, Fox W, Radhakrishna S. The diet, physical activity and accommodation of patients with quiescent pulmonary tuberculosis in a poor South Indian community. A four-year follow-up study. Bull World Health Organ. 1966;34(4):553-71.
7. Kamat SR, Dawson JJ, Devadatta S, Fox W, Janardhanam B, Radhakrishna S, et al. A controlled study of the influence of segregation of tuberculous patients for one year on the attack rate of tuberculosis in a 5-year period in close family contacts in South India. Bull World Health Organ. 1966;34(4):517-32.

This report was the last of a series of nine publications from the Tuberculosis Chemotherapy Center, concerning various aspects of ambulatory chemotherapy. It showed that the close family contacts of patients treated at home were at no additional risk of developing TB, provided the patients received effective chemotherapy. The major risk to the contacts resulted from exposure to the patient before diagnosis.

8. Andrews RH, Devadatta S, Fox W, Radhakrishna S, Ramakrishnan CV, Velu S. Prevalence of tuberculosis among close family contacts of tuberculous patients in South India, and influence of segregation of the patient on early attack rate. Bull World Health Organ. 1960;23(4-5):463-510.

The findings of this study indicated that the major risk for contacts of TB patients being treated at home laid in exposure to the infectious case before diagnosis. Children under 7 years of age, particularly vulnerable to infection should be considered for management with chemoprophylaxis or by Bacillus Calmette-Guérin (BCG) vaccination, or by both measures.

Bacillus Calmette–Guérin Vaccination Trials

1. Trial of BCG vaccines in south India for tuberculosis prevention: first report--Tuberculosis Prevention Trial. Bull World Health Organ. 1979;57(5):819-27.

This report presented the findings of the first 7.5 years of follow-up to study the protective effect of BCG vaccination in a controlled community trial near Madras in South India. BCG vaccines and placebo were allocated randomly to about 260,000 individuals, of whom 115,000 were definitely tuberculin negative at the time of vaccination. Incidence of infection was high in the study population; bacillary disease was more frequent among initial tuberculin reactors. The distribution of new cases of bacillary TB among those not infected at intake did not show any evidence of a protective effect of the BCG vaccines.

2. Fifteen year follow up of trial of BCG vaccines in south India for tuberculosis prevention. Tuberculosis Research Centre (ICMR), Chennai. Indian J Med Res. 1999;110:56-69.

A large-scale community-based double-blind randomized controlled trial was carried out in Chingleput district of Tamil Nadu to evaluate the protective effect of BCG against bacillary forms of pulmonary TB. Over 280,000 individuals were vaccinated with BCG or placebo by random allocation. The entire population was followed up for 15 years; the incidence rates in the three "vaccination" groups were similar confirming the complete lack of protective efficacy in adults and a low level of overall protection.

The results of this study were highly disturbing being contrary to the earlier beliefs in BCG efficacy.

3. Velayutham B, Thiruvengadam K, Kumaran PP, Watson B, Rajendran K, Padmapriyadarsini C. Revisiting the Chingleput BCG vaccination trial for the impact of BCG revaccination on the incidence of tuberculosis disease. Indian J Med Res. 2023;157(2-3):152-9.

A systematic review and meta-analysis had reported that BCG vaccination protects against pulmonary and extrapulmonary TB for up to 10 years. Therefore, results of the Chingleput BCG vaccination were reanalyzed. Retrospective data analysis showed that BCG revaccination in a community offered modest protection against the development of TB disease at the end of 15 years. The observations require further evaluation.

Miscellaneous Tuberculosis Studies

The Ministry of Health and Family Welfare, Government of India regularly brings out India TB Reports providing information of current TB data and other TB-related research activities. A large number of clinical and/or experimental studies, case-reports, reviews, and meta-analyses by Indian investigators are also regularly published which contribute to one or the other aspect of the subject. A major breakthrough research is still awaited.

Multidrug-resistant Tuberculosis

1. Indian Council of Medical Research. Prevalence of drug resistance in patients with pulmonary tuberculosis presenting for the first time with symptoms at chest clinics in India. Part I. Findings in urban clinics among patients giving no history of previous chemotherapy. Indian J Med Res. 1968;56:1617-30.
2. Indian Council of Medical Research. Prevalence of drug resistance in patients with pulmonary tuberculosis presenting for the first time with symptoms at chest clinics in India. Part II. Findings in urban clinics among all patients' with or without history of previous chemotherapy. Indian J Med Res. 1969;57:823-35.
3. Sharma SK, Mohan A. Multidrug-resistant tuberculosis. Indian J Med Res. 2004;120:354-76.

Both the above stated reports and the review highlighted the threat of multidrug-resistant tuberculosis (MDR-TB) in India.

4. Udwadia ZF, Amale RA, Ajbani KK, Rodrigues C. Totally drug-resistant tuberculosis in India. Clin Infect Dis. 2012;54(4):579-81.

The report on extreme and total drug-resistance from Mumbai had raised a huge concern for TB control program in India. A number of new treatment strategies were planned and implemented.

Nontubercular Respiratory Diseases

Asthma and Chronic Obstructive Pulmonary Disease

Most of significant respiratory publications on nontubercular lung diseases from India are restricted to epidemioclinical studies on prevalence, risk factors and/or clinical spectrum. We have listed here some of the large multicenter studies or those including a large data.

1. India State-Level Disease Burden Initiative CRD Collaborators. The burden of chronic respiratory diseases and their heterogeneity across the states of India: the Global Burden of Disease Study 1990-2016. Lancet Glob Health. 2018;6(12):e1363-e1374.

The study was a part of the Global Burden of Diseases (GBD), Injuries, and Risk Factors Study 2016. Using all accessible data from multiple sources, the authors assessed heterogeneity in the burden of COPD and asthma across the states of India from 1990 to 2016. They also assessed the contribution of risk factors to disability-adjusted life years (DALYs) due to COPD and compared the burden of chronic respiratory diseases in India against the global average in GBD 2016. It was concluded that India has a disproportionately high burden of chronic respiratory diseases and contributes to the overall disease burden and the high rate of health loss from them.

2. Jindal SK, Aggarwal AN, Gupta D, Agarwal R, Kumar R, Kaur T, et al. Indian study on epidemiology of asthma, respiratory symptoms and chronic bronchitis in adults (INSEARCH). Int J Tuberc Lung Dis. 2012;16(9):1270-7.

(Detailed Report available as an Indian Council of Medical Research, New Delhi publication)

The multicenter, population study was undertaken at field sites in 12 districts in different parts of India to determine the nationwide population prevalence of and risk factors for asthma and chronic bronchitis (CB) in adults with the help of a standardized validated questionnaire. Advancing age, smoking, household environmental tobacco smoke exposure, asthma in a first-degree relative, and use of unclean cooking fuels were associated with increased odds of asthma and CB. The national burden of asthma and CB was estimated at respectively 17.23 and 14.84 million.

3. Jindal SK. A field study on follow up at 10 years of prevalence of chronic obstructive pulmonary disease and peak expiratory flow rate. Ind J Med Res. 1993;98:20-6.

This was one of the first follow-up field study on patients of COPD with respect to smoking habits and lung function assessment. It was concluded that though the overall trend of prevalence of COPD in different groups did not change, those with an initial airways obstruction had deteriorated significantly more than those with normal initial peak expiratory flow rate (PEFR).

4. Jindal SK, Malik SK. Smoking index - a measure to quantify cumulative smoking exposure. Lung India. 1988;6:195-6.

Smoking index was designed for the first time to quantify cumulative smoking in view of the errors with the commonly used pack-year. Smoking index is now widely for clinical and research purposes.

Air Pollution

1. Pande JN, Bhatta N, Biswas D, Pandey RM, Ahluwalia G, Siddaramaiah NH, et al. Outdoor air pollution and emergency room visits at a hospital in Delhi. Indian J Chest Dis Allied Sci. 2002;44(1):13-9.
2. Balakrishnan K, Ramaswamy P, Sambandam S, Thangavel G, Ghosh S, Johnson P, et al. Air pollution from household solid fuel combustion in India: an overview of exposure and health related information to inform health research priorities. Glob Health Action. 2011;4.

Biomass Exposed Nonsmokers

1. Padmavati S, Pathak SN. Chronic cor pulmonale in Delhi: a study of 127 cases. Circulation. 1959;20:343-52.

   This was perhaps the first report on high incidence of chronic bronchitis and cor-pulmonale in women attributed to prolonged exposure to domestic cooking-fuels.

2. Salvi SS, Barnes PJ. Chronic obstructive pulmonary disease in non-smokers. Lancet. 2009;374(9691):733-43.
3. Agrawal S. Effect of indoor air pollution from biomass and solid fuel combustion on prevalence of self-reported asthma among adult men and women in India: findings from a nationwide large-scale cross-sectional survey. J Asthma. 2012;49(4):355-65.
4. Behera D, Balamugesh T. Indoor air pollution as a risk factor for lung cancer in women. JAPI. 2005;53:190-2.
5. Jindal SK, Aggarwal AN, Jindal A, Talwar D, Dhar R, Singh N, et al. COPD exacerbation rates are higher in non-smoker patients in India. Int J Tuberc Lung Dis. 2020;24(12):1272-8.

Nonsmoker COPD at 15 centers across India was more commonly observed in women exposed to biomass fuels and was characterized by higher rate of exacerbations and higher healthcare resource utilization.

6. Salvi SS, Brashier BB, Londhe J, Pyasi K, Vincent V, Kajale SS, et al. Phenotypic comparison between smoking and non-smoking chronic obstructive pulmonary disease. Respir Res. 2020;21(1):50.

Nonsmoker COPD is more commonly seen in younger subjects with equal male-female predominance and is predominantly a small-airway disease phenotype with less emphysema, preserved lung diffusion, and a slower rate of decline in lung function.

7. Jindal S, Jindal A. COPD in Biomass exposed nonsmokers: a different phenotype. Expert Rev Respir Med. 2021;15(1):51-8.

Interstitial Lung Diseases

1. Singh S, Collins BF, Sharma BB, Joshi JM, Talwar D, Katiyar S, et al. Interstitial Lung Disease in India. Results of a Prospective Registry. Am J Respir Crit Care Med. 2017;195(6):801-13.

Of a total of 1,084 patients from 27 Indian centers across 19 cities, hypersensitivity pneumonitis was the most common new-onset ILD followed by connective tissue disease (CTD)-ILD and idiopathic pulmonary fibrosis. Diagnoses varied between site investigators and experts, emphasizing the value of MDD in ILD diagnosis.

2. Singh S, Collins BF, Sharma BB, Joshi JM, Talwar D, Katiyar S, et al. Hypersensitivity pneumonitis: Clinical manifestations - Prospective data from the interstitial lung disease-India registry. Lung India. 2019;36(6):476-82.
3. Dhooria S, Sehgal IS, Agarwal R, Muthu V, Prasad KT, Kathirvel S, et al. Incidence, prevalence, and national burden of interstitial lung diseases in India: Estimates from two studies of 3089 subjects. PLoS One. 2022;17(7):e0271665.

Data of 2,005 consecutive subjects with ILDs included in a registry between March 2015 and February 2020 were analyzed retrospectively. Sarcoidosis was the most common ILD subtype followed by connective tissue disease-related ILDs, idiopathic pulmonary fibrosis, and hypersensitivity pneumonitis.

4. Jindal SK, Malik SK, Deodhar SD, Sharma BK. Fibrosing alveolitis: a report of 61 cases seen over the past five years. Ind J Chest Dis Allied Sci. 1979;21:177-82.

This was the first report from India on Idiopathic Pulmonary Fibrosis, called Cryptogenic Fibrosing Alveolitis in the earlier days.

Sarcoidosis

1. Gupta SK, Mitra K, Chatterjee S, Chakravarty SC. Sarcoidosis in India. Br J Dis Chest. 1985;79(3):275-83.
2. Madan K, Sryma PB, Pattnaik B, Mittal S, Tiwari P, Hadda V, et al. Clinical Profile of 327 patients with Sarcoidosis in India: An Ambispective Cohort Study in a Tuberculosis (TB) Endemic Population. Lung India. 2022;39(1):51-7.
3. Muthu V, Gupta N, Dhooria S, Sehgal IS, Prasad KT, Aggarwal AN, et al. Role of cytomorphology in differentiating sarcoidosis and tuberculosis in subjects undergoing endobronchial ultrasound-guided transbronchial needle aspiration. Sarcoidosis Vasc Diffuse Lung Dis. 2019;36:209-16.

Bronchiectasis

1. Dhar R, Singh S, Talwar D, Mohan M, Tripathi SK, Swarnakar R, et al. Bronchiectasis in India: results from the European Multicentre Bronchiectasis Audit and Research Collaboration (EMBARC) and Respiratory Research Network of India Registry. Lancet Glob Health. 2019;7(9):e1269-e1279. Erratum in: Lancet Glob Health. 2019;7(12):e1621.

The Indian bronchiectasis registry is a multicenter, prospective, observational cohort study. It included 2,195 adult patients with CT-confirmed bronchiectasis. Previous TB was the most frequent underlying cause and *Pseudomonas aeruginosa* was the most common organism in sputum culture in India. Patients with bronchiectasis in India have more severe disease and have distinct characteristics from those reported in other countries.

2. Dhar R, Singh S, Talwar D, Murali Mohan BV, Tripathi SK, Swarnakar R, et al. Clinical outcomes of bronchiectasis in India: data from the EMBARC/Respiratory Research Network of India registry. Eur Respir J. 2023;61(1): 2200611.

Allergic Bronchopulmonary Aspergillosis

1. Agarwal R, Sehgal IS, Muthu V, Dhar R, Armstrong-James D. Allergic bronchopulmonary aspergillosis in India. Clin Exp Allergy. 2023;53(7):751-64.
2. Agarwal R, Sehgal IS, Dhooria S, Muthu V, Prasad KT, Bal A, et al. Allergic bronchopulmonary aspergillosis. Indian J Med Res. 2020;151(6):529-49.
3. Agarwal R, Sehgal IS, Muthu V, Denning DW, Chakrabarti A, Soundappan K, et al. Revised ISHAM-ABPA working group clinical practice guidelines for diagnosing, classifying and treating allergic bronchopulmonary aspergillosis/mycoses. Eur Respir J. 2024;63(4):2400061.

In the last two decades, most research on allergic bronchopulmonary aspergillosis (ABPA) has been published from India. The prevalence and clinical presentation may differ in India from that reported elsewhere in epidemiology, clinical, and radiological characteristics. Various publications from India have yielded valuable insights into the practices associated with the diagnosis and management of ABPA in India.

Lung Function Tests and Spirometry

Several publications on normal standards of spirometric parameters and other lung function tests in Indian subjects have appeared in the last few decades. Most of this work has been nicely summarized and analyzed in the Joint Indian Chest Society-National College of Chest Physicians (India) guidelines for spirometry. Some other novel studies which have made important observations are listed here:

1. Malik SK, Jindal SK, Jindal V, Bansal S. Peak expiratory flow rate in healthy adults. Ind J Chest Dis. 1975;12:166-71.

2. Aggarwal AN, Gupta D, Jindal SK. Comparison of Indian reference equations for spirometry interpretation. Respirology. 2007;12(5):763-8.
3. Aggarwal AN, Gupta D, Behera D, Jindal SK. Comparison of fixed percentage method and lower confidence limits for defining limits of normality for interpretation of spirometry. Respir Care. 2006;51(7):737-43.
4. Das DK, Chakraborty C, Bhattacharya PS. Automated Screening Methodology for Asthma Diagnosis that Ensembles Clinical and Spirometric Information. J Med Biol Eng. 2016;36:420-9.
5. Bhattacharyya P, Saha D, Paul M, Ganguly D, Mukherjee B, Roy Chowdhury S, et al. Two chair test: a substitute of 6 min walk test appear cardiopulmonary reserve specific. BMJ Open Respir Res. 2020;7(1):e000447.

Lung Cancer

1. Jindal SK, Malik SK, Dhand R, Gujral JS, Malik AK, Datta BN. Bronchogenic carcinoma in Northern India. Thorax. 1982;37:343-7.
2. Jindal SK, Malik SK, Bedi RS, Gupta SK. Risk of Lung cancer in patients with old tuberculosis. Lung India. 1986;4:59-61.
3. Jindal SK, Malik SK, Datta BN. Lung cancer in Northern India in relation to age, sex and smoking habits. Europ J Respir Dis. 1987;70:23-8.
4. Behera D. SC17. 03 Lung cancer in India: challenges and perspectives. J Thorac Oncol. 2017;12(1):S114-5.
5. Singh N, Aggarwal AN, Gupta D, Behera D, Jindal SK. Quantified smoking status and non-small cell lung cancer stage at presentation: analysis of a North Indian cohort and a systematic review of literature. J Thorac Dis. 2012;4(5):474-84.
6. Singh N, Aggarwal AN, Gupta D, Behera D, Jindal SK. Unchanging clinico-epidemiological profile of lung cancer in north India over three decades. Cancer Epidemiol. 2010;34(1):101-4.
7. Parikh PM, Ranade AA, Govind B, Ghadyalpatil N, Singh R, Bharath R, et al. Lung cancer in India: Current status and promising strategies. South Asian J Cancer. 2016;5(3):93-5.

Miscellaneous

1. Udwadia FE, Joshi VV. A study of tropical eosinophilia. Thorax. 1964;19(6):548-54.
2. Sharma SK, Kumpawat S, Banga A, Goel A. Prevalence and risk factors of obstructive sleep apnea syndrome in a population of Delhi, India. Chest. 2006;130(1):149-56.
3. Sharma SK, Ahluwalia G. Epidemiology of adult obstructive sleep apnoea syndrome in India. Indian J Med Res. 2010;131:171-5.
4. Mehrotra AK, Swami S, Soothwal P, Feroz A, Dawar S, Bhangoo HD. Pulmonary Vasculitis: Indian Perspective. Indian J Chest Dis Allied Sci. 2016;58(2):107-19.
5. Bambery P, Sakhuja V, Gupta A, Behera D, Kaur U, Bhusnurmath SR, et al. Wegener's granulomatosis in north India. An analysis of eleven patients. Rheumatol Int. 1987;7(6):243-7.

Joint Guidelines/Consensus Statements/Position Statements Published by Different Indian Societies

Pulmonary Infections

1. Gupta D, Agarwal R, Aggarwal AN, Singh N, Mishra N, Khilnani GC, et al. Guidelines for diagnosis and management of community- and hospital-acquired pneumonia in adults: Joint ICS/NCCP(I) recommendations. Lung India. 2012;29(Suppl 2):S27-62.
2. National Tuberculosis Elimination Program. Guidelines for diagnosis and treatment of tuberculosis. Central TB Division of Government of India. [online] Available from

https://tbcindia.mohfw.gov.in/guidelines/ [Last accessed September, 2025].
3. Sharma SK, Ryan H, Khaparde S, Sachdeva KS, Singh AD, Mohan A, et al. Index-TB guidelines: Guidelines on extrapulmonary tuberculosis for India. Indian J Med Res. 2017;145(4):448-63.
3. Dhar R, Ghoshal AG, Guleria R, Sharma S, Kulkarni T, Swarnakar R, et al. Clinical practice guidelines 2019: Indian consensus-based recommendations on pneumococcal vaccination for adults. Lung India. 2020;37(Supplement):S19-S29.
4. Dhar R, Ghoshal AG, Guleria R, Sharma S, Kulkarni T, Swarnakar R, et al. Clinical practice guidelines 2019: Indian consensus-based recommendations on influenza vaccination in adults. Lung India. 2020;37(Suppl 1):S4-S18.

Spirometry

Aggarwal AN, Agarwal R, Dhooria S, Prasad KT, Sehgal IS, Muthu V, et al. Joint Indian Chest Society-National College of Chest Physicians (India) guidelines for spirometry. Lung India. 2019;36(Suppl 1):S1-S35.

Asthma and Chronic Obstructive Pulmonary Disease

1. Agarwal R, Dhooria S, Aggarwal AN, Maturu VN, Sehgal IS, Muthu V, et al. Guidelines for diagnosis and management of bronchial asthma: Joint ICS/NCCP (I) recommendations. Lung India. 2015;32(Suppl 1):S3-S42.
2. Gupta D, Agarwal R, Aggarwal AN, Maturu VN, Dhooria S, Prasad KT, et al. Guidelines for diagnosis and management of chronic obstructive pulmonary disease: Joint ICS/NCCP (I) recommendations. Lung India. 2013;30(3):228-67.
3. Katiyar SK, Gaur SN, Solanki RN, Sarangdhar N, Suri JC, Kumar R, et al. Indian Guidelines on Nebulization Therapy. Indian J Tuberc. 2022;69 Suppl 1:S1-S191.
4. Jindal SK, Pawar S, Hasan A, Ghoshal A, Dhar R, Katiyar SK, et al. Scoring System for the Use of Nebulizers in the Primary Care Settings: An Expert Consensus Statement. J Assoc Physicians India. 2023;71(6):89-92.
5. Guleria R, Dhar R, Mahashur A, Ghoshal AG, Jindal SK, Talwar D, et al. Indian Consensus on Diagnosis of Cough at Primary Care Setting. J Assoc Physicians India. 2019;67(1):92-8.

Interstitial Lung Diseases

1. Singh S, Sharma BB, Bairwa M, Gothi D, Desai U, Joshi JM, et al. Management of interstitial lung diseases: A consensus statement of the Indian Chest Society (ICS) and National College of Chest Physicians (NCCP). Lung India. 2020;37(4):359-78.
2. Rajan SK, Cottin V, Dhar R, Danoff S, Flaherty KR, Brown KK, et al. Progressive pulmonary fibrosis: an expert group consensus statement. Eur Respir J. 2023;61(3):2103187.

Sleep Apnea Syndrome

1. Sharma SK, Katoch VM, Mohan A, Kadhiravan T, Elavarasi A, Ragesh R, et al. Consensus & evidence-based INOSA Guidelines 2014 (first edition). Indian J Med Res. 2014;140(3):451-68.
2. Sharma SK, Katoch VM, Mohan A, Kadhiravan T, Elavarasi A, Ragesh R, et al. Consensus and evidence-based Indian initiative on obstructive sleep apnea guidelines 2014 (first edition). Lung India. 2015;32(4):422-34.

Pulmonary Interventional Procedures

1. Mohan A, Madan K, Hadda V, Tiwari P, Mittal S, Guleria R, et al. Guidelines for diagnostic flexible bronchoscopy in adults: Joint Indian Chest Society/National College of chest physicians (I)/Indian association for bronchology recommendations. Lung India. 2019;36(Supplement):S37-S89.

2. Mohan A, Madan K, Hadda V, Mittal S, Suri T, Shekh I, et al. Guidelines for endobronchial ultrasound-transbronchial needle aspiration (EBUS-TBNA): Joint Indian Chest Society (ICS)/Indian Association for Bronchology (IAB) recommendations. Lung India. 2023;40(4):368-400.
3. Chawla RK, Kumar M, Madan A, Dhar R, Gupta R, Gothi D, et al. NCCP-ICS joint consensus-based clinical practice guidelines on medical thoracoscopy. Lung India. 2024;41(2):151-67.
4. Christopher DJ, Gupta R, Thangakunam B, Daniel J, Jindal SK, Kant S, et al. Pleural effusion guidelines from ICS and NCCP Section 1: Basic principles, laboratory tests and pleural procedures. Lung India. 2024;41(3):230-48.
5. Dhooria S, Agarwal R, Sehgal IS, Aggarwal AN, Goyal R, Guleria R, et al. Bronchoscopic lung cryobiopsy: An Indian association for bronchology position statement. Lung India. 2019;36(1):48-59.

Respiratory Failure and Critical Care

1. Chawla R, Dixit SB, Zirpe KG, Chaudhry D, Khilnani GC, Mehta Y, et al. ISCCM Guidelines for the Use of Non-invasive Ventilation in Acute Respiratory Failure in Adult ICUs. Indian J Crit Care Med. 2020;24(Suppl 1):S61-S81.
2. Mani RK, Amin P, Chawla R, Divatia JV, Kapadia F, Khilnani P, et al. Guidelines for end-of-life and palliative care in Indian intensive care units' ISCCM consensus Ethical Position Statement. Indian J Crit Care Med. 2012;16(3):166-81.

Miscellaneous

1. Munje R, Chawla R, Chetambath R, Christopher DJ, Dhar R, Ghoshal AG, et al. Position statement of the Indian Chest Society on reinstatement of the Respiratory Medicine department in undergraduate medical colleges in India. Lung India. 2023;40(6):487-9.
2. Behera SK, Das S, Xavier AS, Selvarajan S, Anandabaskar N. Indian Council of Medical Research's National Ethical Guidelines for biomedical and health research involving human participants: The way forward from 2006 to 2017. Perspect Clin Res. 2019;10(3):108-14.
3. Indian Council of Medical Research. (2017). National Ethical Guidelines for Biomedical and Health Research involving Human Participants. [online] Available from https://ethics.ncdirindia.org/asset/pdf/ICMR_National_Ethical_Guidelines.pdf [Last accessed September, 2025].

Sources

1. Jindal SK. Research in clinical sciences. Indian J Chest Dis Allied Sci. 2011;53:175-82.
2. Mathur R, Thakur K, Hazam RK. Highlights of Indian Council of Medical Research National Ethical Guidelines for Biomedical and Health Research Involving Human Participants. Indian J Pharmacol. 2019;51(3):214-21.
3. Dasgupta A, Fernandes L, Chopra V, Rajkumar P. Barriers to building an effective workforce for respiratory research in India: A survey of American Thoracic Society Methods in Epidemiologic, Clinical, and Operations Research India 2017 participants. Lung India. 2018;35(2):184-6.
4. Hess DR. Research and Publication in Respiratory Care. Respir Care. 2023;68(8):1171-3.
5. David Price Guy Brusselle Nicolas Roche Daryl Freeman Alison Chisholm. Real-world research and its importance in respiratory medicine. Breathe 2015 11(1): 26-38;
6. Sharma BB, Singh S, Sharma KK, Suraj KP, Mahmood T, Samaria KU, et al. Methodology of Seasonal Waves of Respiratory Disorders survey conducted at respiratory outpatient clinics across India. Lung India. 2020;37(2):100-6.
7. Abdel-Aal A, Lisspers K, Williams S, Adab P, Adams R, Agarwal D, et al. Prioritising primary care respiratory research needs: results from the 2020 International Primary Care Respiratory

Group (IPCRG) global e-Delphi exercise. NPJ Prim Care Respir Med. 2022;32(1):6.
8. Branson RD, Kallet RH. Creating a Process of Research in Respiratory Care. Respir Care. 2021;66(8):1363-4.
9. Fröhlich E. Animals in Respiratory Research. Int J Mol Sci. 2024;25(5):2903.
10. Chaudhuri S, Todur P, Nileshwar A. Research in respiratory care. Indian J Respir Care. 2020;9:1-4.
11. Pierson DJ. Research and publication in respiratory care. Respir Care. 2004;49:1145-8.
12. National Research Council (US) and Institute of Medicine (US) Committee to Review the NIOSH Respiratory Disease Research Program. Respiratory Diseases Research at NIOSH: Reviews of Research Programs of the National Institute for Occupational Safety and Health. Washington (DC): National Academies Press (US); 2008. 2, Evaluation of the Respiratory Diseases Research Program.
13. Kapoor A. Quality Medical Research and Publications in India: Time to Introspect. Int J Appl Basic Med Res. 2019;9(2):67-8.
14. Ravisankar NP, Singh R, Gurjar M. Collaborative Research in Critical Care Medicine: A Way Forward to High-impact Publications from India. Indian J Crit Care Med. 2023;27(12):869-70.
15. Gogtay NJ. Medical research in India: Fit and fine or frail and vulnerable? Natl Med J India. 2022;35:129-31.

CHAPTER

22

Pulmonary Stalwarts of Modern Era

A large number of physicians and surgeons have significantly contributed to the development of respiratory medicine and medical practices in India in the last 100 years or so. We are listing a few whose contributions are generally acknowledged. Some of these notes have been written by their students or friends who personally knew them, better than the authors of this book.

Pre-Independence Era

Tuberculosis (TB) and other chest infections had dominated the scenario in the late 19th and early 20th centuries. The specialty of *respiratory medicine* was not separately recognized. Many physicians and surgeons had distinguished themselves with extensive clinical services in this area. Some of the early pioneers who made significant contributions to the understanding and treatment of TB in India included DN Palmer, GC Roy, ML Sarkar, KN Purohit, and BC Roy. They all worked on epidemiological and clinical spectrum as well as different treatment strategies. Dr Purohit also held leadership roles in various TB-related organizations including the Indian Tuberculosis Association and the National Tuberculosis Institute. Dr ML Sarkar established the Calcutta School of Tropical Medicine in 1920.

DN Palmer, a British physician who worked in India during the early 20th century, was a renowned expert on TB. He worked at the Tuberculosis Hospital in Madras where he conducted research on epidemiology of TB in India, studying the disease's prevalence, distribution, and transmission patterns. He also developed treatment protocols for TB that were tailored to the Indian context. These emphasized the importance of rest, nutrition, and sanitation in TB treatment. Palmer advocated for the establishment of TB sanatoria, the use of X-rays in diagnosis, and the implementation of public health measures to prevent TB transmission. His work on TB had a lasting impact on the country's approach to TB control and treatment.

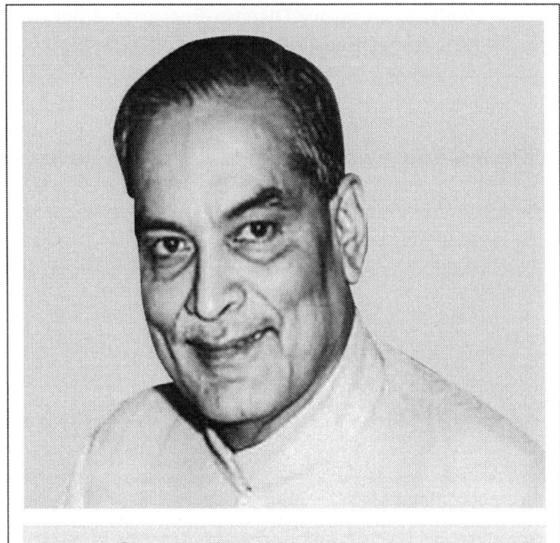
Bidhan Chandra Roy

Bidhan Chandra Roy (1882–1962) became a household name in the medical community. He was a renowned Indian physician, politician, and

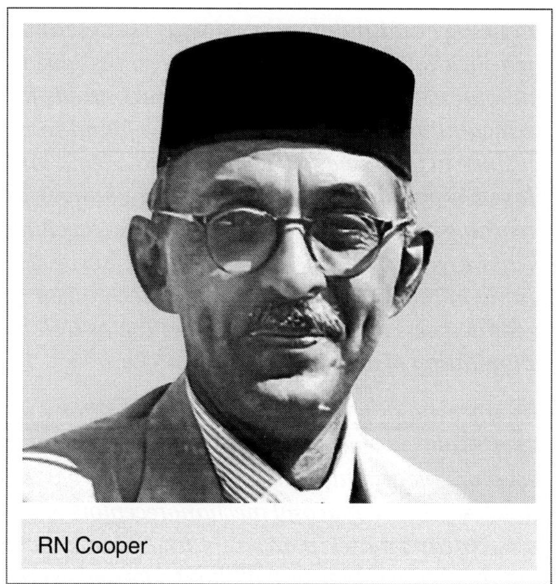
RN Cooper

later the Chief Minister of Bengal. He was also a social worker who made significant contributions to the field of TB. Dr Roy established several TB clinics in Kolkata (then Calcutta) and other parts of India, providing access to TB diagnosis and treatment for thousands of patients. He also raised awareness about the disease through public lectures, writings, and media campaigns. Dr Roy's contributions to TB control and treatment in India were recognized with several awards and honors, such as the *Padma Vibhushan*, India's second-highest civilian honor, in 1961.

Rustam Nusserwanji Cooper is another prominent name that stands out during this period. Cooper is credited with the introduction of modern rigid bronchoscopy techniques as an Honorary Surgeon and Head of the Department of Surgery at King Edward Memorial (KEM) Hospital, Mumbai (earlier Bombay). Besides being an accomplished surgeon, he was an extraordinary individual who was widely revered by patients and admired by the medical fraternity. He had also started the *Charak Clinic* for the poor. He possessed an eclectic collection of books on subjects ranging from comparative religious philosophies to biographies. He was a keen student of the history of medicine and felt strongly that we must remain aware of the trials of those who advanced medicine over the millennia underwent and applaud their achievements. The Bombay municipal authorities had commemorated his contributions with the RN Cooper Hospital in Juhu. He was a founder of the Indian Association of Surgeons and became the first Indian to be conferred membership of the American Association of Surgeons. He was a great surgeon and a greater gentleman who lived an extraordinary life with humility and kindness.

Other notable pioneers included AJS Mehta for research on TB control, MD Goyandka and SK Basu for pulmonary physiology research, RV Rajam for work on lung cancer, and ST Achar for pioneering pediatric pulmonology in India. Contributions by these pioneers helped the introduction of modern diagnostic and treatment techniques and lay foundations of medical research and education. They shaped India's health care system and inspired future generations of medical professionals.

Post-Independence Era—20th Century

Rapid strides were made in all fields in medicine after 1947 for several reasons, which have been discussed earlier. A number of pioneer clinicians, teachers, and research workers were now available in different fields. TB remained a dominant problem, and hence the focus of attention in respiratory medicine in the first few decades after India's independence. However, there were others who began taking interest in nontubercular diseases, especially asthma, chronic bronchitis, and nontubercular lung infections. The pool kept expanding as we progressed in time.

Autar Singh Paintal remains one of the most eminent scientist in basic sciences and a renowned physiologist who gained an international recognition for his discovery of J receptors in the juxtacapillary areas of the lung.

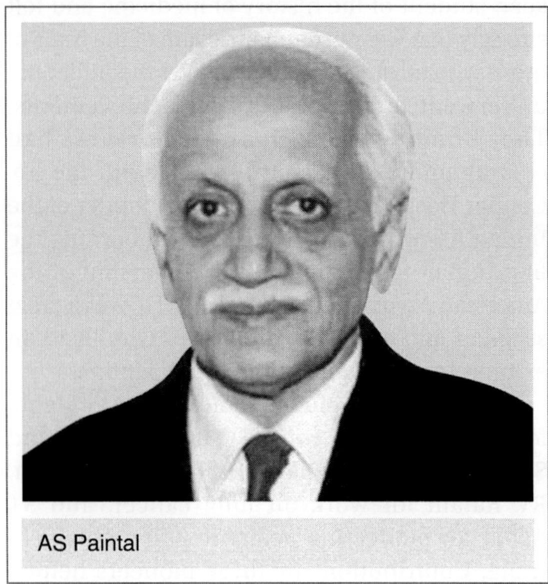

AS Paintal

Prof SK Chhabra, a former Director-Professor of Pulmonary Medicine at Vallabhbhai Patel Chest Institute writes gloriously about Dr Paintal:

Born in 1925 in the small town of Mogok, Myanmar (erstwhile Burma), he moved to India during the World War II to pursue higher studies. With a love for research in basic sciences, he shunned a career in clinical medicine and opted for postgraduation in Physiology. Subsequently, he obtained his PhD from the University of Edinburgh. He joined the Vallabhbhai Patel Chest Institute as an Assistant Director where in 1954 he made the important discovery of J receptors. After a brief stint at the AIIMS, N. Delhi as a senior faculty, he returned to Vallabhbhai Patel Chest Institute in Delhi as Director. Later, he also served as the Director General of the Indian Council of Medical Research (ICMR) contributing to the promotion of medical research and guiding health policies in India.

Dr Paintal developed and perfected single-fiber recording techniques, which were a major advancement in electrophysiology in the 1950s. His most notable contribution is the discovery of type J receptors in the lungs and their role in exercise physiology and pulmonary edema. He described their location in the lungs just next to the alveoli and pulmonary capillaries (the name J stands for juxtacapillary). These receptors were found to be sensitive to pulmonary congestion and edema and played a crucial role in modulating changes in breathing patterns with afferent impulses travelling in nonmyelinated fibers of the vagus nerve. He also hypothesized their role in the mechanism of breathlessness in pulmonary congestion as well as in limitation of exercise.

His other major works included identification and description of sensory receptors such as atrial B receptors, ventricular pressure receptors, gastric stretch receptors, mucosal mechanoreceptors of the intestine sand muscle pain receptors. A little-known fact about him is that even without a formal degree or training in electronic engineering, he learnt to build small circuits and repair his equipment or improvise and build small instruments for his research.

The Government of India conferred the much-coveted Padma Vibhushan in 1981 for his contributions to medical science. One of the most distinguished scientists of the world in the field of Physiology, his contributions and impact on neurophysiology are sometimes discussed as "Pre-Paintal era" versus "Post-Paintal era".

Acutely concerned about the declining standards of scientific ethics, he and several others who were similarly alarmed by the situation in the country founded the Society for Scientific Values. Throughout his career, Dr Paintal was a mentor and inspiration to many young scientists. His dedication to teaching and research fostered a culture of inquiry and innovation. He supervised numerous doctoral students and postdoctoral researchers, many of whom have gone on to make significant contributions to physiology and medicine.

Paintal's legacy is one of excellence and pioneering contributions to physiology. His discoveries have shaped our understanding

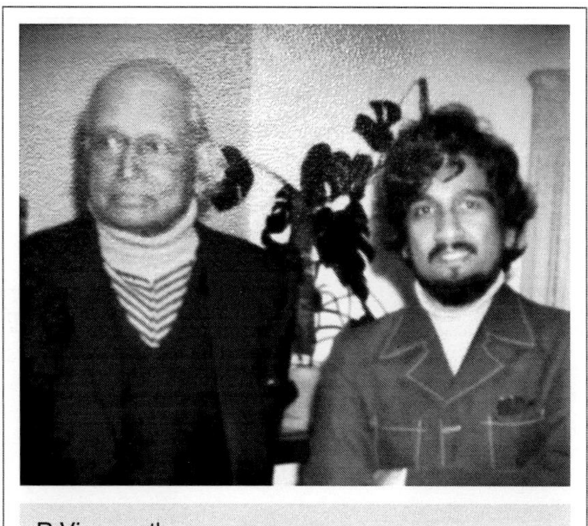

R Viswanathan

of neurophysiology and cardiorespiratory physiology.

Other stalwarts of Paintal's period included Surinder Pal Pamra, a renowned Indian pulmonologist and Founder-Director of National Institute of Tuberculosis and Respiratory Diseases, New Delhi. He had contributed significantly to India's national TB control programs. He was an exceptional clinician, researcher, and mentor who dedicated his life to advancing respiratory health care in India. Purushottam Kashinath Sen was a renowned Indian cardiothoracic surgeon and medical educator. He had pioneered modern cardiothoracic surgical techniques and established AIIMS Delhi's cardiothoracic department. Two eminent chest physicians and researchers born in Tamil Nadu included KV Thiruvengadam and R Viswanathan. They made significant contributions to the field of respiratory medicine including TB and nontubercular diseases in India. Raman Viswanathan was in several ways the lead pulmonary physician and teacher who remained as Director of the Vallabhbhai Patel Chest Institute at the University of Delhi and mentored a large number of students in chest diseases. Dr Basil Varkey, a Professor Emeritus in the USA shares his personal encounter with Professor Raman Viswanathan in following words:

"I met Dr Raman Viswanathan, for the first time at the XXIV World Congress of IUAT at Brussels, Belgium in September of 1978. He was one of the presenters on a half day oral presentations and his short paper was on the results of TB treatment. (I share with you the first thought that occurred to me on seeing Dr Viswanathan presenting his 15 minute (10 minute presentation and 5 minute for questions) at Brussels. Why was this professor of iconic status, nearly 80 years of age, presenting this paper instead of a junior colleague or a trainee/mentee?) During the break time I introduced myself to him and he advised me that he was planning a trip to the US in early 1979 and I gave him my contact information. In the spring of 1979 I got a call from him. I then invited him to speak our noon conference at the Matousek Auditorium. As I was then the Associate Director of the Medicine Residency Program I was able to secure an honorarium for his lecture. I also booked a hotel room at a nearby location but he expressed his desire to stay at my house. He stayed with us in our modest house the night before the lecture. Dr Viswanathan for all his fame and stature was a undemanding and charming guest.

The auditorium was packed with residents, interns and students, and faculty as well. For most in the audience it was the first time they were attending a lecture from a visiting Indian professor. Professor Viswanathan in his tailored dark suit and piercing eyes and confident posture cut an imposing figure. He opened his lecture on "Tropical Eosinophilia" with the lines "When I did this work and published on this subject most of you here were not born." and with a smile he added "you were just a gleam in your parents' eyes". With that he won over all of the audience who listened to him with rapt attention.

We received a very nice letter of thanks from Dr Viswanathan from Ohio and later after he had returned to New Delhi."

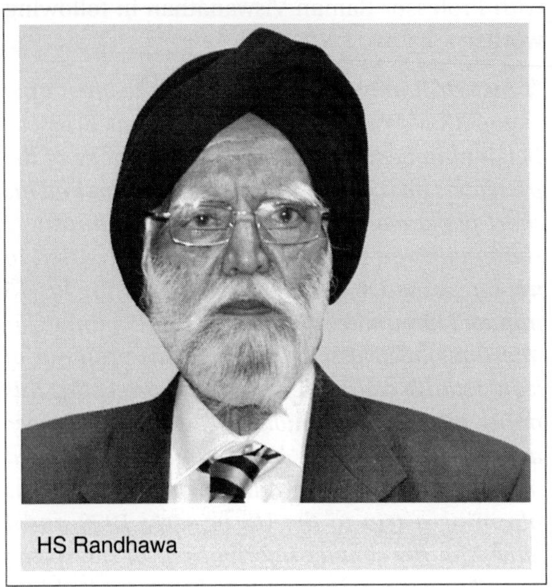
HS Randhawa

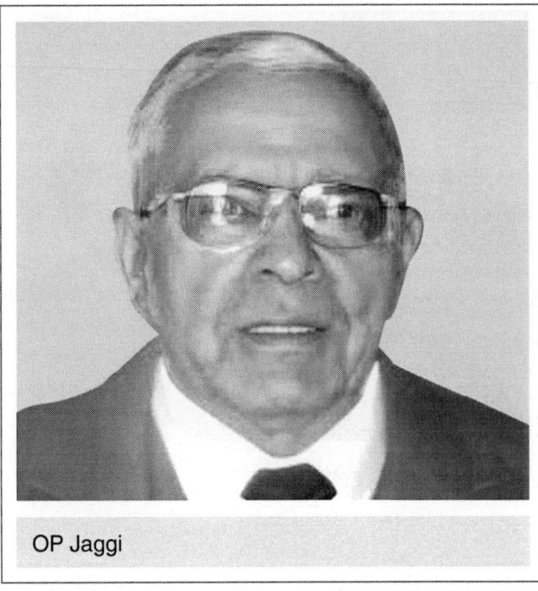
OP Jaggi

During this period, there were several other eminent teachers and research workers at Vallabhbhai Patel Chest Institute at the University of Delhi who significantly contributed in different areas of chest medicine. HS Randhawa, regarded as the doyen of medical mycology in India, focused his research on the etiopathogenesis of invasive and hypersensitivity diseases of the respiratory tract due to fungi and actinomycetes for over five decades. He had a major interest in epidemiology, development of novel laboratory diagnostic techniques, and immuno-diagnosis of respiratory and systemic mycoses. He is globally known for the discovery of *Candida viswanathii* and several other fungi of clinical interest. A new environmental fungus, *Cryptococcus randhawai*, was named after him in view of his significant mycological contributions.

OP Jaggi who had been the Director of the Vallabhbhai Patel Chest Institute, Delhi was the author of over 70 books including an authoritative 18-volume series on History of Science and Technology in India. He wrote on a variety of subjects including the Healing Systems—Alternatives and Choices, Medicine in Medieval India, Yogic and Tantric Medicine, Indian System of Medicine, and Science in Modern India. SK Jain is another doyen who has made immense contributions to cardiorespiratory physiology offering integration of physiology into the clinical disciplines of pulmonary and critical care medicine. His research areas included lung receptor physiology and lung function testing. His research into various aspects of bronchial asthma, chronic obstructive pulmonary disease (COPD), interstitial lung diseases, and lung function tests has contributed immensely to the fields of epidemiology, pathophysiology, and pathogenesis of these diseases.

Professor Man Mohan Singh was a well-known figure and a much sought-after teacher. Dr Ashok Shah, a former Professor at Vallabhbhai Patel Chest Institute describes Dr Singh as a doyen in the field of TB to which he devoted more than half a century of his life. "*Dr Singh, who first worked as a Senior Medical Officer at the Tuberculosis Clinic, better known as "Pili Kothi" became Delhi's first State Tuberculosis Officer of Delhi. Later, he assumed charge of the Rajan Babu Tuberculosis Hospital, Delhi, the largest tuberculosis hospital in Asia as the Medical Superintendent and Senior Consultant in Chest Diseases. He took voluntary*

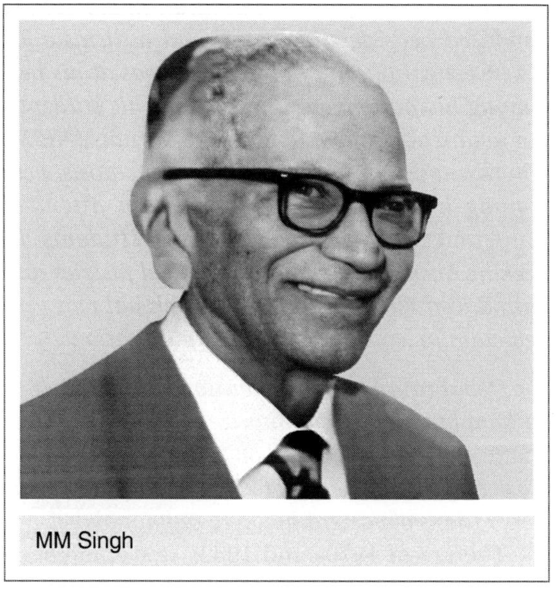
MM Singh

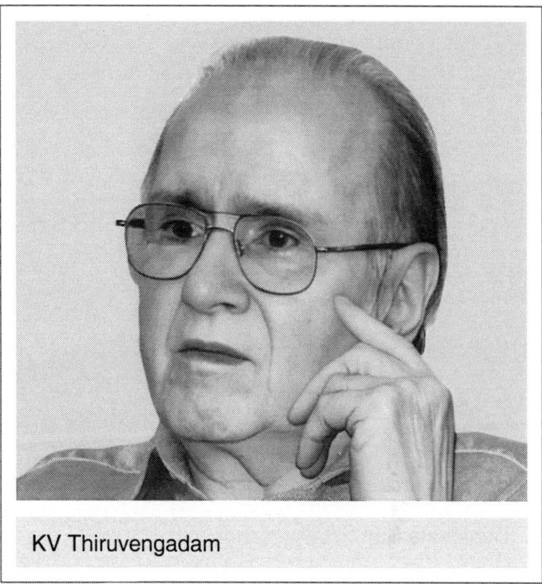
KV Thiruvengadam

retirement in 1985 to take charge as the Director of the renowned New Delhi Tuberculosis Centre, managed by the Tuberculosis Association of India.

The RBTB Hospital was a part of the training program of the DTCD students of the University of Delhi who were allotted to the Vallabhbhai Patel Chest Institute. When the Institute started the MD (Tuberculosis and Respiratory Diseases) of the University of Delhi in the late 70s Dr Singh and RBTB Hospital played a crucial role. He was also appointed as Honorary Professor by the University of Delhi. Dr Singh was the force behind the Delhi TB Association as well as the Tuberculosis Association of India (TAI). He was deeply involved with the Delhi TB Association for nearly half a century and was the Vice-Chairman of the TAI. Prof Singh was also a much published author. When he took over the Indian Journal of Tuberculosis, he made it his mission to get it indexed with the Index Medicus/ Medline. He succeeded in getting the more than 50-year-old Journal indexed which was a major feather in his cap. He remained the Editor until his demise.

For his distinguished contribution toward furthering Indo-Japan relations, Dr Singh was honored by the Government of Japan with the Order of the Rising Sun, Gold Rays with Rosette. It is the second most prestigious Japanese decoration after the Order of the Chrysanthemum. Dr MM Singh was a father figure to many respiratory physicians in India and will be remembered as a passionate teacher and researcher by all those associated with the specialty of pulmonology in India".

KV Thiruvengadam was an eminent chest physician and internist who mentored students in medicine and chest diseases such as asthma and allergies for over 40 years. He was honored with the "Distinguished Chest Physician" award by the Indian Chest Society.

Debabrata Sen was another legendary Professor from Kolkata who also served as Director of IPGMER, Kolkata from 1990 to 1996. Dr Aloke Ghoshal, Medical Director, National Allergy Asthma Bronchitis Institute and Past President, Indian Chest Society, pays tributes to Prof Sen:

"Those were the budding days of Pulmonology in India. The specialty and the department bore the name of tuberculosis and chest diseases. While tuberculosis was the immediate formidable

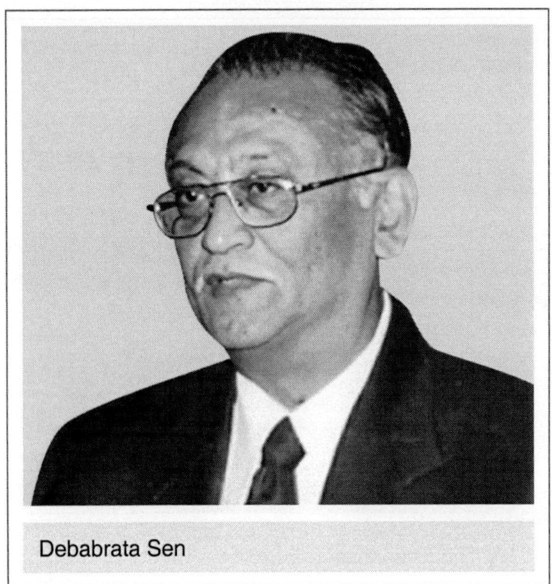
Debabrata Sen

national menace, pulmonology had started to spread its wings to the future. Dr Sen seamlessly covered the fissure, if any, of the diverging interests and shaped the future of pulmonary medicine in Eastern India. Pulmonology was in search of an identity and here was the person to represent it. He was always conversant with the scopes and widening horizons of pulmonology but never undermined the importance of knowing tuberculosis and tuberculosis control. His students loved his magnetic personality, deep medical knowledge, and compassion for humanity.

Immensely popular among his patients, his brilliance in clinics and care for the ill earned him the nickname of "Devata Sen". But what he really imparted to his students and generations thereafter was the rational scientific approach in medicine. His history-taking was like following an Agatha Christie novel; his patient examination looked like drawing a picture. As a result he converted many potential internists, surgeons, and gynecologists to pulmonary medicine.

There were also some unexplained facets of his personality. He epitomized the old "gurukul" values—secrecy and aversion to publicity. In spite of constantly updating himself on advances, he espoused bedside clinics and had a distaste for an investigation-all approach. He was at his best among his patients and then, with his students. An avid reader of contemporary journals (NEJM, Thorax and Indian Journal of Tuberculosis were among his daily reads), he seldom attended conferences. He encouraged his students in seeking answers to their own clinical puzzles and introduced them to clinical research but was very reluctant in lending his name to publications.

Dr Debabrata Sen's contributions are difficult to fathom but may be summarized by saying that he made pulmonology stand on its feet in Bengal and Eastern India and attracted the best of successive generations of postgraduates to pulmonology".

The era of 1970s and 1980s saw emergence of several eminent medical and chest physicians who contributed immensely to the development of *pulmonary medicine* in both TB and nontubercular diseases from different parts of India.

Kishore Chandra Mohanty was a towering chest physician who actively fought against TB in his lifetime. Dr Nikhil Sarangdhar, one of his students remembers him in the following word:

"A doyen of and a leading light to many of the TB workers in India, he led the campaign against TB. Originally hailing from Orissa, he mostly served in Mumbai as Honorary TB specialist and Professor at the department of TB and Chest diseases at the Grant medical college and Sir J J Group of hospitals, Bombay, and later the K J Somaiya Medical College. He founded the Mumbai district anti-TB society and the TB clinics under the Bharatiya Arogya Nidhi and Muslim Ambulance Society trusts, Mumbai, offering free TB treatment services with second-line anti-TB drugs. He was a pillar of strength to the TB association of India for decades. In the battle against TB, he was a General who led from the front for five decades. He was also a dedicated environmentalist, educationist, social reformer, and a nationalist. He travelled 29 times to

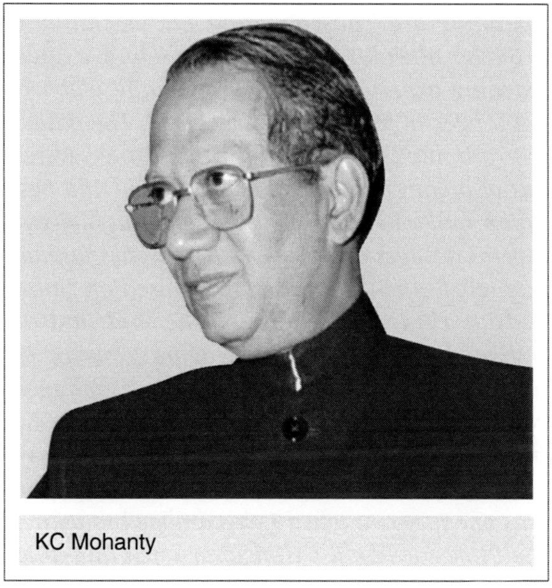

KC Mohanty

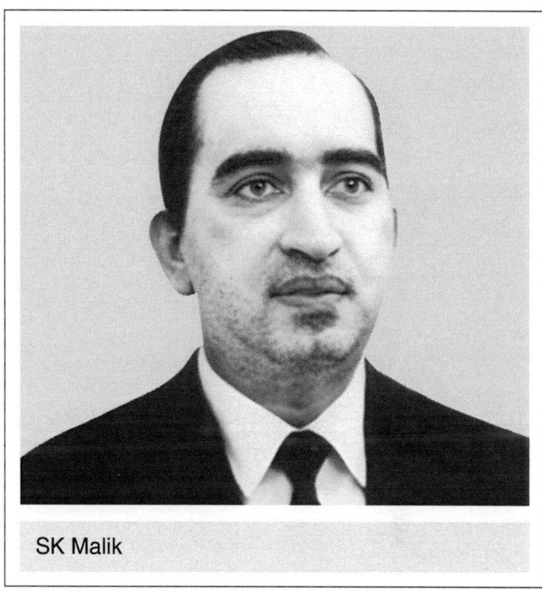

SK Malik

the North-East and established the TB associations of Arunachal Pradesh and Sikkim and the North-East TB association for 8 states.

He was a strict disciplinarian but also gave many opportunities to his generations of students. He used to dress in a classical "bandh-gala" suit and was very fond of fountain pens, of which at least four could be found every time in his shirt pocket. Let me share a small anecdote which provides an interesting glimpse into his personality. On two occasions, once during a trip to the Mount Mary fair at Bandra, Mumbai, and the second during the Hornbill festival at Dimapur, Nagaland, we visited the local stalls and found everything a bit expensive. However, on both occasions he encouraged us to purchase the local products from the same stalls at the prices, saying that "Few rupees extra will not make much difference to us, the native citizens pay a lot for the stalls and often they have to live and support their families on their earnings from this one festival for the entire year, and, therefore, we should feel proud to support their livelihood.

Suresh Malik was another eminent chest physician at the Postgraduate Institute of Medical Education and Research, Chandigarh who pioneered a number of clinical studies on nontubercular lung diseases, in particular on tobacco smoking, domestic air pollution, and chronic bronchitis. He moved from the United States to India with a keen commitment to establish respiratory medicine at par with other sister superspecialties of general medicine. Unfortunately, his life was cut short due to a progressive illness, but he was an iconic pulmonologists for many of us from Chandigarh. I personally owe a lot to him for his guidance and support through thick and thin. In several ways, he laid the foundation for the *first* postdoctoral (DM) program in pulmonary medicine in India which we could subsequently start in 1989 after his demise.

Professor Jitendra Nath Pande was Dr Malik's contemporary colleague at the All India Institute of Medical Sciences, New Delhi who served as Professor and Head of the Department of Medicine. His areas of interest included pulmonary physiology, intensive care, clinical epidemiology, and clinical decision analysis. He contributed immensely to the investigation of

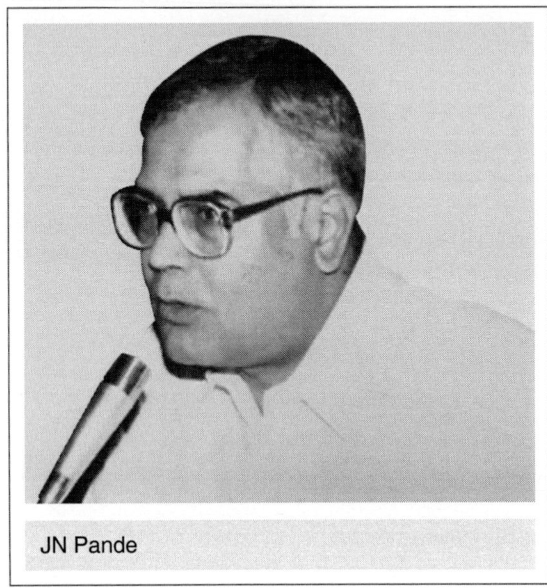

JN Pande

Bhopal Gas Tragedy in 1986. Prof SK Sharma, who closely worked with Dr Pande, writes about his impressions:

"I was closely associated with Professor Pande since the time I joined his Unit in the Department of Medicine. He was the epitome of a great teacher, clinician, and researcher. All these qualities made him very popular among his colleagues, students, and patients. He was a gifted teacher and had an art of abridging patient's clinical details and laboratory investigations and one used to relish his analytic power during clinical discussions in ward rounds, ICU rounds, and in the outpatient department. He always used to encourage his junior faculty and residents to make presentations in clinical combined rounds and clinical grand rounds at AIIMS, New Delhi and used to dominate discussion on any topic and used to contribute very constructively. Besides professional association with Prof Pande, I personally consider myself a lucky person to be mentored by him. He had a great influence in shaping my career. He trained me in pulmonary physiology especially lung mechanics and cardiopulmonary exercise physiology, fiberoptic bronchoscopy, and the technique of broncho-alveolar lavage. Once I had a great learning experience from Prof Pande when he got a referral from Cardiology ward. The patient was admitted in ICCU and was getting severely out of breath while lying down supine and both junior and senior residents on night duty injected several dosages of intravenous diuretics without any relief. After evaluating him based on simple bedside clinical examination, he said that the patient has bilateral diaphragmatic weakness and instructed me to arrange an esophageal catheter with an esophageal balloon and a gastric balloon in the afternoon after the OPD hours. We could confirm the diagnosis with this study. That was one moment when I was amazed to witness the Professor Pande's clinical acumen and quick responses in making a diagnosis. He often told me to develop skills to make a diagnosis the moment patient enters the room. Later, he entrusted me with the responsibility of establishing sleep laboratory in the department of Department of Medicine.

Jointly working together we had several firsts to our credit, we described for the first time acute respiratory distress syndrome (ARDS) in miliary tuberculosis, recruitment of lymphocytes and its subsets from peripheral blood to the disease sites in tuberculosis and sarcoidosis, description of a comprehensive large series of sarcoidosis. Professor Pande was an enthusiastic researcher as well. After rounding in the OPD, wards, ICU in the forenoons, we used to work together in the afternoons performing lung mechanics, cardiopulmonary exercises in the respiratory research laboratory. Professor Pande was always a great support in academics and research for me. When I was senior resident, he was the one who helped me in writing my first publication. I must admit that Professor Pande had outstanding writing skills as well. Professor Pande will always be remembered for his commitment toward clinical care, teaching, and medical research".

P Ravindran stands as a towering figure in the history of pulmonary medicine in Kerala, where his contributions shaped the field profoundly. *Dr C Ravindran,* a Senior Consultant and Pulmonologist in Calicut, briefly writes about him as follows:

"P Ravindran spearheaded the initiative to establish Departments of TB and Chest Diseases as independent departments, which catalyzed the growth of similar departments across Kerala's medical colleges. His efforts led to the approval of the DTCD course in 1977, followed by the MD (TB and Respiratory Diseases) program in 1984 at Trivandrum and Calicut Medical Colleges, setting the stage for comprehensive pulmonary education state-wide. Under his leadership, Pulmonary Medicine departments across Kerala were equipped with advanced diagnostic and therapeutic tools. He also pioneered Kerala's first allergen manufacturing center and introduced an applied allergy and immunology clinic, significantly advancing the field. He established a Clinical Epidemiology Unit in Trivandrum. This was later upgraded to the Clinical Epidemiology Resource and Training Center (CERTC), which trained medical faculty and offered an MPhil program in clinical epidemiology. He served as the chief editor of Lung India, and his academic leadership extended to several different roles, including the Presidency of the Indian Chest Society, reflecting his influence on pulmonology".

Lucknow was one important place which produced quite a few chest physicians and teachers in chest medicine. Professor BK Khanna was one such doyen who steered the department

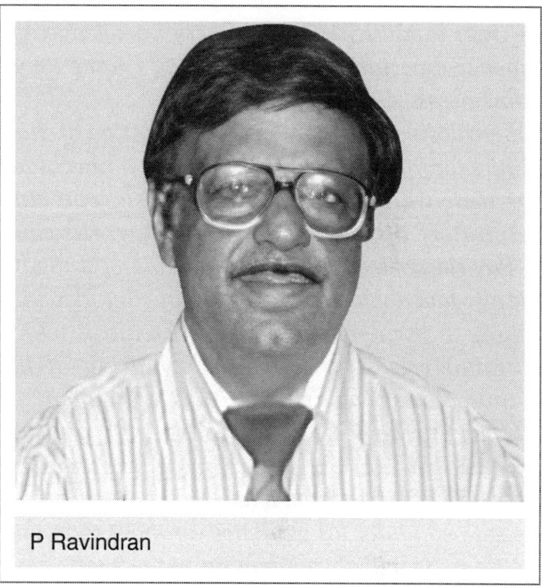

P Ravindran

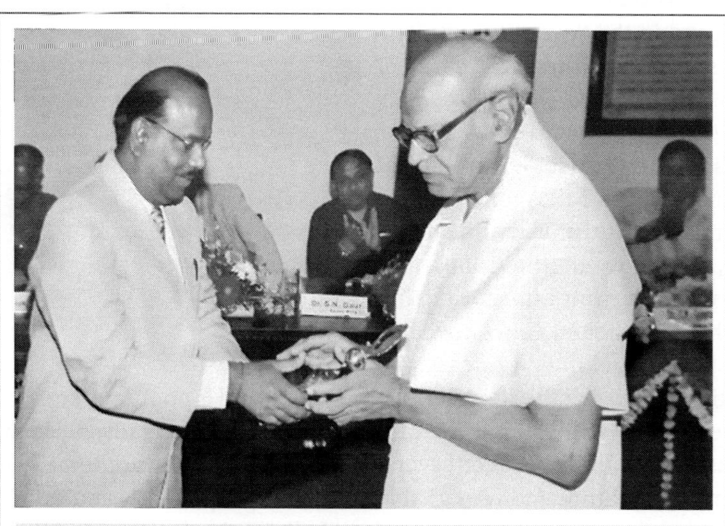

Prof BK Khanna (being felicitated by Dr Rajendra Prashad)

at King George's Medical College, Lucknow for about three decades. Prof Rajendra Prashad, the former Director of Vallabbhai Patel Chest Institute Delhi and Institute of Medical Sciences and Research, Saifai, who was one of his students informs that Dr Khanna was instrumental to start pulmonary function laboratory, allergy clinic, and rigid and flexible bronchoscopy in the department of TB for the first time in the state of Uttar Pradesh. *"He was a very knowledgeable teacher especially in tuberculosis. I have never come across such a brilliant teacher especially in tuberculosis. He laid down the foundation of short clinics for final year MBBS students; a novel idea for their training about tuberculosis, common respiratory diseases, and chest X-Ray. His chest X-Ray classes were very popular among students. He also laid down the foundation of nontubercular wards in the department of tuberculosis which ultimately lead to the transformation of the Tuberculosis Department to Department of Pulmonary Medicine. Apart from being a clinician par excellence, he was a passionate teacher and a very able administrator. It has been my privilege to be trained under his guidance for more than four decades. He will always remain in the hearts of all the students who were taught by him. While paying tribute to him one of his students wrote "Professor Khanna" was a legend in the field of tuberculosis and chest diseases. I do not find any genius of his stature in this subject. Whatever pulmonary radiology we know, all credit goes to him."*

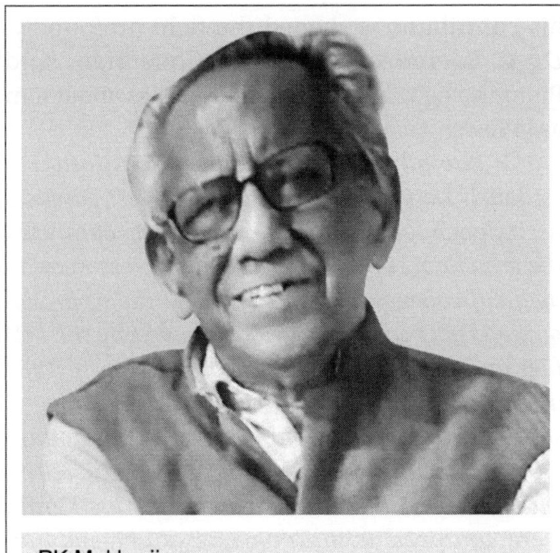
PK Mukherji

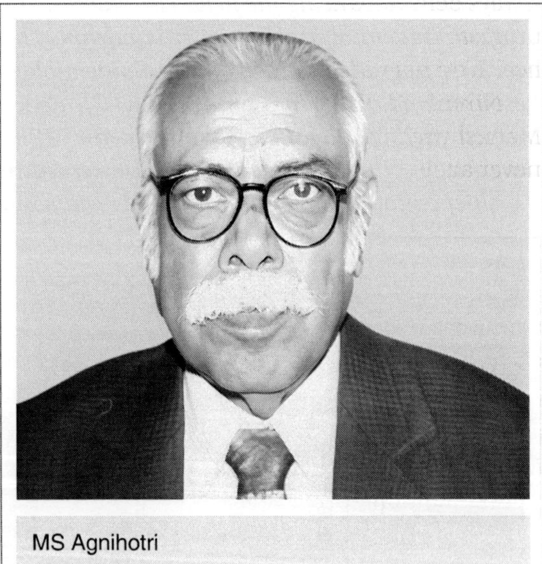
MS Agnihotri

Prof Rajendra Prashad also writes about Professors PK Mukherji and MS Agnihotri who made significant contributions while at KG Medical College, Lucknow in the 1980s and 1990s. Mukherji was instrumental in starting Associations of Chest Physicians, Lucknow also called as Chest Club of Lucknow for academic and social activities which is still running. He was a thorough gentleman with a very pleasant personality. Dr Prashad has fondly recalled several instances of his very firm nature and remarkable decisions. Similarly, another doyen, MS Agnihotri had laid down foundation of Allergy Clinic as early as 1970 and is popularly known as father of Allergy in State of Uttar Pradesh. He was the first to think about oral immunotherapy, initiated the same for allergic patients, and popularized the subject of allergy in the state of Uttar Pradesh. He also developed a pollen calendar for North India. He had also developed a lot of interest in Ayurveda in latter part of his career and propagated Ayurveda and Yoga in Bronchial Asthma and other Allergic diseases. All his students remember him for his teaching, administrative and managerial qualities.

Prof Ashok Anant Mahashur was another leading figure from Mumbai who with SR Kamat was instrumental in establishing the first *intensive respiratory care unit* and transformed the department into a world-class center for respiratory medicine. He introduced several innovations such as bronchoscopy, advanced pulmonary function testing, the Environmental Pollution Research Centre, and several others. He was also instrumental in setting up the department of Chest diseases at T N Medical College and B Y L Nair hospital, Mumbai along with Dr G S Parihar during the 1980s. Dr Mahashur possessed a futuristic approach far ahead for his time and always believed that Respiratory Medicine should progress by leaps and bounds beyond the public health domain of TB.

Nikhil Sarangdhar, who had also seen Mahashur from close quarters, shares that he never allowed his illness to affect him and always faced life with great strength, enthusiasm, and an infectious smile. Abha Mahashur, daughter in law of Dr Mahashur, describes him *"as an ocean of knowledge which he kept expanding with his tireless efforts and eagerness to learn and stay updated. He was a voracious reader, keen observer, and a visionary in pulmonary medicine. He strongly believed that focus in life should be in being productive, progressive, and futuristic. He stayed relevant all across his life as he constantly evolved with time and generation. From an intense political conversation with elderly, an intelligent scientific discussion with medical personnel to a totally entertaining fun ride with kids, he was everyone's favorite. He was a selfless soul and "a true teacher" in all sense. His teaching skills were exceptional where he would go to an extra mile to teach his students, for which he is still remembered by all. A student achieving any accomplishment would fill his chest with pride. He took responsibility of his students. Those were the days when conventional teaching came with a lot of strictness and rules. He was passionate about the Respiratory ICU setup by him at the Seth G S Medical College and K E M Hospital, Mumbai. The evening hours at our*

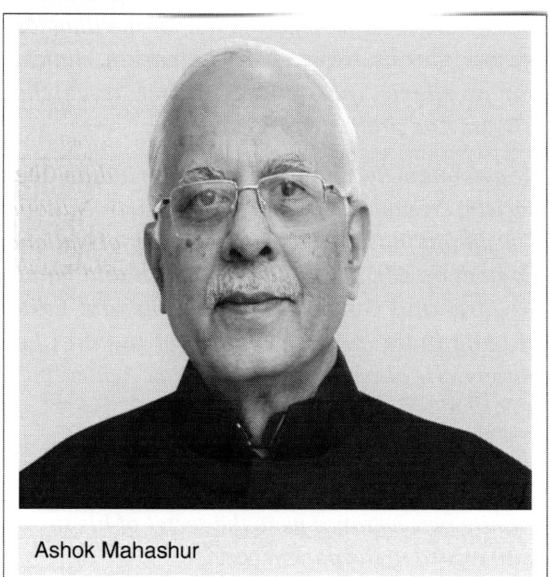

Ashok Mahashur

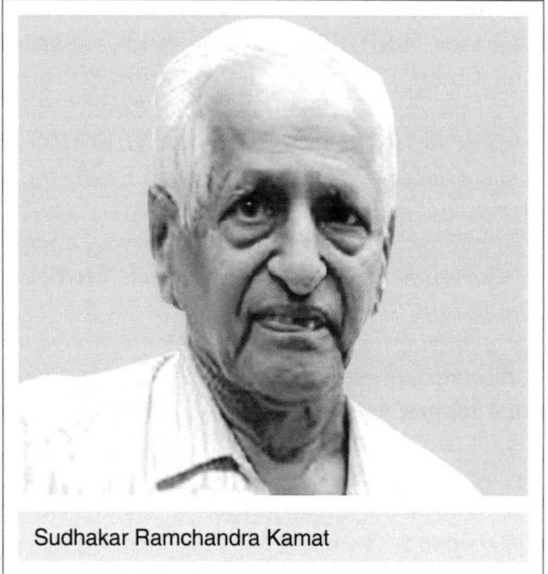

Sudhakar Ramchandra Kamat

residence were like a curfew situation where the whole house would maintain a pin drop silence for a phone call at our landline at sharp 9 PM. Those few minutes would be a strict no talking zone here and a super stress zones for his registrars on call there at ICU. He was a disciplinarian in working hours and a guardian round the clock, thus all his students bonded with him on different levels and kept touch with immense love and gratitude even after migrating from his gurukul. He was like a giant tree loaded with fruits which kept bending down with the weight of knowledge, life experiences, and humility who kept giving shade to all those who approached.

He was truly a "Bheeshma Pitamah" of pulmonary medicine who witnessed the evolution of our field, worked hard to excel in practice, and had an eye for future. He touched every soul he met, he inspired every mind he taught, and he loved every heart he was surrounded with."

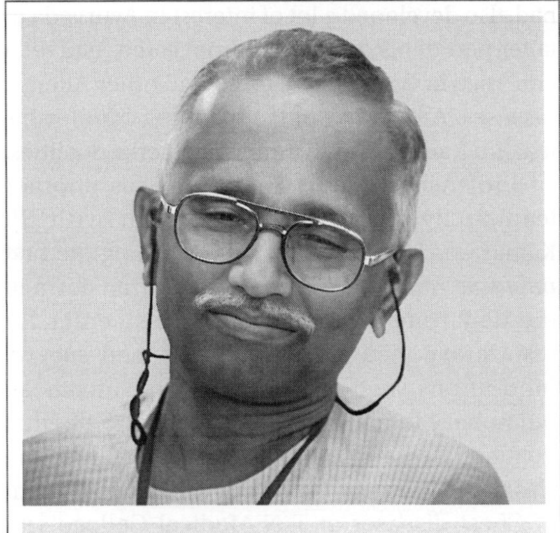

CN Deivanayagam

CN Deivanayagam, was a veteran pulmonologist of India who was a Professor of Thoracic Medicine, Madras Medical College and later Dean of TAMARAI (now Sri Ramachandra Medical College and Research Institute, Chennai, Tamil Nadu). Vijayalakshmi Thanasekaran, Former Emeritus professor of TB and Chest Diseases, SRIHER, Chennai and a Senior Consultant Pulmonologist pays her tributes: *"CN Deivanayagam will be remembered forever, because in 1991 when many found HIV/AIDS as a social stigma, he was the first in South India to conduct an autopsy in an HIV/AIDS patient and publish it in Lung India. He created a ward at Government Hospital of Thoracic Medicine, Tambaram, Chennai in 1993, exclusively for PLHA (people living with HIV/AIDS). This has grown into a recognized center of excellence in patient care, training, and research in HIV/AIDS. It is the largest health care center for HIV/AIDS patients in Asia. Even before antiretroviral drugs were available free of cost for AIDS patients in government hospitals, Dr Deivanayagam treated these patients with non-antiretroviral allopathic medicines along with alternative medicines and presented his work at XIII International AIDS Conference in Durban, South Africa. In 1980, Dr Deivanayagam initiated the indigenous preparation of sweat chloride analyzer, iontophoresis equipment, along with engineers of IIT Madras and used it for pilocarpine iontophoresis sweat chloride test for the diagnosis of cystic fibrosis. He was a disciplinarian, clinician par excellence, passionate teacher, researcher, scholar, and prolific writer.*

He was one of the founder members of Indian Chest Society, President of Indian Chest Society, National Consultant in HIV and AIDS, Member of National Council on AIDS, Ministry of Health and Family Welfare, and Government of India and Editor of Lung India (Official Journal of Indian Chest Society). He also received the Lifetime Achievement Award of Indian Chest Society in 2012.

He also contributed to Tamil Literature and Peace initiatives. Infinite patience, infinite purity, and infinite perseverance were the secret of his success with regard to the patient care".

Current Era

A number of medical teachers and eminent clinicians have continued to make headlines in their respective areas of pulmonary and critical care practice for their contributions in the current era since the last part of the 20th century to date. They have adopted the latest medical techniques and interventions in respective fields. It is futile to make a list of the stalwarts of the present era which we leave for the authors of the future to reminisce. Undoubtedly, a long innings of Jagdev Singh Guleria, a former Dean and Professor of the All India Institute of Medical Sciences, New Delhi, is highly significant for his continued commitment to chest medicine through mentoring a large number of students as an eminent general physician, cardiologist, and pulmonologist. Farokh Udwadia is another renowned physician who established critical care as a model service in Mumbai and promoted bedside medicine.

Udwadia is more known for his stress on bedside medicine. As an Emeritus Professor of Medicine at Grant Medical College and the JJ Group of Hospitals, he has taught medical students for over five decades. Besides critical care medicine and respiratory disease, Udwadia has addressed other critical issues related to medical, social, and cultural history. He has written several books on medicine and allied subjects. His book "Man and Medicine" is like an epic on history of medicine. Another publication, "*Tabiyat*—Medicine and Healing in India" was another masterpiece. His research and interpretation has always been guided by history, tradition, art, literature, and science.

The last half a century has also seen the emergence of women pulmonary physicians in India even though only a fewer women had opted for respiratory medicine in the past. Sivaramakrishna Iyer Padmavati, who passed away in 2020, was among the first few women cardiologists in India. Her work on chronic bronchitis and cardiopulmonary disease in Indian women due to long-term exposures to smoke from domestic fuel combustion of solid fuels was well ahead of time. Now, a number of pulmonary medicine departments have a significant number of female faculty members. Uma Mohan K, one of my own former students and now Professor at St

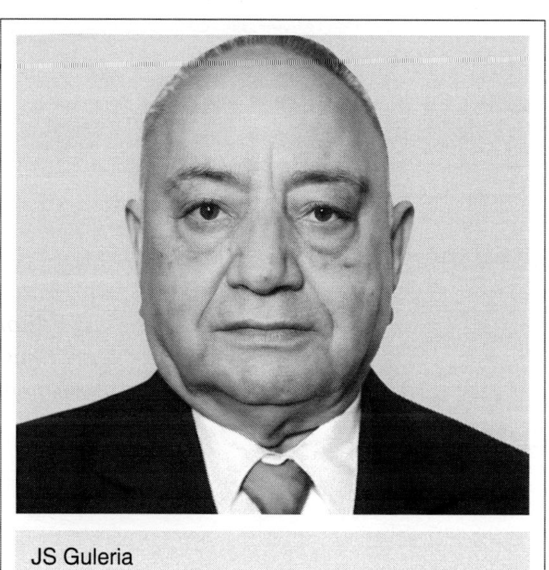

JS Guleria

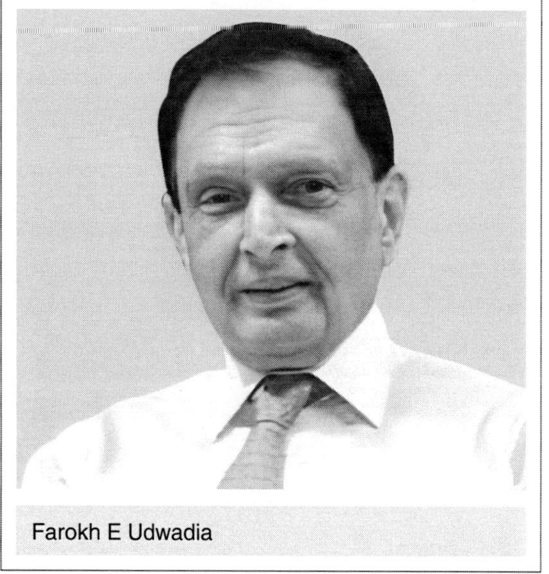

Farokh E Udwadia

John's Medical College, Bengaluru, writes about her journey:

"When I ponder about the origin of my fascination for pulmonary medicine, the carousel of memories stops at this photograph shot during my residency; I am fortunate to be in the same frame as these titans in pulmonology, SK Jindal, D Behera, D Gupta, and AN Aggarwal. They have accomplished the daunting task of starting the first superspecialty program in pulmonary medicine in India. Each of our four mentors was immersed in impactful research in important fields like airway diseases, sarcoidosis, and lung cancer. We flourished in the warm glow of their tutelage during our stint in PGI as the rock-solid foundations for lifelong learning and research were laid!"

The number of women members of Indian Chest Society has almost doubled from 14% in the past to 27% for the present. We also see an increased presence of women in the intervention and critical care areas. Undoubtedly, the trend is likely to continue in the future. Sooner than later, we are likely to see their greater participation in teaching and research fields.

There are several eminent contemporary pulmonologists, physicians, surgeons, and basic scientists who continue to significantly advance the developments in different fields of respiratory medicine. It is difficult for me to summarize their contributions for the present. I, therefore, leave it for the future authors of history on the subject.

The gaps in technology between the Indian and Western medical practices are practically reduced to negligible. Undoubtedly however, there remains a significant nonuniformity of medical services attributed to regional, political, and economic differences and disparities. There are also significant gaps in original and basic research in different fields. Translational research directed to the issues, problems, and solutions of problems relevant to the country are lacking. There is also an inadequate attention given to general medical perspectives. Most of these gaps require greater inputs at different levels of health care. It is for the future to judge the ongoing developments, contributions of pulmonologists of different hues, and the role of the current leadership.

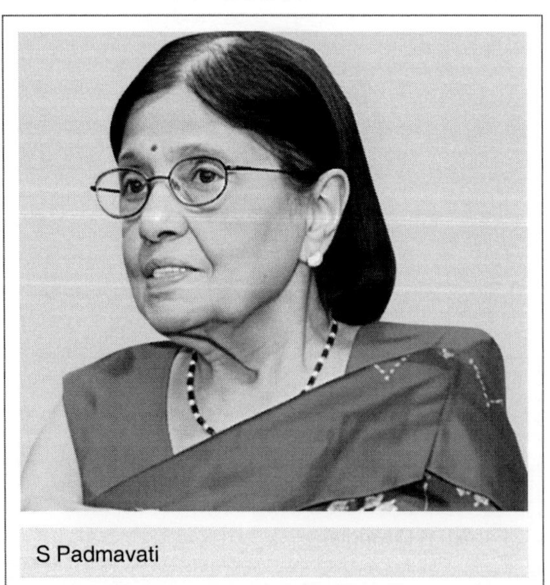
S Padmavati

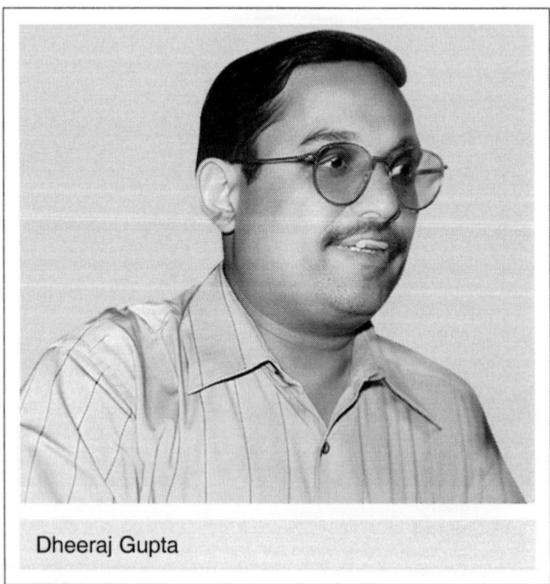
Dheeraj Gupta

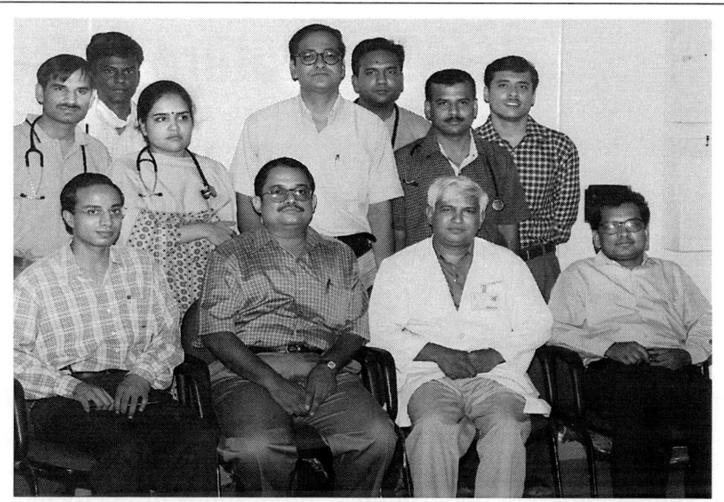

Faculty of Pulmonary Medicine (PGIMER, Chandigarh) 1999–2002
Sitting (left to right): Ashutosh Nath Aggarwal, Dheeraj Gupta, Surinder Kumar Jindal, Digamber Behera
Standing (left to right): Surinder Kumar, Balamugesh T, Uma Maheswari K, Ashutosh Ghosh, Rajesh Gupta, Mahendran Chetty, Pralay Sarkar

Sources

1. Jindal SK, Shankar PS, Vijayan VK, Kamat SR, Deivanayagan CN. Down the memory lane: Lung India three decades. Lung India. 2012;29(3):205-11.
2. Anshu, Supe A. Evolution of medical education in India: The impact of colonialism. J Postgrad Med. 2016;62(4):255-9.
3. Thippanna G. History of respiratory medicine. Lung India. 1997;15(3):125-8.
4. Marfatia M. (2022). A surgeon and a gentleman. [online] Available from https://www.mid-day.com/news/opinion/article/a-surgeon-and-a-gentleman-23232178 [Last accessed September, 2025].
5. Thanasekaraan V, Krishnaswamy UM. Leading women pulmonologists in India: Beacons of change. Respirology. 2022;27(4):311-3.
6. Padmavati S, Pathak SN. Chronic cor pulmonale in Delhi: A Study of 127 Cases. Circulation. 1959;343-52.

Personal notes by:

SK Chhabra on Autar Singh Paintal
Basil Varkey on R Viswanathan
Ashok Shah on MM Singh
Aloke Ghoshal in Debabrata Sen
SK Sharma on JN Pande
Rajendra Prashad on BK Khanna, PK Mukherji and MS Agnihori
Nikhil Sarangdhar on K.C. Mohanty
Abha Mahashur and Niknil Sarangdhar on AA Mahashur
V Thanasekaraan on CN Deivanayagam
C Ravindran on P Ravindran
Uma Mohan K on her Residency days

The Future of Respiratory Medicine in India

Thomas Frieden in his 2005 title "The World is Flat: A Brief History of the Twenty-first Century" argues that the recent globalization has ushered an era of global competition and opportunity allowing individuals and companies worldwide to compete and collaborate more easily than ever before. Although Frieden primarily talked about the flattened field in economic activities, the same applies in all other areas. In medicine and science where scientific aptitudes are different and developments are rather fast; it also demands adaptation through innovations and continuous education.

Respiratory medicine is only one small area which is no different from other medical fields. The progression is not just linear but occurs on a logarithmic scale. Some of the new discoveries are rather sudden and unexpected which make a predictable future as uncertain. Extensive applications of microchips in medical devices and the introduction of artificial intelligence (AI) in medicine have completed altered the scenario of new developments. Gordon Moore, the co-founder of Intel corporation in 1965 had anticipated that roughly every 2 years, the number of transistors on microchips will double suggesting that computational progress will become significantly faster, smaller, and more efficient over time. Moreover, the "super atomic" material could lead computer chips that are hundreds or thousands of times speedier than those available today.

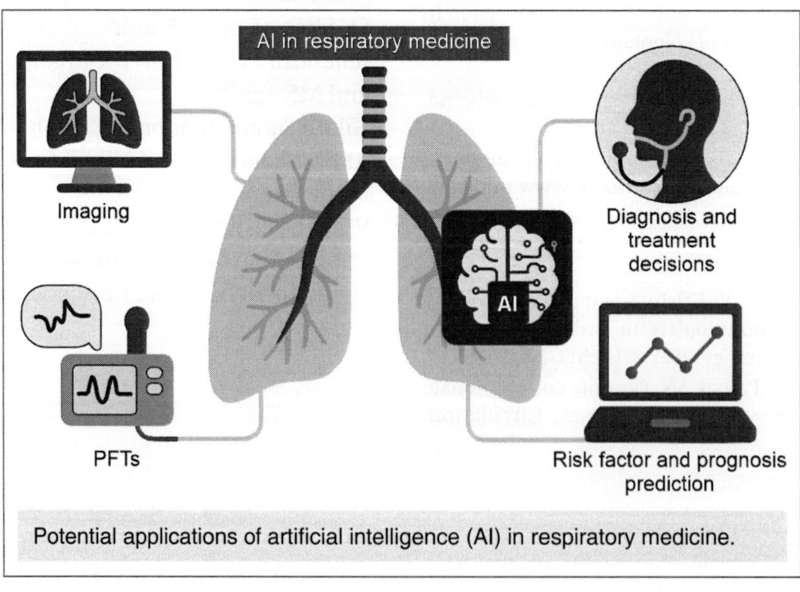

Potential applications of artificial intelligence (AI) in respiratory medicine.

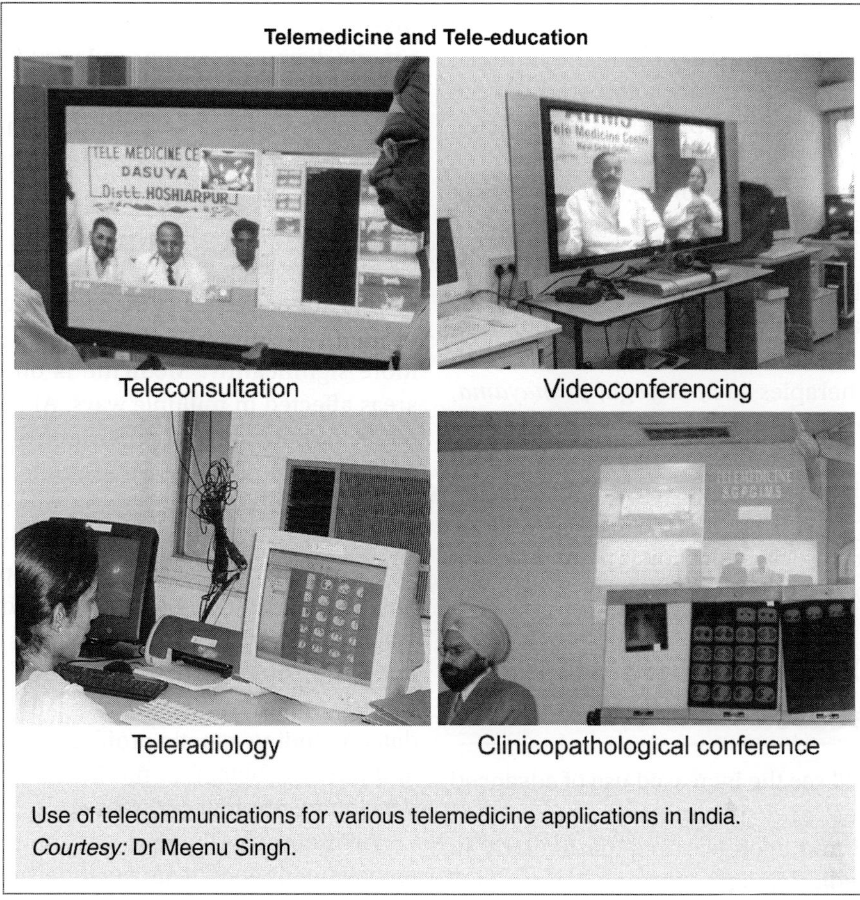

Use of telecommunications for various telemedicine applications in India.
Courtesy: Dr Meenu Singh.

Emerging Trends in Medicine in India

In general, the developments of technology in India run parallel to those that happen elsewhere in the world. The future of respiratory medicine in India therefore will not be different. Digital health is already changing the practice of medicine. One can expect a more rapid progress in the future. It includes telemedicine, AI-powered diagnostics, and mobile health applications. Other important developments include the rapid expansion of personalized medicine which involves the use of tailored treatments based on genetic profiles and biomarkers. Identifying genetic markers helps to predict disease susceptibility, treatment response, and assists in classifying patients into specific phenotypes to guide treatment decisions. It also includes precision treatments with targeted therapies for specific diseases. Regenerative medicine for degenerative disorders with use of stem-cell therapies and tissue engineering is another area which will expand further.

A lot of research work is happening in the world in the fields of cellular and molecular biology, cell signaling and communication, gene expression and regulation, as well as epigenetics and chromatin remodeling. Other areas of research interest in the specialty include lung development and regeneration; immunology and inflammation; and respiratory physiology, biophysics, and respiratory neurobiology. There is a relative lack of a translational approach of basic research in respiratory medicine in India. Basic research which involves the study of the fundamental biological processes underlying respiratory health and seeks to understand the underlying mechanisms of diseases is rather sporadic and individualistic.

Simultaneously, integrative treatment strategies will also become more prominent, not only in India but also in several other countries. Combining conventional medications with alternative therapies such as *yoga, pranayama,* acupuncture, mindfulness-based interventions, and herbal drugs will continue to fancy and benefit a significant segment of population. The current expansion of *"Patanjali"* ayurvedic pharmacy and "yoga" education is pointer to their growing popularity.

Future Diagnostic Strategies for Lung Diseases

The future will see the increased use of advanced technologies and innovative approaches involving AI and deep learning, particularly in analyzing medical images such as X-rays and CT scans. Deep learning algorithms used to detect and classify various lung diseases are trained on large datasets to improve their accuracy and effectiveness. Computer-aided detection (CAD) systems will also be employed to help doctors diagnose lung diseases more accurately and quickly. These systems use machine learning algorithms to analyze medical images and detect abnormalities.

Telemedicine and remote monitoring will become more prevalent enabling patients to receive remote advice. This is particularly useful for patients with chronic lung diseases who require regular monitoring and treatment. Point-of-care diagnostics will become increasingly important for use particularly in rural areas where access to healthcare facilities is limited. Portable and handheld devices will be used to diagnose diseases at the point-of-care. Point-of-care genetic diagnosis for tuberculosis (TB) is already being done under the National TB Elimination Programme. Biomarkers and genomics will also play a greater role in diagnosing lung diseases.

Artificial Intelligence

Artificial intelligence is transforming all spheres of life. It is going to influence the future even more significantly. Medicine is one of the key areas affected in multiple ways. AI in respiratory medicine finds applications in both diagnostic and management plans. As an example, AI-powered algorithms can analyze chest X-rays and CT and MRI scans to diagnose respiratory diseases with greater accuracy. AI can also identify patterns and make interpretations of lung function tests and diagnose respiratory diseases such as asthma and chronic obstructive pulmonary disease (COPD). More fundamentally, AI can analyze patient data, including genetic profiles, medical history, and lifestyle factors, to predict the likelihood of developing respiratory diseases.

Artificial intelligence can help in disease management and create personalized treatment plans based on individual patient characteristics. This type of personalized treatment plan can help to improve treatment outcomes. AI can also be useful for disease monitoring with the help of AI-powered sensors and wearable devices can remotely monitor patients' respiratory health, thus enabling early detection of disease exacerbations. AI-driven decision support systems can therefore provide healthcare professionals with real-time guidance on diagnosis, treatment, and management of respiratory diseases.

Artificial intelligence also helps in research and development since it can rapidly analyze large datasets to identify new insights into respiratory diseases. It can also aid in the discovery of new treatments by analyzing molecular structures and predicting potential therapeutic effects. AI-powered chatbots and virtual assistants can facilitate virtual consultations, improving access to respiratory care through tele consultation. AI-driven platforms can provide personalized education and support to patients, empowering them to manage their respiratory health effectively.

Artificial Intelligence Concerns

There are also several potential risks and concerns associated with AI use. There are data-related risks which include those related to data quality and privacy concerns as well as data-security breaches. AI algorithms are only as good as the data they are trained on. Poor data quality can lead to biased or inaccurate results. Electronic health records and other medical data are sensitive and vulnerable to cyberattacks. Moreover, unauthorized access to medical data can compromise patient confidentiality and trust.

Artificial intelligence-associated algorithmic risks include bias in decision-making and perpetuation of existing biases and disparities in healthcare, particularly if they are trained on biased data. Complex AI algorithms can be difficult to interpret, making it challenging to understand the reasoning behind their decisions and lack of transparency. Dependence on technology and over-reliance on AI can lead to decreased critical thinking skills among healthcare professionals which may potentially result in serious clinical risks associated with misdiagnosis as well as delayed diagnosis. AI-generated treatment plans may not account for individual patient needs or complexities, may fail to detect or respond to critical patient safety issues, such as allergic reactions or medication errors.

Importantly, there are serious regulatory and liability risks. The rapid development and deployment of AI in healthcare has outpaced regulatory frameworks, creating uncertainty and potential liability. As AI assumes greater role in healthcare decision-making, questions arise about liability in cases of adverse outcomes or errors. AI-generated medical discoveries or inventions may also raise complex intellectual property issues. Finally, there are serious societal risks. The increasing use of AI in healthcare may displace certain jobs or tasks, particularly those involving data analysis or routine decision-making. Its use may exacerbate existing health disparities if not designed or implemented with equity in mind. Over-reliance on AI can lead to decreased human interaction and empathy in healthcare, potentially compromising patient care and satisfaction.

Challenges in Respiratory Medicine

A rising respiratory disease-burden is a major concern. Currently, diseases of the respiratory system constitute the largest disease burden accounting for 15.3% of all prescriptions for total patients with diseases in India. Upper respiratory tract infections alone, the largest type of respiratory disease constituted 27% of the share in 2024. COPD is one of the fastest-growing respiratory diseases in India, accounting for 6% of all respiratory diseases. India accounted for 32% of the global disability-adjusted life years (DALYs) from chronic respiratory diseases, despite having only 18% of the world's population. State-wise, the burden of chronic respiratory diseases varies with the highest rates of age-standardized DALYs from COPD and asthma found in relatively less developed states in north India.

Air-pollution is an important issue which is unlikely to resolve in near future in spite of the significant efforts on the part of the government and other agencies. Environmental health with a focus on air pollution, climate change, and lung health continues to pose challenges now and in the near future. India is expected to see a rise in chronic respiratory diseases, such as COPD and asthma, due to factors such as air pollution, smoking, and changing lifestyles. The trend of continued increase in diseases such as asthma and COPD is likely to aggravate even further, at least for a decade or so. India's rapidly growing economy and urbanization have led to increased air pollution, which exacerbates respiratory diseases. Further, climate change is expected to worsen air quality, heat stress, and other environmental factors that can impact respiratory health.

On the other hand, India's healthcare infrastructure is rather inadequate, particularly in rural areas, making it difficult for people to access quality respiratory care. There is a shortage of skilled healthcare professionals, including pulmonologists and respiratory therapists. Socioeconomic disparities make it even more difficult to handle the respiratory diseases which disproportionately affect vulnerable populations, such as the poor, women, and children. Tobacco use and smoking are major risk factors for respiratory diseases which are more significant in the vulnerable populations. There is a need for indigenous innovations and solutions tailored to India's unique healthcare challenges. But India's research funding for respiratory diseases is limited, hindering the development of new treatments and diagnostic tools. There is greater need for leveraging digital health technologies such as telemedicine and mobile health applications, to improve access to respiratory care. India can also utilize data analytics and surveillance to better track respiratory diseases, identify trends, and inform policy decisions. A multifaceted approach is required to address these challenges. It involves government initiatives, healthcare infrastructure development, research and innovation, and community engagement.

Tuberculosis and Other Respiratory Infections

Presently, India has a high burden of TB and the disease remains a significant public health challenge. According to recent estimates, India accounted for 27% of the global TB cases, with approximately 2.8 million reported cases in 2022. The National TB Elimination Programme is already in force. It is expected that the disease burden will significantly diminish although total elimination is unlikely in the near future. The number of multidrug-resistant cases seems to grow and will continue to pose problems of management. It is, however, expected that the number will diminish with effective treatment strategies being enforced.

The gap between estimated and reported TB cases in India has increased approximately 1.9 times, highlighting the need for improved diagnostic services and reporting mechanisms. India reported 64,400 cases of drug-resistant TB in 2022, which poses a significant challenge to TB control efforts. Despite a decline in TB-related mortality, India still accounts for a significant proportion of global TB deaths, with an estimated 331,000 deaths in 2022. To address these challenges, India will need to strengthen its TB control efforts, including improving diagnostic services, expanding access to treatment, and promoting awareness and education about TB prevention and control.

It is difficult to define the true burden of respiratory infections which remain a major concern. Respiratory illnesses generally follow seasonal patterns, with surges during the winter and monsoon seasons. The emergence of new viral mutations significantly impacts the future trends. The last COVID-19 pandemic tells the importance of remaining vigilant and prepared to handle any such potential episode in the future. It is important to introduce robust surveillance system and preparedness measures to mitigate the impact. India is adopting a "One Health" approach to address the problem focusing on the inter connectedness of human, animal, and environmental health.

Bronchial Asthma

The burden of asthma in India over the next decade is a pressing concern. With approximately 35 million people currently suffering from asthma, India has one of the largest asthma populations in the world. Many asthma cases remain undiagnosed or misdiagnosed, leading to inadequate treatment and poor health outcomes. Moreover, India's healthcare infrastructure is often inadequate, particularly in rural areas, making it difficult for people to access quality care. Exposure to air pollution, biomass fuel, and tobacco smoke contributes to the development and exacerbation of asthma. The problems are likely to persist in the near future. While there is not a specific projection for the next decade, the global asthma prevalence is expected to increase, and India's large population and growing urbanization will likely contribute to this trend.

Asthma Burden

Overall, addressing the burden of asthma in India will require sustained efforts to improve healthcare infrastructure, increase awareness and education, and reduce environmental risk factors. The Indian government has launched initiatives like *Ayushman Bharat Yojana,* which provides free treatment to hospitalized patients at government and selected private hospitals. Efforts to reduce exposure to biomass fuel and improve air quality are underway, such as the distribution of liquid petroleum gas connections to poor families under *PM Ujjwala Yojana project.*

Inhalation Therapy

Inhalation therapy is the key to asthma management and will continue to remain so. Advancements in inhaler technology and nano-technology are likely to improve drug delivery and efficacy. Patient adherence will be greater with development of user-friendly inhalers, smart inhalers and patient education to treatment plans. Smart devices equipped with sensors and digital platforms monitor patient adherence, track dosages, and provide real-time feedback on inhaler technique. Researchers are also exploring the use of nanoparticles to improve drug delivery efficiency and reduce side effects. This technology can target specific areas of the airways, maximizing therapeutic effects while minimizing systemic exposure.

Inhaler-free Era

While future developments in inhalational therapy are expected to improve the treatment, personalized medicine and "inhaler-free era" are also on the horizon. New delivery mechanisms, such as RNA-interference (RNAi), to provide more effective and convenient treatment options are being explored for the treatment of asthma. These therapies work by silencing specific genes that contribute to inflammation and airway constriction. Some key RNAi therapies for asthma include ARO-RAGE, small interfering RNA (siRNA) therapies, and microRNA (miRNA) therapies. RNAi therapies can reduce inflammation and airway remodeling, leading to improved lung function and reduced symptoms. They can target specific genes involved in asthma, reducing the risk of side effects and improving treatment efficacy.

These treatments can be administered via subcutaneous injections, which can provide sustained release of the therapeutic agent or administered intravenously, allowing for rapid distribution throughout the body. Targeted delivery mechanisms with nanoparticles can be engineered to target specific cells or tissues, allowing for precise delivery. Lipid-based delivery systems, such as liposomes, can be used to deliver therapeutics to specific cells or tissues. Cell-penetrating peptides or antibodies can be used to deliver RNAi therapeutics directly into specific cells or tissues. Work is already going on in an RNAi therapeutic targeting respiratory syncytial virus infection, which can exacerbate asthma and TD101 which act on the transforming growth factor-beta (TGF-β) pathway involved in airway remodeling.

Personalized Treatments

Future management strategies involve a multifaceted approach. Personalized medicine will play a crucial role, with treatments tailored to individual patients' needs. Precision medicine will help identify specific biomarkers for asthma, enabling early diagnosis and targeted treatments. For instance, eosinophils are important in predicting treatment responses and driving treatment choices. Digital health technologies involving mobile apps, wearable devices, and telemedicine platforms to enable real-time monitoring, improve adherence to treatment plans, and enhance patient-physician communication are already in use. Their role is going to expand enormously.

Genetic testing will enable physicians to tailor treatment plans to individual patients' needs, optimizing asthma management, and minimizing adverse reactions. Noninhaler therapies may potentially replace or complement traditional inhaler therapy for certain patients. Biologic therapies are already in use and more are being developed to target specific inflammatory pathways in asthma. New oral therapies are also being investigated for their potential to treat asthma.

Noninhaler therapies are easier for patients to use and improve adherence to treatment plans. They may offer improved efficacy or faster onset of action compared to traditional inhalers. Noninhaler therapies may have different side effect profiles compared to inhalers, potentially reducing local side effects like throat irritation. But noninhaler therapies may be associated with systemic side effects, which could be a concern for some patients. New noninhaler therapies, especially biological agents, may be more expensive than traditional inhalers, potentially limiting accessibility for some patients. Noninhaler therapies may also require more frequent monitoring and titration to optimize dosing and minimize side effects.

In conclusion, while noninhaler therapies hold promise, inhalers will likely remain a vital part of asthma management for the foreseeable future. A personalized approach, considering individual patient needs and preferences, will be essential in determining the best treatment strategy.

Chronic Obstructive Pulmonary Disease

India is expected to face a significant burden of COPD in the next decade. The estimated prevalence is alarming, with over 57 million people suffering from obstructive airway diseases. India will likely have the third-highest economic burden of COPD globally, after China and the US, from 2020 to 2050. The economic burden is estimated to be significant, with costs expected to rise to $8 billion by the end of 2016. India accounts for 20% of the annual worldwide COPD mortality, with an age-standardized death rate of 64.7 per 100,000 population. The country's large population, urbanization, and air pollution contribute to the increasing burden of COPD.

To address the growing burden at the national level, it is essential to focus on prevention and management strategies such as smoking cessation, air pollution control, increasing the use of clean energy sources, and promoting sustainable transportation. It is also important to improve access to healthcare services for early detection and treatment. Unlike for asthma, there are fewer new developments in management strategies. The new goal-post for COPD management is to achieve disease stability which includes comprehensive treatment to control symptoms, reduce lung function decline, improve quality of life, and prevent exacerbations. The digital technologies such as the wearable devices to monitor lung function are sometimes helpful to detect an exacerbation and start early treatment. Similarly, AI can help analyzing data to predict exacerbations and optimize treatment plans.

Future Management Strategies

Treatment strategies for COPD involve a multifaceted approach using multiple medications, such as bronchodilators, corticosteroids, and phosphodiesterase-4 inhibitors, to achieve better symptom control. New inhalers with feedback mechanisms to ensure proper usage and reduce side effects are going to play a significant role as in case of asthma. There is no immediate likelihood of any targeted or personalized medicine approach in COPD. The new development areas primarily include new combinations, new delivery mechanisms and exploring alternative delivery methods (such as dry powder inhalers and soft mist inhalers).

Pulmonary rehabilitation implementing exercise and education programs to improve lung function, overall health, and quality of life is likely to find a greater role in future along with pharmacotherapy. Alternative therapies incorporating yoga, *pranayama,* acupuncture, herbal drugs, and mindfulness-based interventions to reduce symptoms and improve well-being will continue to stay for a significant number of patients. Surgical options including lung volume reduction and lung transplantation will find an increased space in COPD management in India in future.

Interstitial Lung Disease

The burden of interstitial lung disease (ILD) in the next decade in India is difficult to assess since ILD itself is a syndromic diagnosis which encompasses a large number of diseases of various etiologies. Undoubtedly however, the likely burden of ILD over the next decade is a pressing concern because of the noticeable and significant increase in trend in recognition of these diseases. This is driven by advancements in diagnostic technologies such as improved imaging techniques and use of biomarkers. Moreover, there is a growing awareness among healthcare professionals. Factors such as environmental exposures, occupational hazards, and genetic predisposition in a country with a growing economy and large population will likely play a significant role in shaping the epidemiology of ILD in India.

Future treatment options for ILD are promising, with several expected breakthrough therapies. Besides the antifibrotic and immunomodulatory drugs, there is ongoing work on targeted therapies that focus on specific molecular pathways. These therapies have shown potential in reducing fibrosis and improving lung function. Stem-cell and gene therapy are also being explored to repair or replace damaged lung tissue. Gene therapy approaches including gene editing and gene expression modulation can be used for specific genes involved in ILD, such as targeting the TGF-β pathway to reduce inflammation and fibrosis or restoring surfactant protein which is critical for lung health. Both viral vectors (such as adenovirus and lentivirus) and nonviral carries such as nanoparticles and liposomes are being investigated to carry the genes to the lungs. Gene therapies may be combined with other treatments, such as antifibrotic medications, to enhance efficacy. Gene therapies may also be tailored to individual patients based on their unique genetic profiles identified with help of genetic markers to predict disease susceptibility and treatment response.

Digital health technologies find similar applications for ILD management as for other respiratory diseases. Similarly, integrative treatment strategies using multiple medications and pulmonary rehabilitation will find increased use in management. Alternative therapies incorporating yoga, acupuncture, and other interventions are helpful to reduce symptoms and improve well-being. Lung transplantation for end-stage disease is already expanding in India. Both the numbers and outcomes of treatment are rapidly increasing.

Respiratory Cancers

There is already a large burden of respiratory cancers in India which is expected to rise significantly in the future. According to recent estimates, India's reported cancer incidence in 2022 was around 19–20 lakhs, with the real incidence being 1.5 to 3 times higher than reported cases. The economic burden of cancer in India is also substantial, with estimated gross domestic product (GDP) losses ranging from US$ 11 billion in 2020 to US$ 36–40 billion by 2030. A high proportion of cases continue to be detected at late stages, making treatment more challenging. India has a poor cancer detection rate of 29%, with only 15% and 33% of breast, lung, and cervical cancers being diagnosed in stages 1 and 2, respectively. In particular, lung cancer is a significant concern with a rising incidence and mortality rate. Other respiratory cancers, such as those affecting the trachea, bronchus, and pleura, also contribute to pose a growing burden.

There are rapid developments in the strategies for management of cancers. Noninvasive liquid biopsies enable monitoring of disease progression or response to therapy without the need for traditional tissue biopsies. Current and future management strategies for lung cancer focus on personalized treatment approaches, incorporating cutting-edge technologies and innovative therapies. Next-generation sequencing (NGS) technology provides detailed genetic profiles of tumors to decide treatment strategies. Personalized medicine plays a crucial role, with treatments tailored to individual patient characteristics which results in enhancement of efficacy and minimization of side effects. Molecular testing is gaining increasing importance in identifying specific genetic mutations and biomarkers, guiding treatment decisions. Targeted treatments and immunotherapy, including with checkpoint inhibitors are now used to combat tumors with specific genetic mutations. A multidisciplinary approach is essential in managing lung cancer, involving a team of experts, including oncologists, surgeons, radiologists, and pathologists. More such multidisciplinary "Tumor Boards" are likely to emerge in India as is the practice elsewhere in the world.

Respiratory Critical Care

Critical care is a rapidly expanding field in India both in the corporate and the public sector. Future strategies for management will involve a multifaceted approach. New innovations in oxygen therapy and assisted ventilation are useful in enhancing patient comfort and outcomes. Introduction new protocols and devices in critical care also result in prohibitive costs which are unaffordable for a large segment of patient-population in India. This is an important issue which remains to be dealt by the health administrators.

Telemedicine and remote monitoring, personalized medicine, respiratory physiotherapy, and pulmonary rehabilitation are as relevant in critical care as in other areas of respiratory care. In an interesting article, "Critical care medicine in the 21st century: from CPR to PCR", the authors make strong case for these two historical paradigms of cardiopulmonary resuscitation and polymerase chain reaction to summarize how critical care medicine began, and how it could mature in the years to come with incorporation of molecular biology in critical care.

In all probabilities, the future developments in respiratory medicine in India will follow the overall progress as elsewhere in the world. Newly introduced diagnostic tests, medical treatments, inventions, and surgical options will be available sooner than later. But disparities in the level of care and costs are likely to persist for a significant period of time. It is important for different stakeholders, especially the health industry, to appreciate the differences in the applications of new discoveries and developments in clinical practice. The gaps in local and global research are likely to continue in the near future. Serious and concerted efforts are required to fill the gaps. This is not just essential to compete with the rest of the world but necessary to discover and design solutions and strategies relevant for the local population.

Sources

1. Moore GE. Cramming more components onto integrated circuits. Electronics. 1965;38(8):114-7.
2. Honkoop P, Usmani O, Bonini M. The Current and Future Role of Technology in Respiratory Care. Pulm Ther. 2022;8(2):167-79.
3. Al-Anazi S, Al-Omari A, Alanazi S, Marar A, Asad M, Alawaji F, et al. Artificial intelligence in respiratory care: Current scenario and future perspective. Ann Thorac Med. 2024;19(2):117-30.
4. India State-Level Disease Burden Initiative CRD Collaborators. The burden of chronic respiratory diseases and their heterogeneity across the states of India: the Global Burden of Disease Study 1990-2016. Lancet Glob Health. 2018;6(12):e1363-74.
5. Singh V, Sharma BB. Respiratory disease burden in India: Indian chest society SWORD survey. Lung India. 2018;35(6):459-60.
6. GBD 2019 Chronic Respiratory Diseases Collaborators. Global burden of chronic respiratory diseases and risk factors, 1990–2019: an update from the Global Burden of Disease Study 2019. EClinicalMedicine. 2023;59:101936.
7. DrugsControl Media Services. (2024). Sales In The Respiratory Market Reached Rs 1,638 Crore In November 2024. [Online] Available from https://drugscontrol.org/news-detail.php?newsid=41044 [Last accessed September, 2025].
8. Directorate General of the Health Services. (2024). National Tuberculosis Elimination Programme. [online] Available from https://dghs.mohfw.gov.in/national-tuberculosis-elimination-programme.php [Last accessed September, 2025].
9. Bendre AD, Peters PJ, Kumar J. Tuberculosis: Past, present and future of the treatment and drug discovery research. Curr Res Pharmacol Drug Discov. 2021;2:100037.
10. Lee A, Xie YL, Barry CE, Chen RY. Current and future treatments for tuberculosis. BMJ. 2020;368:m216.
11. Jindal SK. Koch's postulates—Pitfalls and relevance in the 21st century. Ind J Tuber. 2018;65:6-7.
12. Merchant SA, Shaikh MJS, Nadkarni P. Tuberculosis conundrum—current and future scenarios: A proposed comprehensive approach combining laboratory, imaging, and computing advances. World J Radiol. 2022;14(6):114-36.
13. Jindal SK. Caring for respiratory disease in India in the COVID era. Expert Rev Respir Med. 2021;15:959-61.
14. Monoson A, Schott E, Ard K, Kilburg-Basnyat B, Tighe RM, Pannu S, et al. Air pollution and respiratory infections: the past, present, and future. Toxicol Sci. 2023;192(1):3-14.
15. Charriot J, Vachier I, Halimi L. Future treatment for asthma. Eur Respir Rev. 2016;25(139):77-92.
16. Peter RM. (2025). The future of asthma treatment: is a cure possible? [online] Available from https://www.labiotech.eu/in-depth/future-asthma-treatment/ [Last accessed September, 2025].
17. Calhoun WJ, Chupp GL. The new era of add-on asthma treatments: where do we stand? Allergy Asthma Clin Immunol. 2022;18:42.
18. Shah-Neville W. (2024). Promising cure for COPD: Is a breakthrough treatment within reach? [online] Available from https://www.labiotech.eu/in-depth/copd-cure-breakthrough-treatments/ [Last accessed September, 2025].
19. Cona LA. (2024). Advancements in COPD Treatment: A Promising Cure. [online] Available from https://www.dvcstem.com/post/promising-cure-for-copd [Last accessed September, 2025].
20. Bang AA, Bang S, Bang A, Acharya S, Shukla S. Recent Advances in the Treatment of Interstitial Lung Diseases. Cureus. 2023;15(10):e48016.
21. The Lancet. (2022). Digital technology and the future of interstitial lung diseases. [online] Available from https://www.thelancet.com/series/digital-technology-and-ILD [Last accessed September, 2025].
22. Cristian SS, Rivera-Ortega P. Present and future perspectives in early diagnosis and monitoring for progressive fibrosing interstitial lung diseases. Front Med (Lausanne). 2023:10:1114722.
23. Sotiropoulou V, Karampitsakos T, Katsaras M, Papaioannou O, Tsiri P, Sampsonas F, et al. What is new in the treatment of interstitial lung diseases. Pneumon. 2023;36(2):1-9.
24. Singh N, Agrawal S, Jiwnani S, Khosla D, Malik PS, Mohan A, et al. Lung Cancer in India. J Thorac Oncol. 2021;16(8,):1250-66.
25. Ramnath N, Ganesan P, Penumadu P, Arenberg D, Bryant A. Lung cancer screening in India:

Preparing for the future using smart tools & biomarkers to identify highest risk individuals. Indian J Med Res. 2024;160(6):561-9.
26. Sathishkumar K, Chaturvedi M, Das P, Stephen S, Mathur P. Cancer incidence estimates for 2022 & projection for 2025: Result from National Cancer Registry Programme, India. Indian J Med Res. 2022;156(4&5):598-607.
27. Tirupakuzhi Vijayaraghavan BK, Nainan Myatra S, Mathew M, Lodh N, Vasishtha Divatia J, Hammond N, et al. Challenges in the delivery of critical care in India during the COVID-19 pandemic. J Intensive Care Soc. 2021;22(4):342-8.
28. Villar J, Méndez S, Slutsky AS. Critical care medicine in the 21st century: from CPR to PCR. Crit Care. 2001;5(3):125-30.
29. World Critical Care and Anesthesiology Conference. (2025). Future Scenario of Critical Care in India. [online] Available from https://criticalcongress.episirus.org/future-scenario-of-critical-care-in-india/ [Last accessed September, 2025].
30. Munje R, Chawla R, Chetambath R, Christopher DJ, Dhar R, Ghoshal AG, et al. Position statement of the Indian Chest Society on reinstatement of the Respiratory Medicine department in undergraduate medical colleges in India. Lung India. 2023;40(6):487-9.
31. Dasgupta A, Fernandes L, Chopra V, Rajkumar P. Barriers to building an effective workforce for respiratory research in India: A survey of American Thoracic Society Methods in Epidemiologic, Clinical, and Operations Research India 2017 participants. Lung India. 2018;35(2):184-6.
32. Jindal SK. Leadership in medicine. Ind J Chest Dis Allied Sci. 2014;56:69-70.
33. Jindal SK. Integrated Clinical Data into Clinical Practice. Indian J Chest Dis Allied Sci. 2019;61:117-8.
34. Jindal SK. Research in clinical sciences. Indian J Chest Dis Allied Sci. 2011;53:175-82.

INDEX

F

G

H

I

O

P

T

U

V

W

X

Y

Z